Health Care Systems
in World Perspective

health administration press

M2240 School of Public Health
The University of Michigan
Ann Arbor, Michigan 48109
(313) 764-1380

Lewis E. Weeks, Ph.D.
Editor

The Press was established in 1972 with the support of the W. K. Kellogg Foundation as a joint endeavor of the Association of University Programs in Health Administration (Washington, D.C.) and the Cooperative Information Center for Hospital Management Studies (The University of Michigan).

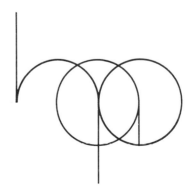

MILTON I. ROEMER, M.D. is Professor of Health Services Administration in the School of Public Health at the University of California, Los Angeles. He was Research Professor of Administrative Medicine at Cornell University 1957-62 and Associate Professor of Social and Administrative Medicine at the Yale Medical School 1949-51. After qualifying in medicine in 1940, he earned the M.A. degree in sociology and the M.P.H. in public health. From 1943 to 1949 he served in the United States Public Health Service on rural health and federal-state relations. He was Chief of the Social and Occupational Health Section of the World Health Organization (Geneva, Switzerland) 1951-53 and Director of Medical and Hospital Services, Province of Saskatchewan (Regina, Canada) 1953-56. Dr. Roemer is a Diplomate of the American Board of Preventive Medicine and Public Health (1949) and a fellow of the American Public Health Association (in which he was Chairman of the Medical Care Section 1956-57). He serves as consultant to the World Health Organization, International Labour Office, U.S. Public Health Service, USAID, and several voluntary health organizations. In 1974 he was elected to the Institute of Medicine of the National Academy of Sciences.

Health Care Systems
in World Perspective

Milton I. Roemer, M.D.

University of California
Los Angeles

Health Administration Press
Ann Arbor
1976

Library of Congress Cataloging in Publication Data

Roemer, Milton Irwin, 1916-
    Health care systems in world perspective.

    Bibliography: p.
    1.   Medical care.   I.   Title.
RA411.R56   362.1   75-36706
ISBN 0-914904-13-2

Contents

Foreword

Health services all over the world at present find themselves in a fruitful, also often painful process of adjusting to new scientific insight, technological advances, and to changing political and humanitarian ideologies.

In this context one can often hear statements along these lines: "National experience gained in health services cannot be transferred to other countries," or "Methods which have given excellent results in one country cannot as a rule be applied with success elsewhere."

Such views are frequently stated in blunt and simple form—as if generally accepted—regardless of whether one discusses the organizational structure, the administration, the quality control system, the financing or, most important, the functions of health services.

The background for this attitude is clear enough. Health services in any given country are an integral part of the political, economic, and administrative structure of the country concerned, and can therefore only be understood within this frame. The main principles which govern national life in general, from power structure to interpersonal relationships, reflect themselves also in the health services. As a matter of fact, one way of classifying health service systems throughout the world into categories is to relate them to the dominant political and economic philosophies. But this self-evident fact does not justify the negative attitude towards exchange of experiences noted above.

Firstly, of course, there exists an *international armamentarium* of "tools" available to health services all over the world, in the form of health personnel, equipment and building standards, medical know-how in diagnosis, treatment, and rehabilitation, methodology in research, etc. It is, in my opinion, of great value to study, on a comprehensive basis, to what extent it has been possible to apply current medical science and technology in existing health services.

Secondly, health services may be characterized as a "flexible" sector of society. Collective solutions for solving health problems may, for example, be found in countries where the individualistic approach is the traditional one. This holds true perhaps especially for the *financing* of health services, but also for their organizational structure and administration. One may express the same thought in other words: due to the positive and noncontroversial goal of health services one is more free than in other sectors to test and apply methods which differ from the basic philosophy or ideology of the country concerned. As a matter of fact, health services may sometimes serve as a lever to achieve more rational and humanitarian approaches also in other sectors of society.

Under any circumstances, even the most skeptical health administrator, sociologist, or politician is willing to draw conclusions from the *unsuccessful* experiments and experience in other countries. Negative findings are frequently as rewarding as the positive ones.

Much more could be said in favor of comparative studies of health services. Let me point to just one more reason why international exchange of data in this field is more important in our days than perhaps in any period before us. With a certain amount of simplification it may be stated that there exist four main categories of countries in the world today: 1) industrialized countries with a predominantly free enterprise or market economy; 2) industrialized countries with a centrally planned economy; 3) underdeveloped countries in possession of natural resources in high demand (oil, minerals, or other raw materials or sources of energy); and 4) underdeveloped countries poor in natural resources.

The majority of the peoples of the world live in countries in categories 3 and 4. No one should close his eyes to the fact that we are witnessing the broadest and deepest revolution in the history of mankind: this majority of mankind has become conscious of its dismal life situation and is unwilling to accept it. Promotion of health, prevention, and treatment of disease is a fundamental part of their just demands. It is essential that they should as far as possible avoid the unsatisfactory solutions, and outright mistakes and failures from which so many countries before them have suffered—and still suffer.

Milton I. Roemer is one of the very few contemporary medically trained scientists who has consistently and tenaciously addressed himself to comparative studies of health services, and to surveys which may be used for such comparison. Since he has been doing this for more than twenty-five years and in countries representing all the main categories existing at present, the selected papers published in this collection provide invaluable material for forming a picture of the current situation; they also present the reader with important parts of the history of the development of health philosophy and health services since the Second World War. While improved material standards of living correctly have been credited with a major positive impact upon morbidity and mortality, question marks are now cropping up. Indeed, more and more "manmade" pathogenic agents, not only biophysical but also psycho-social and socioeconomic, are being identified. In other words, economic growth in the traditional sense does not always result in improved health. On the contrary, this situation has not only confronted health services of conventional types with new and challenging tasks, but also has blurred the former delineation between health and social welfare services.

For much too long a time studies of the type found in this volume could only count on a very limited number of readers—specialists in health administration and the like. It is a credit to international health workers like the author that research in this field has now become "in," and attracts interest in much wider circles—not only at the academic, but also at the administrative, political, and executive levels. The rising cost of medical care, the increasingly complex nature of preventive, curative, and rehabilitative health activities, the necessity of planning for the optimal utilization of available resources, the need for establishing priorities, the attempts to mobilize to a greater extent the local community and the individual for a more active role in the promotion and maintenance of health — these have all become questions of importance and urgency, on which different national experiences can offer useful lessons.

KARL EVANG, M.D.
Director General of Health Services,
Norway (1939-1972)

Oslo, Norway
26 October 1975

Preface

This collection of 30 papers is intended to provide perspective on the variety of health care systems operating throughout the world. It represents work done by the author over the last 25 years, mainly through field studies sponsored by the World Health Organization, but also by the Pan American Union, the U.S. Peace Corps, research grants from the U.S. Public Health Service, or in other ways. Assignments of the International Labour Organization or voluntary bodies in Canada, Venezuela, or the United States provided the basis of certain papers.

All but four of the papers have previously appeared in either published or processed form, but many of them are not easily accessible. More important, it seemed of possible value to assemble them in a format and order which might give greater meaning to the development, the structure, and dynamics of the varied health care systems of the world. Accordingly, from about 70 papers or monographs produced over the years, based mainly on field studies in some 45 countries on all the continents, these 30 papers have been selected in the attempt to present a balanced account.

Obviously, the several chapters represent the viewpoint of one person, and this has its advantages and shortcomings. As for the latter, the accounts may be presented with a certain bias—the bias of someone who, with a background of public health study and work, regards health services as a social right more than a market commodity (although in most countries it is treated, to some extent, as both). As for its advantages, there may be, it is hoped, some internal consistency and rationale in the analysis of countries with very different political, economic, and social structures. Others, viewing the same facts, might interpret them differently, but that task I must leave to them. In the selected bibliography at the end, there are listed numerous works by other observers of differing viewpoints.

As mentioned, these papers have been written over the course of 25 years; yet the organization of health services is obviously a very dynamic process.

One could not hope to produce a truly up-to-date account of the health care system in all countries today without a large staff, continuously at work. In brief introductory statements to each chapter, I have tried to draw the reader's attention to some of the most significant changes occurring since the paper was written. Still, even some "out-of-date" accounts may have historical value, not only for the countries or the health problems involved, but also for temporal perspective on current happenings in other countries, like the United States, where today's events are like those a generation ago in Europe.

Unlike a number of excellent books on international health, this one is not focused exclusively on the developing countries or on those nations which have adopted certain important social devices, like social security. While certainly not complete or encyclopedic, it attempts to give the reader some glimpses of all kinds of country—developing and industrialized, capitalist and socialist. It also examines certain facets of health service—like disease-specific campaigns, ambulatory care, or hospitals—across all types of country. No pretense, of course, is made to coverage of all the important facets of health services.

This combined approach inevitably results in some repetition. A relatively detailed account of the current structure of health services in Malaysia, for example, naturally includes reference to its health centers. At the same time a world review of organized ambulatory services makes references to Malaysia's health centers. Crucial health care system models like the British or the Soviet, or sectors of them, are mentioned in several places. The apparent duplication, however, is hopefully justified by presentation of these facts in different contexts. Perhaps this may sharpen perspective on certain issues, as well as reinforcing the learning of whatever this book has to teach.

The volume is organized in five parts. First is a background section, intended to provide an overview of the world's health care systems along dimensions of time (development) and space. Part two is on the developing countries, analyzing problems and practices in selected countries of Latin America, Asia, and Africa. Part three is devoted to industrialized (I prefer this term to "developed"—since no country is fully so) countries, as seen in Western Europe, North America, Australasia, and the Soviet Union. Part four examines a number of specific health programs or problems as handled throughout the world. Manpower, facilities, or processes like social insurance are explored in the diverse manners by which they are applied in different national settings. Finally, in part five, general interpretative papers are presented on issues that have special, often controversial significance in the world today, especially in the United States.

After these papers there is a General Bibliography of the writings of health scholars who have studied the world and published about it, especially in English. The many gaps which will be evident in the main text will doubtless be filled by consulting these works, as well as numerous differing points of view.

This volume may perhaps be of use as a textbook in university courses on international heath or comparative health care systems. Perhaps it might serve as a reference source. Hopefully, it will stimulate others to produce further accounts of health care systems of the world in greater depth and sophistication. Hopefully also it may provide some background to social policy decision-makers in this or other countries who sometimes view a health service problem as though there were only one possible solution to it.

Finally, I should like to acknowledge my debt to the World Health Organization, the International Labour Organization, the Pan American Union, and several United States federal agencies for providing me the opportunity of making these studies of health care systems of other nations. To the national governments of these countries, and to countless health workers and citizens in them also goes my gratitude for providing me with so much information and guidance. For the interpretations of this knowledge, or for errors in transmitting it, of course, the author must take responsibility. My principal hope is that the fallacies in reporting or in judgment may not be too numerous, and that the principal impact may be that all of us, of every nationality, will realize that we have much to learn from each other in developing health care systems to better meet the health needs of mankind.

MILTON I. ROEMER

Los Angeles, California
June 1976

Part One

Background and Overview

Chapter I
Historic Development of Worldwide Health Service Systems

A trend toward increasing social organization of health services has been evident since ancient times and in all parts of the world. The shape taken by this organization varies with the social, political, and economic context of different nations at different time periods. Everywhere, however, the organization involves in varying degrees both (1) the mobilization of economic support for health services and (2) the rationalized provision or delivery of those services for certain populations or to tackle certain disease problems—to achieve greater equity and effectiveness.

In this first chapter, a worldwide view is taken of these organizational trends—briefly for early times and in somewhat more detail for the period since World War I (about 1920) up to 1959. Significant trends since 1959—for example, the extension of the concept and role of "health centers" or the rise of the percentage of gross national product devoted to health purposes—will be discussed in later chapters. This text was published originally under the title "World Trends in Medical Care Organization" in Social Research (Vol. 26, 1959, pp. 283-310). It is reprinted here by permission.[1]

For at least a century there has been a trend throughout the world toward the social organization of health services. As the scope of medical and related services has widened with expanding knowledge, larger and larger segments of the total health field have been subjected to collective controls, mainly through actions of government. Collectivization has been applied both to the systems of economic support for health services and to the patterns of provision or delivery of those services. The effect has been to make more health services available to more people.

The forms that this process of social organization or collectivization of health services have taken vary with the changing political and economic situations in different countries. In fact, the general political setting is the major determinant of these forms, despite the frequent claims of the health professions about being masters of their own fate.

A review of world trends in this field may be helpful in giving perspective on current events in the United States and the likely course of health affairs in the future.

EARLY COLLECTIVE MEASURES FOR HEALTH

The earliest societies known showed social or group consciousness of the need for health services. Medicine men or shamans, whose duties were to drive away evil spirits believed to cause disease, were usually held in high esteem and were often supported by collective gifts from the tribe. Ancient Babylonia developed legal codes for the practice of surgery, specifying rewards or punishments depending on the outcome of the procedure and the social class of the patient. The Hebrews formulated dietary and other sanitary laws for the collective protection of nomadic tribes.

The city-states of classical Greece appointed physicians to serve the poor, and these positions were coveted for their prestige and remuneration. In ancient Rome, physicians were attached, as servants, to the great latifundia, serving the family of the land-lord and to some extent treating the local slaves. Surgeons were attached to the Roman legions, and there were military hospitals. The aqueducts and sewers of Rome obviously required organizational genius.

In medieval Europe the Church was the major organized power, and monasteries were the main repositories of medical knowledge. The monks and priests sometimes attempted to heal the sick. Feudal estates had lay healers attached to the household, for the benefit of the lord and his family; as in Rome, the local serfs were also treated, partly because of their economic value. With the Renaissance, the rise of the universities—which trained physicians systematically—and the growth of cities, doctors broke away from the feudal manors and set up shop in the cities as "free" practitioners.

In Elizabethan England, responsibilities were placed on the towns and other local authorities for aid to the "worthy poor." Medical services of a sort were among these social responsibilities, given by a doctor appointed by the Overseer of the Poor. In the larger cities, like Paris and London, hospitals were organized for the sick poor—places of refuge for the old, the destitute, and the disabled who would otherwise beg and die on the streets. The Church took the first action, and later the city governments.

As classes of journeymen or craftsmen grew in the cities, guilds were formed, whose functions included collective aid to the sick. A disabled brother would be helped financially, and the cost of medicines and doctor fees would be paid. The insurance idea grew not only among tradesmen, but in Central Europe among all residents of a particular duchy or village. By the midnineteenth century these "voluntary health insurance" schemes were commonplace among the lower economic classes of Europe.

With rising industrialization in Western Europe, cities grew at a phenomenal rate and, within them, slums. The working class began to organize, socialist philosophy was formulated, and humanitarianism emerged as a social doctrine. Reports were made on the sordid condition of the poor in London and, motivated by the desire to reduce epidemic disease which might spread to all classes, the English Parliament enacted the first public health laws, around 1848. Similar "sanitary awakening" occurred in Germany and France a few years later. Governmental police powers were invoked to assure safe water supplies, to isolate and quarantine cases of infectious disease, to vaccinate against smallpox. The "rights" of the individual were suppressed in the interests of preventing disease in the mass.

In 1865 czarist Russia, with the abolition of serf-dom, established the system of "zemstvo" medicine. For the first time a large peasant population received medical care as a public benefit, financed through taxes paid by the people to the zemstvo or district authority. Doctors were engaged on a salary, and auxiliaries or "feldshers" were trained, to extend the capacity of the small supply of physicians. The quality and quantity of services were meager, but the principle of medical service as a collective function, rather than a matter for private purchase, was established.

In Germany the social-democratic forces were growing and threatening conservative leadership. To steal their thunder, the Conservative premier, Prince Otto Bismarck, introduced in 1883 the first law making insurance compulsory for disability compensation and for medical care costs. Workers of low income were required to be members of "Krankenkassen" or group sickness funds, to which a large number already belonged on a voluntary basis. Upper income persons were exempt. Soon other countries followed suit, England not until 1911 under the middle-of-the-road Liberal, Lloyd George. There were various limitations regarding the persons covered by these "compulsory health insurance" schemes and the benefits provided. The British system, for example, financed only the services of general medical practitioners and drugs—not specialists, hospitalization, or dental care.

Gradually, coverage under the health insurance programs extended to persons of higher income and specified occupations. Benefits also widened, to include more types of medical service. Health insurance was part of the whole social security movement for pensions for the aged and assistance to the poor. Unemployment insurance and family allowances were to come later. The concept of employer liability for industrial accidents gradually emerged in all industrialized countries, including the United States after 1910. Workmen's compensation laws provided cash replacement of wage loss, when disability was due to an accident on the job (later when it was due to occupational diseases), and necessary medical care. The struggles against the old legal doctrines of "master-servant relations" and "assumption of risk" are a saga of social conflict leading finally to the assignment to management of responsibility for industrial hazards.

As European nations took control over the economically backward stretches of Asia and Africa, colonial medical systems were established. Designed originally to protect the European settlers and military forces sent out to hold the colony for the mother country, these systems were slowly extended to the native populations. Because expenditures for such welfare services were to be kept to a minimum, economical and efficient patterns were employed: typically, doctors and auxiliary personnel on salary, working not from private offices but from strategically placed dispensaries and hospitals. These schemes hardly scratched the surface of the enormous disease problems in the tropics, but they provided a pattern of highly organized health service on which the present systems in India, most of Africa, Indonesia, and other former European colonies are built.

In the industrialized countries, government assumed responsibilities for certain diseases of a serious, chronic nature which were at the same time threats to the community. Mental disease was so regarded after the early nineteenth century, especially after Philippe Pinel, in the wake of the French Revolution, succeeded in separating the insane from the criminal and destitute. Mental hospitals began to be operated everywhere by government. In the late nineteenth century, first in Germany (1859) and then elsewhere, tuberculosis received similar recognition, with special sanatoria established by voluntary societies and later by cities and provinces. In the twentieth century the treatment of venereal disease also became a social responsibility.

Development in the United States recapitulated in many ways worldwide developments, telescoped into a shorter span of years. Systems of limited medical care for the poor were organized in the colonial period, after the Elizabethan pattern. In 1750 the first hopital was established for the sick poor, in Philadelphia. Merchant seamen were important for the economic progress of the young republic, and a special hospital service was established for them in 1798 under the federal government. Public health boards were organized in a few of the larger cities after 1800 to meet emergency situations, but the first full-time technical staff for disease prevention was not organized by a state until after the Civil War, in Massachusetts in 1869. Small health insurance schemes were associated with isolated mines and railroad construction projects in the late nineteenth century. By the time of the First World War the United States had its institutions for mental disease and tuberculosis, operated by governments, its local schemes for medical relief of the poor, its organized health departments, and its community hospitals—usually nongovernmental but collectively constructed and operated.

It is obvious that up to the First World War a great deal of organization of health servies had already occurred throughout the world. Collective action had been taken for various segments of the population or for various phases of total health service which were believed beyond the capacity of the individual. In the main, nevertheless, the procurement of medical care on a world scale was still regarded more as a personal than a social responsibility.

THE INTERWAR PERIOD

With the end of the First World War a sharp spurt occurred in the conception of social responsibility for health. In almost all countries new legislation was passed to expand social security systems. The International Labour Organization was founded on the slogan "peace through social justice," and set out to promote health insurance programs.

One of the most far-reaching sequelae of the war was the Russian Revolution and, with it, the inauguration of the Soviet system of health services. For the first time there was established in an independent country a system of complete medical service, under which personal health care—both preventive and curative—was offered to everyone without charge. All physicians and other health workers became employees of the state, and all hospitals and other medical facilities became governmentally owned and operated. The whole system was centrally controlled and organized, including the manufacture of drugs, the education of medical and related practitioners, and the promulgation of research. Great emphasis was placed on preventive medicine.

In the socialist society of the Soviet Union, health service became a deliberate goal of government, not based on a conception of police power against sanitary violations or straining to offer minimum interference in the private world of medical practice. Unlike the colonial systems, which were also publicly organized, there was continuous expansion in quantity and quality of services. The improvements over conditions in czarist Russia were ten- and twentyfold in health personnel and medical facilities.

As a direct outcome of the First World War, military medicine in nearly all the warring powers achieved a high state of development. This is, in effect, a completely socialistic system of health service, applied to millions of men under arms. The experience was bound to have continuing influence, and after 1920 most of the Western powers set up elaborate systems of medical service for veterans. In the countries with basic health insurance systems these special veterans' services were limited to care of war-connected disabilities. In the United States, without a health insurance framework, political pressures led to extension of benefits to the much larger category of non-service-connected disabilities. A great network of special hospitals was constructed, with salaried medical personnel, to provide services for veterans.

In all countries increased medical knowledge led to the growth of medical specialism. With it, the cost of medical care rose sharply. For the noninsured upper and middle classes in the industrialized countries, a type of specialist developed, giving elegant service. London had its Harley Street, New York its Park Avenue. For most of the world population, however, specialist services had to be given in hospitals, in the wards or in institutional outpatient departments.

As a result, there was a large and steady expansion of hospitals under governmental auspices. Except in the United States and Canada, where the local "voluntary" hospital became the predominant pattern, general hospitals everywhere came under increased public control. In Scandinavia, Great Britain, New Zealand, Mexico, India, and elsewhere, salaried full-time hospital specialists were engaged—with sharp separation from the general practitioner who treated the patient outside the hospital. Even in France and Germany, where private specialists did most of the hospital work, the attending staffs were small and select. The great majority of patients were "ward cases" not paying private fees; instead the specialist received an "honorarium" or part-time salary for his service in the hospital on an annual basis.

In the United States, on the other hand, hospitals developed mainly as the "workshop" of the private physician, and he usually collected private fees for his services to patients. General practitioners and specialists alike had hospital "privileges." But with specialists mainly in private office practice (rather than attached to hospitals), a new pattern developed: the group medical clinic. This American phenomenon was started originally by the Mayo brothers in a Minnesota village in 1887. After the First World War the idea took hold and sprouted. It represented a new social form of medical practice, in which a type of technical collectivism replaced purely individual enterprise.

To a great extent the social organization of medical services continued to take the form of voluntary societies directed to specific health objectives. In Catholic countries like Italy and Belgium, such organizations, associated with the Church, were particularly numerous and influential. In these countries, and in Holland as well, almost the whole public health program was operated by voluntary societies—one for child health, another for tuberculosis, another for maternity, and so on. But government came increasingly to control these societies, through large financial grants made condi-

tional on meeting certain standards. In South America, many hospitals established originally by churches were gradually taken over by governments.

During the interwar period the health insurance systems of Europe took a further spurt in coverage and benefits. France inaugurated its program in 1928. With the doctors in this traditionally individualistic country in a firm bargaining position, an indemnity pattern of medical fees was established, constituting the least possible "interference" by the state in the doctor-patient relationship. The social insurance idea spread east and west, with Japan requiring compulsory health coverage for certain occupational groups in 1922 and Chile (the first Latin American country) in 1924.

The Pan-American Sanitary Bureau had been organized in 1905, largely under United States influence, with its headquarters in Washington, D.C. This was Teddy Roosevelt's era of "the big stick," and the PASB was the "soft voice" that went with it. Between the wars this agency spread the gospel of sanitation and hygiene to the semifeudal economies of South and Central America. A groundwork was laid for later public health expansion.

The Great Depression of the 1930s had widespread influences on the organization of health services. In Europe the social forces generating welfare programs had matured a generation earlier, but in the United States it took the grim thirties to lead to governmental reform. Under the New Deal the Social Security Act was passed, in 1935, part of which provided federal grants to the states for public health services. The entire public health movement gained tremendous impetus. Under the pressures of economic depression, hospital financing faced a crisis, and the Blue Cross movement came to the rescue. These voluntary insurance schemes for financing hospital care were, in a sense, an American counterpart of the European development of public hospital systems.

A series of bills were introduced in the United States Congress for federally sponsored medical care insurance. Although none passed, they served as continuous threats, in the face of which conservative groups decided to capitulate on lesser issues. There is no doubt that the program of federally supported hospital construction, enacted in 1946, resulted from the pressures created by the various Wagner-Murray-Dingell bills. The same was true for the expanded programs of industrial hygiene, tuberculosis control, and cancer research, which emerged in these years. Improved medical services for the indigent were developed everywhere, under the welfare authorities.

The interwar period, then, saw continued ad-

vances in the social organization of health services throughout the world. The approach was often piecemeal, but the direction was clearly toward subjecting larger and larger sectors of health need to public control. The extent was obviously greater in countries with strong socialist or social-democratic movements.

SECOND WORLD WAR AND AFTER

The First World War had been to "save the world for democracy," but not everyone took the slogan seriously. With the rise of fascism and the Axis powers, the Four Freedoms of the Second World War became objectives in deadly earnest. Even before the war was over, nations drew up their "postwar" plans—the goals for which the war was being fought. High on the agenda of the democratic nations were plans for extension of health services.

Out of wartime Britain came the famous Beveridge Report on "Social Insurance and Allied Services," which called, among other things, for

> . . . a comprehensive national health service [which] will ensure that for every citizen there is available whatever medical treatment he requires, in whatever form he requires it, domiciliary or institutional, general, specialist or consultant, and will ensure also the provision of dental, ophthalmic and surgical appliances, nursing and midwifery, and rehabilitation after accidents.

It is interesting to observe that Sir William Beveridge, like Lloyd George and Otto Bismarck before him, was a conservative statesman, and moreover, that his plans were very similar to proposals being made by the Medical Planning Commission of the British Medical Association.

The British National Health Service, finally set underway in 1948 by the Labour government, provides virtually complete health service, curative and preventive, to every resident of the British Isles. Nearly all hospitals were taken over by the government, and all hospital specialists placed on salary. To satisfy various special interests, an unwieldy administrative structure was established, with separate authorities for hospital, general practitioner, and public health services. In recent years the Conservative government has introduced partial charges for drugs and some other items. The Service, nevertheless, establishes the principle of health care as a citizen right. The retention of private office practice for general practitioners is obviously a compromise with the past, which may become gradually modified as neighborhood health centers are constructed. The chief reason for the snail's pace in construction of these public buildings has been the cold war, with

its enormous military expenditures and consequent curtailment of spending for welfare purposes.

Extension of social insurance has occurred in every Western European country since World War II. In France, health coverage was extended to nearly the entire population, although the indemnity payment system was retained. A Ministry of Social Security took direct control of the whole system from the former semiautonomous insurance societies. In the immediate postwar period (under a coalition government including the extreme left) the most sweeping occupational health legislation of any Western European country was enacted in France. For the first time, every employer was required to establish an industrial health service—not only to prevent occupational diseases and accidents, but to promote proper job placement and general health protection of the workers. The entire public health system in France was greatly strengthened.

The hospital systems in Scandinavia, which had long been outstanding, were markedly expanded. Sweden in 1948 enacted, under the Social Democratic regime, legislation to extend its voluntary health insurance scheme to the entire population. But the effective date was postponed. Sweden had been neutral in the war and its people did not suffer. Pressure for "economies" and the opposition of the medical profession were stronger than public demands for health service. Again and again the effective date was postponed, and it was not until 1955 that, with modifications, the legislation was effectuated, requiring health insurance protection for 100 percent of the Swedish population. Norway established universal coverage for its health insurance system in 1957.

Even in the defeated Axis countries, medical care insurance was extended after the war. But the autonomous insurance societies in West Germany, Austria, and Italy were very strong, and the relatively conservative Christian-Democratic regimes in these countries had no intention of disturbing them. Thus, while insurance coverage was extended, there was no nationalization of the social insurance system under direct government control, as in both Britain and France. Public health services, under direct government supervision, were expanded, but only slightly.

In Eastern Europe, where the prewar monarchies or oligarchic regimes had kept social welfare programs to a minimum, the destruction of fascism wrought the greatest changes in health service. In Poland, Hungary, Bulgaria, Roumania, Albania, and Yugoslavia, coalition governments, with strong Communist participation, won control. Limited programs of health insurance for industrial

workers—a very small percntage of the national population—had been operating in these countries; medical services for the vast peasantry had been extremely poor. The Communists soon gained complete control, and steps were taken to make health services available to everyone as a public benefit, so far as resources would permit. The legislation passed was based essentially on the Soviet model. Even after Yugoslavia broke its relations with the other countries of Eastern Europe, it retained the basic pattern of health service, with salaried personnel working out of governmental centers. Private practice declined to low levels. In 1948, when Czechoslovakia's government became Communist-controlled, similar health measures were enacted there.

The reorganization of health services in these Eastern European countries was not easy. Large numbers of doctors had been killed, since many were Jews. Others, having been members of middle class, propertied families, fled to the West with the victory of the Communist regimes. Many more doctors and nurses had to be trained, and destroyed hospitals rebuilt. Health centers had to be established everywhere. The results, according to British and French observers who have traveled in these countries, have been impressive. While there are still personnel shortages, health services have been extended to the remotest villages. Clinics for complete medical care (not merely for first aid) are found in the larger factories. There is unified administration of all preventive and curative services, with local citizens' committees theoretically having a voice in policy formation.

The Soviet Union health system, too, had to rebuild its physical structures after the war. Thousands of doctors, feldshers (medical assistants), nurses, and technicians were trained, and hundreds of new hospitals and health centers were built. The extension of organized health services to the rural villages continued. Strange to Western ears is the fact that country doctors are paid higher salaries than city doctors of the same training, since their living conditions are more humble and their responsibilities greater. Starting as a primitive, underdeveloped country in 1918, the Soviet Union today has more physicians per 1,000 population than the United States. Their training, however, like that of all European doctors, is shorter than that of American doctors.

The postwar movement toward social organization of health services has been dynamic in nearly all countries. Even before its independence was granted, India launched its Health Survey and Development Committee, whose four-volume report in 1946 called for a completely governmental health service, very much along the lines of the Soviet system. The Bhore Report, named for the chairman of the Committee, contemplates integrated public health and hospital administrative units, with salaried personnel providing everyone with free service. Under the Congress party, with its middle class professional and business leadership, progress toward this goal has been slow. A medical care insurance plan has been started among certain workers in the large cities (Bombay, Calcutta, Delhi), the medical and nursing schools have been strengthened, and good work has been done in specific fields like malaria control. Health services to India's hundred millions in the villages still remain primitive, but there is no question about the intention, once economic resources are stronger, to develop a completely socialized system of medical services.

The Union of South Africa had its national commission which likewise recommended a socialized health system, much emphasis being placed on health centers. Under the Conservative government, with its apartheid policy, which took over control a few years after the war, these recommendations were not implemented. A number of demonstration health centers for the African Negroes were developed, however, and the public hospital system was expanded. For the upper income white population in the Union, medical service remains essentially a private matter.

Other parts of the British Commonwealth reacted differently to postwar demands for the Four Freedoms. New Zealand had instituted a system of medical care insurance in 1938, covering the entire population regardless of individual insurance contributions. There were various difficulties in getting the participation of physicians, however, and the program did not go smoothly until after the war. In Australia the Labour government proposed a comprehensive health insurance system, but medical opposition was so strong that only a scheme for high cost drugs was launched. In the 1950s this was extended to include physician's services for old-age pensioners and certain other benefits. Hospital services in Australia have long been predominantly under the public auspices, although there are great differences among the states.

In Canada the Liberal party (ideologically like the Democrats in the United States) was long in control nationally (until 1957), and has theoretically favored national health insurance since 1919. There were repeated postponements, however, for which various reasons were offered. With the election to power of a semisocialist CCF (Cooperative Commonwealth Federation) government in Saskatchewan in 1944, the first compulsory insurance program for health

services on a state-wide or province-wide basis was inaugurated on the North American continent. It was confined to hospitalization, although in one region of the province, with 50,000 people, a comprehensive medical care insurance program was also launched. Local government plans for general practitioner services had held doctors in rural municipalities of the Canadian prairies since 1916. In 1949 the province of British Columbia, despite its much more conservative government, followed Saskatchewan's lead with a hospitalization insurance scheme, and other provinces developed modified plans for public financing of hospital care. Special programs in Canada for cancer and poliomyelitis, for general care to the indigent, for medical services to workmen's compensation cases, and for military veterans were expanded in the postwar period, bringing further segments of medical need under public auspices. By 1956 the federal government passed legislation to share the costs of general hospital care with any province in which the entire population is covered by a public program. In January 1959 this law became universal, bringing general hospital insurance to almost all of Canada.

In the economically underdeveloped countries of Asia and Africa, important strides toward social organization of health services were made in the postwar years. Recently emancipated countries, like Burma and Indonesia, undertook serious reorganization and expansion of their health systems. Since the old colonial governments offered health care— limited as it was—as a public service, the pattern was well established. In these countries, resources in trained personnel, buildings, equipment, and supplies were extremely limited. The Dutch had maintained in the East Indies (Indonesia), for example, one trained physician for about 75,000 persons (U.S. average is one to 750), and most of these were in the larger cities. First steps to improvement therefore required vast programs of training and construction, but no one has questioned the basic necessity of preventive and curative medicine for everyone as a public service.

Even in the persistent colonies there were extensions of health services after the war. The United Nations established a Trusteeship Council which, while getting fewer newspaper headlines than the Security Council, exerted much influence on the conduct of affairs in the "non-self-governing territories." The rumblings in Kenya put the British Colonial Office on its toes, as the discontent in Tunisia stimulated the French. Additional health centers, mobile clinics, and hospitals were established in Africa and the Pacific Islands.

The forces of democracy, literacy, industrializa-

tion, and personal expression are probably at their lowest ebb in the Moslem states of the Middle East. The fellaheen of Egypt and their peasant brethren in Iraq, Syria, Jordan, Saudi Arabia, and other Arab lands are perhaps more firmly ground under the heel of feudalism and ignorance than any other peoples in the world. Despite this, the leaders of even these countries were driven by world forces to expand health services for their depressed millions. A number of modern hospitals and health centers, with salaried medical and technical staffs, were constructed in Egypt. Programs for the control of malaria, trachoma, bilharziasis, yaws, syphilis, and tuberculosis were planned throughout the Arab world.

The new state of Israel was born in 1948, bringing to the Eastern Mediterranean area its first demonstration (with the possible exception of Lebanon) of a modern democracy. In Israel there developed an advanced system of health service under the Ministry of Health and the Jewish Labor Federation. In Palestine, under the British mandate, important groundwork had been laid, and the Jewish Labor Federation (Histadruth) had been operating since the early twentieth century. The latter's Kupat Holim (sickness fund) provides insured medical services for two-thirds of the population. While voluntary in coverage, this scheme—unlike any other in the world—gives all its services through salaried physicians working in dispensaries and hospitals.

Occupied Japan naturally came under heavy American influence. Many Japanese labor groups and social insurance experts advocated extension of the old piecemeal health insurance system into an integrated national scheme covering everyone. An American advisory commission, however, advocated continuation of the voluntary system, with local option of the prefectures as to type of coverage. A network of health centers was constructed, on the U.S. pattern of confinement to preventive services.

The revolution in China, bringing a Communist government to power in 1949, naturally brought enormous changes in health service. Even under the Kuomintang regime the government had been committed, at least in theory, to a system of socialized health services. Under the new government, major efforts were extended to reach the goal. Training institutions were expanded, with much stress being put on "middle medical personnel"—health workers trained for only a year or two who, under proper medical direction, could quickly bring some minimum services to the villages. Hundreds of new hospitals and health centers were constructed. Great public education campaigns on hygiene and insect control were launched, with ordinary citizens given responsibilities for local direction. Tens of millions were vaccinated. While some private medical practice continues in the larger cities, nearly all new Chinese graduates have become employees of the socialized health service.

Even though its participation in the war had been slight, Latin America also shared in the postwar expansion of organized health services. Almost every South American republic developed after 1945 a system of health insurance for certain segments of the population. Usually miners and industrial workers were covered, but not agricultural peons or tenants or peasants. While coverage was thus limited to only a small fraction of the population—five or ten percent—the framework has been laid for expansion as industrialization increases. Medical service under the insurance systems is given usually by physicians on part-time salary, working out of special clinics. Public health services have been greatly expanded, largely under the stimulus of assistance from the Institute of Inter-American Affairs, set up as part of President Roosevelt's good neighbor policy. In 1952 Chile, which had been the first American republic to launch a compulsory insurance system, took the important step of expanding and integrating its diverse programs of preventive and curative medicine under unified central direction. Described as its "National Health Service," inspired obviously by the British example, this was one more move toward a systematic public service that would make health care, supported mainly by tax funds, a right of everyone.

CURRENT TRENDS OF IMPORTANCE

Underlying many of the developments of the years following World War II was the inspiration of One World as applied to health—an inspiration made real in the founding of the World Health Organization.

The constitution of the World Health Organization, which came into effect in 1948, was an event of real importance—not because of its lofty definition of health ("a state of complete physical, mental, and social well-being") so widely quoted, but because it set up a practical organization for doing something about it. Unlike the League of Nations Health Division before it, WHO set up its own Assembly and Executive Board, so that it would not be a feather in the larger polical winds. Unfortunately the Cold War had its effect, and in 1950 the Soviet Union and other Communist nations withdrew. Not until July 1955, after the Geneva "summit" conference and the great relaxation of international tensions, did the Soviet Union return to WHO.

Despite these and other difficulties (such as serious controversies between Catholic and other coun-

tries on the birth control issue), important contributions have been made by WHO. Most of all, the Organization has helped to convey to the smaller and the underdeveloped countries the general importance of large investments for health. It has helped to put the health ministry in the larger arena of national affairs, instead of being a second-string activity. Sound technical advice is given by WHO on a score of medical and public health problems. Nationalism and insularity are being reduced, with the result that progressive forces in the health field tend to be fortified in each country.

The "technical assistance" approach to helping the underdeveloped countries of the world has, of course, been promoted by the United Nations as a whole. For many, the idea is accepted chiefly as a bulwark against communism. It is argued that communism thrives simply on suffering, and therefore any technical advancement that will reduce human misery will weaken the Communist movement. By the same token, some leftists oppose all UN and WHO technical assistance efforts on the grounds that they are cloaked with this somewhat negative motive and, moreover, may sometimes help to strengthen the position of reactionary governments.

The fact is that, regardless of motives, the ultimate effect of technical assistance programs must always be progressive and in the direction of social organization of health and related welfare services. The greatest impediment to the liberation of impoverished peoples from backwardness and feudalism is their physical lethargy, fatalism, and lack of hope. Social revolutions, or even modest movements toward democratization, are not made by the apathetic dwellers in mud huts who have no reason to expect a brighter day tomorrow. But when, with technical advances, regardless of their source, these people learn that life need not be dull and hopeless, and untimely death can be prevented, then they begin to move. They demand more worldly goods, more education, and richer experiences from life; they become passionately dissatisfied. This is bound to lead, in the long run, to democratization and increased social organization of all types. This is the ultimate consequence to be expected from the activities of the World Health Organization. While WHO has rather scrupulously avoided direct involvement in the "controversial" issues of medical care planning, there can be no doubt that the long-term effect of its work is to heighten governmental responsibilities for the protection of health and hence the social organization of health services.

From the great accumulation of crippled veterans and civilians left by the war, there has arisen in all the industrialized nations a powerful movement for rehabilitation of the handicapped. The philosophy has become widespread that no human being is beyond redemption, however disabled, and that with patient treatment and encouragement he can be helped to become independent or at least more self-reliant. In Great Britain, Soviet Russia, Scandinavia, Japan, Germany, and the United States many specialized institutions have been developed for this type of service. The "vocational rehabilitation" program in the United States provides special funds for these purposes. In a sense this movement has added another category—the crippling orthopedic disorders—to the list of chronic diseases for which public responsibility is assumed (like tuberculosis, mental disorder, and syphilis). Another sector of health need is thus being transferred from individual to social responsibility.

Along with disabilities due to crippling trauma and disease, there is in all the industrialized countries another class of disabilities that is increasing: the chronic disorders associated with old age. With the reduction of infant mortality rates, the conquest of most epidemic diseases, and the increased longevity of the population, a much greater proportion of the people than formerly are afflicted with heart disease, cancer, rheumatism, diabetes, and other non-bacterial disorders. Being chronic, these diseases require medical care that is expensive and beyond the means of many individuals. Public action, therefore, is deemed necessary—especially in the development of numerous institutions for the aged and chronically ill. General hospital beds are filling up with these "long-term cases," and movements have been stimulated in America and Europe for "home care" of such patients. Geriatrics, a new medical specialty, has emerged.

Medical care programs, in a sense, fight a losing battle. The more effectively health is promoted, the more diseases prevented and lives saved—the more new problems must be faced. Older people, biologically, have more ailments requiring care. The fact that these ailments are expensive to handle has summoned public action, adding further impetus toward social organization of health service.

Hospitalization for chronic and acute disease alike is increasing on a world scale. With advances in science, the capacities of the doctor in an office or on a home call have relatively dwindled. For the best possible diagnosis and treatment of nearly all serious disease, the hospital is the modern place of choice. As a result, hospitals have been multiplied everywhere—in the poorest as well as the richest countries. The hospital has become the ideological and practical center of health service in the community. But hospitals are expensive places to build and operate, and thus are increasingly sponsored by governments.

As a corollary of hospital construction trends, there have evolved in many countries forces for geographic extension of hospital services far and wide. It is basically a drive for rural equality that has led to the movement in Europe, South America, Africa, the United States, and elsewhere for "regionalization" of hospital services. If country-dwellers, they must have access to the same type of hospitals and specialists as city-dwellers. Yet not every village can have the full symphony of medical equipment and skills. The answer, put forward everywhere, is for institutions to function in a cooperative network, with large, complex units at the urban centers and smaller ones at the rural peripheries. Patients with difficult problems may be referred from the outpost toward the center, while consultant services are sent from the center outward.

The regionalization idea requires planning and central control. As demands for agrarian equality grow, governments and (in the United States) voluntary agencies are extending the organization of hospitals along regional lines. The movement inevitably advances overall planning and systematization of health service.

Rural health equality also demands other actions. The maldistribution of doctors between town and country is a feature of almost all countries. But steps are being taken to increase the proportionate numbers of physicians in rural areas. In many of the South American countries a period of service in a rural village is required of all new medical graduates, as a condition of licensure. Turkey and Switzerland have sent young doctors to the rural districts on military duty. In the United States, special fellowships are given by state governments to rural youth, on the condition that they will spend the first few years of their medical practice in rural communities needing a doctor.

The "health center" movement is seen throughout the world. In large measure the health center is a physical structure designed to bring preventive and curative medicine to rural regions. In the United States it has been restricted to a place for housing the local department of public health, but elsewhere it is used also for giving general medical services to the ambulatory patient.[2] The "mobile clinic" is a further expedient widely employed, in the face of personnel shortages, to bring medical services to agricultural people in Africa and South America.

The general stature of public health in the structure of governments has been enhanced in recent years. In the agricultural and underdeveloped countries, large campaigns are being launched against mass endemic diseases like malaria, yaws, yellow fever, and tuberculosis. Great reductions have been made in malaria during the last ten years. Little has been accomplished, however, in improving basic environmental sanitation. Mechanisms of water supply and excreta disposal are part of a family's standard of living, not affected so readily as is the provision of medical care by the construction of a hospital or health center. The housing of peasant families, moreover, is tied up with ancient systems of land tenure, which have been only slightly modified, despite newspaper headlines (in India, Egypt, Italy, and elsewhere) about "land reform" legislation.

In the industrialized countries, on the other hand, environmental sanitation has made great progress, and the diseases of filth have been reduced to very small proportions. As a result the public health movement has shifted its emphasis from the infectious diseases to other spheres. Nutrition, dental hygiene, general health education, and mental health are getting increasing attention—widening the scope of public concern about personal health. In the United States there is concern also for the prevention or at least early case finding of chronic disease—although interest in such activities is by no means universal among public health authorities. The field of "epidemiology" is now defined as the study of the mass distribution and socioenvironmental factors associated with all diseases, not simply with the communicable diseases.

In Europe and the United States there are many proposals by health leaders to broaden the scope of official public health agencies to include administrative authority for all curative services, as well as preventive. While this may seem like a technical detail of jurisdiction, on closer inspection it is seen to be a movement toward integrated social control of all health services to meet public needs most effectively and efficiently.

Within medical practice the growth of specialization has set into play further forces for the social organization of health service. In most of the world, outside of the United States and Canada, specialty service is intimately associated with hospitals, and specialists are usually salaried employees, in the manner of pathologists or radiologists in this country. The worldwide extension of specialization, relative to general practice, therefore, heightens the proportion of doctors working in an organized framework. In the United States, where specialty practice is mainly individualistic, other consequences are seen. As has been mentioned, the high cost of specialty services has generated the organization of more voluntary medical care insurance plans—even by the doctors themselves (Blue Shield plans). To integrate

the provision of various specialist services, the group practice clinic has been developed. The several "specialty board" certifications have introduced a type of superlicensure which, in effect, subjects doctors to greater professional controls.

Along with the specialties in medicine itself, there is seen everywhere an enormous growth of paramedical and auxiliary personnel. Beyond the pharmacist and the nurse, there are laboratory technicians, x-ray technicians, dieticians, physiotherapists, occupational therapists, speech therapists, medical social workers, dental hygienists, opticians, bracemakers, psychologists, and clerks and aides of all types. The complexity of this army of health personnel heightens the need for social organization, for most of these health workers must function as part of an institutional team.

In the underdeveloped countries much use is made of medical auxiliaries for doing work that, in wealthier countries, is done by physicians. They are widely used in Africa, South America, Indonesia, and China. In the Soviet Union, where the current supply of doctors is already high, these "middle personnel" serve to extend a great volume of services to rural people. Under professional direction, auxiliary personnel can mean a sensible economy of medical skills. Without supervision, however, they can only mean substandard services. In India there are thousands of "traditional doctors"—untrained village artisans who practice according to semimagical "systems" of medicine 3,000 years old, systems with some empirical value but quite lacking in scientific foundation. The government permits these healers to practice their art independently, and even supports separate Ayurvedic schools for them. China, on the other hand, is attempting to incorporate its traditional doctors within the overall medical framework, training them to do specific tasks in collaboration with scientific physicians.

To train doctors and auxiliaries, schools of medicine and related disciplines are being everywhere expanded. Outside of the United States these are nearly always under the auspices of government, and in the United States the percentage of governmental support for professional education is steadily rising. With the education of the doctor financed mainly by the public, the claims of the public on the services of the new graduate are naturally great. Physicians engaged in private practice frequently contend that high fees for their services are justified by their personal investments of money and time in their education. They overlook the fact, however, that tuition payments cover only a small fraction of the costs of medical education in the United States, and even less in other countries, the bulk of costs being met from social sources.

The general health consciousness of the public is rising everywhere. Newspapers and magazines in all countries feature news about medical science and, while much reporting is sensationalized or distorted, the effect is to heighten the demands of people for medical attention. Experience in Europe, America, and Asia alike is toward higher volumes of demand for medical services, especially when social programs have removed economic barriers. Despite the need for correction of backlogs of medical neglect, and the consequent high volume of medical service on the initiation of medical care programs, the volume of services does not later fall, but continues to rise. With education and experience in organized medical services, the tendency is toward steadily increasing public demand.

One aspect of this heightened demand for medical services is a preoccupation with mental and emotional problems, seen at its highest level in the United States. Psychiatry has been growing as a medical specialty in all countries, but in the United States psychiatric theory and practice have become an interest of vast numbers of the general population, especially the middle class. There can be no doubt that this tendency is related to the general tensions of a highly competitive society. European observers find the psychiatric influence in American culture to be grotesque, and associate it with basic national fears and insecurities. Despite all this, the expansion of psychiatric concepts in the United States and elsewhere has the effect of widening the sphere of human ills to which medical service may be applied. Since psychiatric treatment, moreover, is usually long and expensive, the need for public financing is enhanced.

With the worldwide increase in demands for medical and related services, the costs have everywhere been rising. The rise since, say, 1900 has been both absolute—in the amount of money spent each year for all health purposes—and relative, that is, in the proportion of total national wealth being devoted to health purposes. Where nearly all health expenditures are budgeted by government, as in Great Britain, this absolute rise in health expenditures is very noticeable, and conservative critics have asked how much a nation can afford for health services. The fact is that, even under current expanded conditions, only about five percent of national income is being spent for all health services in Great Britain and the United States.[3] Some warn, of course, that medical care expenditures should not be permitted to rise so high that a people will not have enough money for food and shelter. Surely such basic human needs should not be compromised by health expenditures,

but this is hardly the realistic issue. The proportion of national wealth being spent on armaments, for example, is far greater than the modest percentage that now supports all public and private expenditures for preventive and curative service. The real issue is how much wastage in the economy can be eliminated, so as to permit further rises in the outlay for positive human purposes. No nation has yet found a maximum in health expenditures, beyond which "extravagance" could be claimed.

THE FUTURE OF HEALTH SERVICE

Current trends throughout the world point clearly to the increasing social organization of all health services. The pattern of collective financing and organized provision of medical and related services will naturally vary in different countries, but the eventual transformation of medical care from a private commodity to a social service cannot be doubted. The battles in the United States about various forms of health insurance are only minor skirmishes that may retard the rate of this transformation, but can hardly affect its final outcome.

One reason for this prediction is that health service, in the larger political context, is not a revolutionary issue. It does not jeopardize the foundations of the social system, as do other issues, like collective bargaining or foreign policy. For this reason it is a highly popular feature in the program of not only liberal but even center and sometimes conservative polical parties in most countries. A very broad area of agreement can be achieved on health goals with the widest sections of the population: witness the support of the National Health Service by the Conservatives in Great Britain or the advocacy of national health insurance by Democratic party leadership in the United States.

In nearly all countries outside of the United States the public character of medical service has come to be taken for granted. There are, of course, areas of debate within the bailiwick of government on administrative patterns. The medical profession often fights rear guard actions based on arguments about the "personal doctor-patient relationship," "free choice of doctor," or the "independence of medicine"— concepts that are reasonable when they are not distorted. But the inclusion of more and more sectors of the health field under social control goes on throughout the world.

One of the important slogans developing in recent years throughout the world is the goal of "positive health." While much philosophical speculation is associated with the phrase, and even some beclouding of basic economic issues like health insurance, its importance is that it implies an almost unlimited horizon for health achievement. Even when important diseases like tuberculosis or cancer are effectively prevented or cured, "positive health" remains to be achieved through ever widening programs of nutrition, housing, physical culture, and general improvement of the physical and social environment.

Another slogan significant for the future is "social medicine," which originated mainly in Europe and has clothed organized health measures in a new dignity. While American medicine has been slow to accept the term, the concepts associated with it have slowly penetrated at least the intellectual sections of American medical education. In its limited sense, "social medicine" refers to all programs of public health and organized medical care, and the study of the social origins of disease. In its broad sense, however, it refers to the application of medical knowledge and leadership to all programs for social betterment—to industrial organization, public housing, education, social relations in the community, and even foreign policy. The goal of health as "physical, mental, and social well-being" implies measures in fields far broader than technical medical services. In the interests of health, if the goal is sincerely sought, reforms are needed in every aspect of social life. As the limits of achievement of purely medical services are reached, through their social organization, the need for further advances through other economic and social measures becomes clearer. In this sense the objectives of "social

medicine," and the very formulation of the concept, represent an ideological advance toward overall social improvement.

Health is by no means the highest goal in any social system, whether democratic-capitalist, feudal-agricultural, or state-socialist. It is often sacrificed for higher goals, especially in the brutalities of war, whether agressive or defensive. Nations will arm to protect their rights, even though death, disease, and suffering must follow, simply because defeat is regarded as the greater evil. The importance of social movements for better health is that, aside from the immediate goal, they focus attention on positive human ends. They stress a value system in which life is the highest good and untimely death the greatest evil. In this sense the worldwide trend toward social organization of health services is also advancement toward a goal of world peace.

NOTES

[1] This chapter, based principally on a study made by the author as a medical consultant for the World Health Organization, was presented as a paper at the Hospital Administrators Development Program at Cornell University, Ithaca, New York, on June 22, 1959. For further detail see "Medical Care in Relation to Public Health," a WHO monograph prepared by the author for use as a working paper at the World Health Assembly of 1957.

[2] For more current information on health centers, see chapter 22.

[3] By 1974, this percentage rose in the United States to nearly eight percent.

Chapter II
A Global View of Financing and Delivery Patterns

Examining the health care systems of the world in the 1970s, one finds a variety of patterns, which could be classified in many ways. One approach is to identify the methods of financing health services, since each of the several possible methods tends to be associated with a certain system of delivery. In most countries, there are mixtures of financing methods, and corresponding patterns by which the services are provided to different population groups. Yet, in nearly all countries there is a trend toward increasingly collectivized financing; with this goes a heightened recognition of health care as a "right" of citizens. Likewise, there is increasing public concern for both efficiency and quality assurance concerning the services provided.

A brief overview of the current scene is presented in this chapter, which was published under the title "Health Care Financing and Delivery Around the World" in The American Journal of Nursing *(Vol. 71, June 1971, pp. 1,158-1,164, copyright June 1971, The American Journal of Nursing Company). Reproduced, with permission, from* American Journal of Nursing.

When we examine the many and diverse systems of health service delivery around the world, we quickly discover that the ways of raising money for financing care are closely related to the patterns by which that care is provided. We can learn a great deal by studying the methods of health care financing in different countries and observing the delivery patterns associated with them.

METHODS OF FINANCING

There are hundreds of ways of financing health services if we consider all the ramifications at different times and social settings. They can, however, be generally classified in a half-dozen types:

- PERSONAL PAYMENT—private purchase of service, from the individual's personal resources, including those he may have borrowed or received from another source (a relative, friend, loan company, and so on). It could also include payment by barter.

- CHARITY—support from funds donated by persons who may or may not become beneficiaries of the service.

- INDUSTRY—provision of services at the expense of an enterprise, supported from its earnings.

- VOLUNTARY INSURANCE—support of services from funds raised through periodic contributions by groups of persons. These funds may be variously sponsored, but the services are supported only for contributors or their dependents.

- SOCIAL INSURANCE—insurance required by law to support certain services to designated beneficiaries. Statutory requirements may set up governmental trust funds or may mandate contributions to various nongovernmental bodies.

- GENERAL REVENUES—support through taxation by local, provincial, or national governmental authority on incomes, land, sales, corporation profits, and the like. Services are not confined to taxpayers.

These six methods of fundraising for health care

are all found in some degree, and in varying mixtures, in the majority of countries of the world. One of the methods may predominate heavily—like general revenues in the Soviet Union or Great Britain or personal payments in the United States. In most countries, however, all six methods are employed, often for the care of different sectors of the population or for an attack on specified diseases.

Personal Payment

Until a few years ago, more than half of the costs of personal health services in the United States were met through individual purchasing in the open medical market. Now, however, voluntary insurance, social insurance, and general revenues have come to support the majority of these costs, particularly hospital costs. Personal payment still carries most of the cost of ambulatory medical care, dental care, and medications.

Under this method, service is provided typically by independent practitioners, and the provider's responsibility is directly to his patient. To a limited extent, service may be delivered through organized resources, such as group practice clinics or hospital emergency rooms.

Even in countries in which general revenues support health services for the bulk of the population—as in most nations of Africa or Asia—personal payment may still play an important part in the care of a few. Thus, in the capital city of a country like Ethiopia or Thailand, one finds a great deal of private medical practice. A small percentage of affluent persons seeing private doctors are preempting a high proportion of the total medical manpower, with enormous resultant inequities.

In Malaysia, which I studied in 1968, I found that about sixty percent of the nation's doctors were in private practice in the various state capital cities. This left forty percent for the governmental services on which about eighty percent of the population depended for their scientific (as opposed to traditional healing) medical care. Moreover, these private doctors are reported to earn two or three times the salaries paid to government doctors.

The personal payment system also supports most of the nonscientific healers throughout the developing world. The fees of village healers are typically low, and often they are paid in goods, but their aggregate amount must be high. Likewise, in all countries self-prescribed drugs are personally paid for. In Latin America, field surveys have shown such outlays to be extremely high, accounting for more than half of all personal expenditures on health service. Obviously, the self-chosen medication is, in large measure, the poor family's medical care.

Charity

Nowhere today does charity predominate as the method of health care support, but in the past it played a substantial role in several nations. In preindustrial Europe, hospitals and even separate dispensaries for ambulatory care were mainly charitable institutions for the care of the poor. They were supported by donations or bequests, although by the eighteenth and nineteenth century governmental subsidies became common.

That charitable pattern was transplanted by the Spanish and Portuguese to Latin America, where *beneficencia* and *santa casa* hospitals became the first organized forms of medical care. However, even when large government grants help support them, these hospitals typically have large, poorly equipped wards, with small staffs of devoted religious sisters. Outpatient facilities are meager. The guiding spirit is not the early preventive treatment, but merciful succor to the destitute, and the icons all around make it obvious that the soul is being served as much as the body.

Religiously supported missions in Africa and elsewhere undoubtedly make a solid contribution at very low cost, but they are rarely models of modern medicine. Often they must be subsidized by government, and they collect fees from patients who can afford to pay.

In some European countries, agencies started by charity have come to be integrated into the public health services. The various "cross societies" in Holland provide maternal and child health services, as well as general visiting nurse care for the homebound sick. They receive government payments for these services, as do similar agencies in Italy and Spain. In Latin America, the typical Red Cross society for ambulance and emergency services was started with private donations, but now is generally supported by large government grants.

In the United States charity is playing a relatively declining role in the health services. There are many agencies for attacking specific diseases—like cancer, multiple sclerosis, or those causing blindness—but the greater part of their charity-raised funds go to research, professional education, and construction, rather than to direct patient care.

A major part of voluntary health donations goes into hospital endowments, whose earnings help to support care of the poor. Also, philanthropic foundations have supported such important innovations in health care as the Rochester Regional Hospital Council (Commonwealth Fund) or the Health Insurance Plan of Greater New York (Rockefeller). Altogether, however, charity accounts for less than five

16

percent of the nation's sixty billion dollar annual health outlay, as of 1970.

Industry

Industrial health service varies greatly and is found to some degree in all countries—capitalist, developing, and socialist—but nowhere is it a predominant method. In countries like Saudi Arabia or Liberia, the health services of British or American oil companies or of the Firestone Rubber Company constitute a model of excellence for the whole coun-'try. Similar comments can be made about the programs of the United Fruit Company in Central America, the Anaconda Copper Company in Peru, or the Standard Oil Company in Venezuela. Workers in these enterprises clearly receive better health care than the national average. Management knows that healthy workers are good business, and if private industry did not take the initiative, good health care would usually not be available. Similar reasoning applied to the isolated mining, lumbering, and railroad developments in the United States of the late nineteenth and early twentieth centuries.

Many developing countries require large corporations, especially those of foreign ownership, to provide minimal health services for workers. This is true of sugar or coffee plantations in Latin America, tea or rubber estates in Asia, cocoa farms or mines in Africa. As social insurance laws are enacted in these countries, their provisions often replace independent management financing.

The industrial services in the developing countries tend to be of much wider scope than in America, providing personal preventive services, environmental sanitation, and general medical care.

Voluntary Insurance

Voluntary insurance was a highly important mode of financing medical care in the eighteenth and early nineteenth centuries throughout Europe. Countless sickness funds, friendly societies, and mutual benefit associations were organized by consumers, either on an occupational or geographic basis, to pay the cost of out-of-hospital medical care. From these, there evolved the mandatory systems that we now define as social insurance or social security.

Today the voluntary health insurance societies of the Western European countries are fully integrated in the social insurance systems. In Germany, France, the Benelux and Scandinavian countries, Italy, and Spain, they have become essentially agents of a governmental system. Most or all persons are required by law to join them and to pay certain contributions, in return for which they gain statutory rights to medi-

cal care and certain other benefits. In addition, the insurance societies may still offer supplementary benefits not required by law, or they may enroll such persons as the self-employed, whose membership is not always compulsory.

The patterns of medical care for the ambulatory patient have been only minimally affected by these European insurance societies. They have made medical care more accessible to people by covering the costs, but have hardly altered the basic patterns of private medical and dental practice and of the private sale of drugs or appliances. There are various forms of surveillance, but the private practitioner remains essentially independent. Hospital services have perhaps been somewhat more affected, with costs shared by government and insurance and certain minimal standards usually imposed by the insurance societies.

In Australia and the United States, we see the operation of voluntary health insurance in a purer form. These are the only remaining industrialized countries of the world in which voluntary enrollment in health insurance plans constitutes a major source of financing. Australia provides government subsidies to the plans to enhance their ability to attract low income persons into membership, a mechanism now being proposed in several bills in the United States Congress. This device has succeeded in getting about seventy-five percent of the population covered, but various deductibles and cost-sharing features have caused increasing discontent in recent years.

In the United States before 1930, only a trivial percentage of the American population held voluntary health insurance. The great depression of 1929-1939, rising costs of medical care, and threat of governmental intervention rapidly stimulated a voluntary insurance movement. However, the major initiative and achievements came not from consumer organizations, but from associations of providers (hospitals and doctors) and from commercial insurance carriers. By 1964, about seventy-eight percent of the American population had some form of private insurance for hospital expenses and lesser percentages had coverage for other medical needs.

The major gaps in coverage were among the poor, the rural people, and the aged. That last gap led to enactment of social insurance for the aged in 1965. As in Europe before us, the voluntary health insurance plans were woven into the social insurance system not as local carriers of financial risk, but as intermediaries for the payment of the fees of doctors, hospitals, and other vendors.

Also as in Europe, the American voluntary health insurance plans, in the main, did very little to change the patterns of medical care delivery. The important exception was among a handful of consumer- or employer-sponsored plans, which altogether reach about six percent of the insured population. In these plans—best known are the Health Insurance Plan of Greater New York and the Kaiser-Permanente Health Plan of the west coast—group medical practice with relatively comprehensive health benefits is offered. The efficiencies achieved by these patterns are now being highlighted for official encouragement in new legislative proposals on national health insurance, under the labels of "comprehensive health service organizations" or "health maintenance oranizations."

Probably the only nation that still depends mainly on nongovernmental health insurance, yet offers services in rather highly organized frameworks, is Israel. Here the Workers Insurance Fund covers about seventy-five percent of this small nation's population for medical care, but the services are not privately rendered as in Western Europe. Instead, the insurance money has been used to establish a network of polyclinics and hospitals where the physicians, dentists, and all other personnel are in salaried employment. The rugged conditions of life faced by new immigrants and the necessity for frugal economic policies evidently induced a pattern of medical care which would encourage maximum benefits per unit of input.

Social Insurance

In Japan, a limited pre-World War II social insurance movement was strengthened after the war by mandatory coverage of nearly the whole population. Here again, however, little was done to modify the patterns of private medical practice.

Likewise in Canada, social insurance has been financing hospital care since 1957 and physician's care since 1968, with little modification of delivery patterns. The program is set up province by province, with the federal government matching about fifty-fifty the money raised through social insurance and other means in each province. Here and there, some group practice clinics have been stimulated, and patterns of hospital finance have also been modified, but the prevailing system of private medicine and autonomous hospitals has been essentially unchanged. The same has applied to Medicare in the United States and also to the workmen's compensation laws in the fifty states.

In only two European countries, so far as I know, has the social insurance device been associated with a wholesale modification of patterns of medical care delivery. These are both socialist or semisocialist nations—Poland and Yugoslavia. After the war and their socialist revolutions, these countries kept the social security concept but, instead of perpetuating the numerous semiautonomous local insurance societies, set up an integrated national system to which industrial employees contributed. The national insurance fund became the principal source of support for a network of health centers, polyclinics, and hospitals staffed by teams of salaried personnel. All insured persons use these resources without charge. Others (about thirty percent of the Polish population) may use them, but have to pay, or they can see private providers.

On other continents, the social insurance financing mechanism has quite a different meaning for health care delivery from that in Western Europe. Social security has been widely applied in Latin American countries, where it usually covers only the ten to fifteen percent of the citizens who are industrial workers. For this sector, mainly in the larger cities, there is typically a separate and well-developed medical service, rendered through a special network of hospitals and health centers. The quality of services in those facilities is usually higher than that available to the noninsured population. There may be separate social security systems for different classes of employed persons—often a more comfortable type of hospital service for white collar, as compared to blue collar, workers.

These are the arrangements in Mexico, Brazil, Peru, and elsewhere. Occasionally, fee-for-service is applied in localities with too few insured workers and dependents to warrant a health center, but organized frameworks are the general rule.

Similar organized facilities under social insurance are found in Iran and Turkey. In Tunisia and India, on the other hand, social insurance finances medical care for certain workers, but the services are obtained through the ministry of health network of health centers and hospitals that serve the general population. The insured workers pay no fees, and they may have priority of access, but they theoretically receive the same quality of service as the general population.

In general, social insurance is believed to have the advantage of fiscal stability, in contrast to other methods of financing medical care. It is not subject to the uncertainties of legislative appropriations, nor to the ups and downs of charity or voluntary enrollment. At the same time, most of the laws give a voice to workers and employers in the administration of the program. And in most countries, the social insurance fund need not fear invasion by other government ministries; it is reserved for benefits to the insured.

General Revenues

In every country of the world, general tax revenues are used for financing certain components of health service. In the United States despite all its emphasis on free private enterprise and voluntary insurance, a wide variety of programs have long been supported from general revenues. Some are for special persons—like veterans, American Indians, merchant seamen, or the poor. Others are for special diseases—like mental disorder, venereal disease, tuberculosis, or crippling conditions in children and rehabilitable adults. The conventional public health services for environmental and personal disease prevention everywhere are supported by general revenues.

In some countries, however, taxation has become the predominant method of financial support for all health services. These may be placed in three groups.

First are the countries that have gone through a period of social insurance financing and reached a point when politically the shift to general revenues seemed simple and safe. These include New Zealand, Great Britain, and Chile. New Zealand introduced its social insurance program in 1939, providing for overall physician's care, hospitalization, drugs for everyone, and dental care for children. All residents were covered, and nearly everyone paid an earmarked health insurance contribution. By about 1965, the program was so firmly established that its support was transferred to general revenues.

Great Britain started its mandatory health insurance for manual workers—but not their dependents—in 1911. General doctor's care and drugs were provided, while hospitalization was supported by combinations of general revenues, voluntary insurance, and personal payments. In 1948, after World War II, the National Health Service was established, assuring virtually complete medical care to everyone, financed about eighty percent from the general treasury. Here substantial changes were made in the organization of services, principally for hospital and specialist care. All hospitals, voluntary and local governmental, were taken over by the central government and assigned to "regional hospital boards." Various regulations were made to induce a better distribution of doctors, to encourage reasonable prescribing of drugs, to stimulate grouping of general practitioners, and to achieve other improvements.

Chile was the first Latin American country to apply the social insurance idea to health care, with a program for manual workers in 1924. After gradual expansion of its coverage and benefits, in 1952 a national health service was legislated. This covered all insured workers and their dependents, along with all low income families (rural and urban) and all children; this was estimated to be about seventy percent of the population.

To provide services, the country was divided into thirteen health zones, in each of which there was established an integrated regional network of health centers, district hospitals, and central hospitals. The great majority of the nation's health personnel work full-time or part-time for the Chilean National Health Service. While social insurance contributions from both workers and employers were continued after 1952, a much larger amount was drawn from general revenues.

A second category of countries dependent mainly on general revenues for their medical care are the great mass of developing nations of Africa and Asia. Some countries of these continents also have social insurance programs, but these affect a very small percentage of the population. Likewise personal payments play an important part, especially in the main cities, as do charitable missions at selected places. But the majority of the people—insofar as they have access to any scientific medical care—get it at health centers and government-owned hospitals staffed by salaried personnel.

The socialist nations make up the third category. The Soviet Union was the first, in 1917, and its model made the most radical changes in patterns of medical care delivery. Covering 100 percent of the population, the Soviet system gives virtually all services through networks of health centers, polyclinics, and rural, district, and provincial hospitals. Unification of preventive and curative services is emphasized. Professional education is controlled by the Ministry of Health rather than the universities, and even the production of all drugs, supplies, and equipment is planned by this ministry. All personnel are salaried civil servants, and new graduates are obligated to spend their first three years of work in an area designated by the government. Remarkably large numbers of doctors, nurses, and middle personnel are trained, and the whole system is planned according to norms designed to meet all reasonable needs in urban and rural areas. Nearly all foreign observers have been impressed with the efficiencies and massive impact of the Soviet health system.

With certain modifications, this system has been emulated by Czechoslovakia, Hungary, Bulgaria, and other Eastern European countries, except Poland and Yugoslavia. It has also been applied largely in Cuba, although the financing mechanism differs between industrial workers and farm people. In

Communist China, the vast rural population is served directly by a governmental system using mainly auxiliary health personnel, while city workers are served through resources attached to factories or in public institutions.

CONCLUSIONS

Are there any general conclusions to be drawn from this review of different methods of health care financing in various political and economic contexts? A few may be warranted.

• In some degree, purely personal payment is found in all countries of the world, but it is much more extensively used where collectivized methods of financing health care are weaker. The greatest volume of health service tends to go to those with most immediate purchasing power, rather than to those with greatest health needs.

• The charitable method has been of generally declining importance, as the costs of good medical care have risen and the resources of government have become far greater than those of private donors. Industrialized nations have increasingly come to reject the moral judgments and social class distinctions often associated with charity financing.

• Industrially supported health services have contributed to the production process by helping to maintain a healthy work force. They are, however, extremely uneven as between small and large enterprises. Increasingly these services have come to be replaced by services supported through voluntary and social insurance.

• In all industrialized societies, voluntary insurance has played a large role historically in enhancing the access of people to medical care and in supporting larger quantities and quality of health personnel and facilities. Yet is has proved unable to reach all the population in need of service, and both its successes and the failures have led almost everywhere to compulsory statutes or social insurance, with widened governmental standards for health protection and more vigorous controls over the costs and quality of medical care.

• Social insurance is really a conservative form of taxation, and in most countries it has been supplemented by some support from general revenues. Everywhere, the population coverage and the scope of health benefits under it have grown wider, and in some countries it has become feasible to shift to general revenue financing without fear of program retrenchments.

• The nature of medical care patterns adopted under general revenue financing depends on the prevailing political ideology and the economic level of the country. In prosperous countries with a long tradition of free enterprise, like Great Britain, private practice remains strong for ambulatory care, but highly organized services develop inside hospitals.

• In most socialist countries, though not all, a full commitment to health care support under general revenues has been made. In these circumstances, private practice tends to die out as public services develop.

• Countries in the developing world tend often to stand between competing ideologies. A growing middle class seeks private care, with pleasant amenities, in the main cities, coopting a relatively large share of the nation's medical resources. But governments are under pressure to extend health care to the massive populations in rural areas and to the poor who have migrated into the cities. "Planning" has become the standard approach to defining priorities.

• On the whole, one can observe throughout the world—in its capitalist-parliamentary, its socialist, and its developing sectors alike—a clear trend toward increasing collectivization of health care financing. With this has evolved an increasing organization of resources designed to enhance both the efficiency and the effectiveness of medical care delivery.

Part Two

Developing Countries

Chapter III
The Disease Picture in
One Developing Country: El Salvador

In the developing countries, with their heavily rural and agricultural populations living under primitive conditions, the incidence and types of disease problem are very different from those in the industrialized countries. Data for one such country–El Salvador, Central America–were assembled as part of a survey conducted in late 1950 and early 1951 under the auspices of the World Health Organization. This survey was designed to plan a comprehensive health program in one rural district of about 100,000 population, referred to, in this chapter, as the "health demonstration area."

While health conditions, as reflected in mortality and morbidity data, have undoubtedly improved in El Salvador since 1950, the account presented is still a reasonably valid reflection of the type of disease spectrum found in most developing countries today. The text is excerpted from A Health Demonstration Area in El Salvador, *an unpublished World Health Organization document produced for the Pan American Health Organization (Washington, D.C., February 1951, pp. 48-73), and reprinted here by permission.*

As in regions throughout the world not previously serviced with good public health organization, specific data on the health status of the population in the demonstration area of El Salvador are not abundant. There are many general ideas, surmises, and speculations made by local people, some of which may have partial validity, and the valiant efforts of the Direccion General de Sanidad in the last few years have brought forward data on specific diseases in certain localities. For the most part, however, an assessment of the health problems of the area must depend on evaluation of data for other parts of the Republic or for El Salvador as a whole. General living conditions through the nation are so similar that application, with caution, of their health records to the demonstration area will probably not entail serious errors. First we may consider death rate data, and then information on morbidity.

DEATH RATES

Crude as they may be, death rates are probably the best measure of health problems currently available. It will be helpful to consider certain basic data for El Salvador, as a whole, before reviewing the more limited data available for the demonstration area.

Interpretation of almost all vital statistical data from El Salvador demands extreme caution. Births and deaths are reported simply to the mayor of each municipality, according to law, but it is generally recognized that many deaths and an even greater number of births are never reported, especially in the rural sections. Causes of death must be extremely inaccurate because of the enormously important fact that about eighty-five percent of all deaths are not attended by a physician. The "cause" is simply entered onto the record by the municipality official, on the basis of the family's explanation and his own judgment. It is obvious that, under such circumstances, any death associated with a fever may be recorded as due to malaria and causes referable to a multitude of internal disorders would be missed. In entirely rural sections, like the demonstration area, the proportion of deaths without medical attendance is even higher, probably close to ninety-five percent.

For El Salvador as a whole, the most recent data indicate a crude death rate in 1949 of 13.0 per 1,000. Compared with the record of the United States of about ten per 1,000, this does not appear extremely high, but it must be recalled that there are far larger proportions of children and smaller proportions of aged persons in El Salvador. If age-adjusted comparisons were made, the differential would undoubtedly be greater. The figure of 13.0 per 1,000 is, moreover, almost certainly an understatement. A separate nationwide death rate has been computed for 1950 from reports of death coming solely from jurisdictions served by health departments (described below), having a combined population of 878,000 (about forty-two percent of the national population); for this "registration area" from which more complete reporting may be expected, the crude death rate was 15.4 per 1,000.

There has undoubtedly been improvement in the overall rate of death in El Salvador in the past fifty years. In the period 1900-1905, the crude death rate for the Republic was reported at about twenty-five per 1,000, which was doubtless an understatement.[1] The downward trend in death rates has been by no means uniform, however. In 1940, the crude rate was reported as 17.5 per 1,000 and in 1943 up again to 20.2 per 1,000.[2] It would be interesting to trace the relationship between the world price of coffee over the years and El Salvador's general death rate.

The latest data giving rates of death, by cause, for the Republic are for 1948. These are shown in table III.1.

In this tabulation, some liberty has been taken in grouping diagnoses in order to highlight major problems which would be obscured if each diagnosis were listed separately. It is to be noted that "all other causes" contributes 37.1 per 100,000 to the total deaths, and if the exact causes were known for these deaths, the proportion of certain diagnoses in the whole list might be altered. The large figure of 31.4 per 100,000 for senility is also to be noted, and the figure of 18.0 for chronic rheumatism which—while undoubtedly a serious cause of disability—is seldom a primary cause of death. The same applies to the helminthic diseases (21.4 per 100,000) which clearly are debilitating but rarely fatal by themselves.

In view of these statistical difficulties, one must be

Table III.1 Major causes of death in El Salvador: 1948	
	Rate per 100,000
All causes	1,430.0
Diarrhea and enteritis, and dysentery	287.1
Diarrhea and enteritis under two years of age	145.8
Diarrhea and enteritis over two years of age	134.1
Dysentery	7.2
Pneumonia, influenza, bronchopneumonia, and bronchitis	148.4
Pneumonia and bronchopneumonia	63.5
Bronchitis	68.5
Influenza	16.4
Malaria	133.2
Accidents, all types	65.1
Diseases peculiar to the first year of life	61.1
Prematurity	9.0
Birth injury	11.6
Congenital debility	40.5
Diseases of the cardiovascular system	40.0
Diseases of the heart	14.8
Intracranial lesions, vascular	13.1
Nephritis	12.1
Pulmonary tuberculosis	38.6
Avitaminosis	38.2
Whooping cough	35.8
Senility	31.4
Other diseases of the digestive tract	30.7
Other infections and parasitic diseases	28.0
Helminthic diseases	21.4
Cancer and other malignant tumors	19.9
Chronic rheumatism	18.0
Syphilis	17.7
Other diseases of the nervous system	16.4
Anemias	9.5
Measles	6.8
All other causes	37.1
Data from the *Anuario Estadistico de la Republica de El Salvador*, 1948, p. 178.	

extremely cautious in deciding which diseases represent the "number one" problems to be tackled by a public health program in El Salvador, and all the more cautious in the demonstration area for which the data are even less reliable. There can be no question, of course, about the overwhelming importance of the infectious and parasitic group of diseases, but the breakdown of categories within this group is not so easy. The actual relative importance, as causes of death, among: (1) dysentery, (2) malaria, (3) tuberculosis, and (4) pneumonia is far from certain. Moreover, outside of childhood, the role of cardiovascular disease and cancer in causing morbidity and deaths is probably greatly underestimated because of the enormous lack of doctors (and these diseases are often difficult for even well-trained physicians to diagnose).

The only data available for the demonstration area as a whole, at this writing, are the overall numbers of deaths for the twelve municipalities. These are available as averages over the five-year period 1945-1949 and are shown in table III.2.

Table III.2

Number of deaths in the demonstration area: average per year during 1945-1949, by municipality

Municipality	Number
Colon	202
Tonacatepeque	155
Ciudad Arce	228
Opico	231
Tocachico	81
El Paisnal	77
Aguilares	57
Guazapa	78
Apopa	153
Nejapa	136
Quezaltepeque	413
San Matias	36
Total	1,833

Since the population of this combination of municipalities is a little under 100,000 at present and has probably varied from about 90,000 upward since 1945, the crude death rate over this period has probably been between nineteen and twenty per 1,000. In the year 1949 there were 1,747 deaths in the area which would yield a current death rate of about eighteen per 1,000. It is likely, therefore, that the overall death rate in the area is higher than for the nation as a whole.

The only data on causes of death within the demonstration area available at this time are for the *municipio* of Quezaltepeque. This municipality has a population of over 16,000, about half of which is in the town and half is entirely rural. It seems likely that the record of deaths for Quezaltepeque is a good reflection of conditions in the entire area, within the general limitations discussed above. In 1949 the crude death rate for Quezaltepeque was 19.9 per 1,000 population. In this tabulation, causes of death

are listed according to the principal categories in the International List of Causes of Death—a method which corrects for some of the statistical difficulties. Rates per 100,000 are, however, not available; the relative importance of different causes is indicated by the percentage distribution shown in table III.3.

Table III.3

Causes of death in Quezaltepeque: 1949, in percentage distribution

International List Category	Percentage
Infectious and parasitic diseases	49.3
Respiratory tract diseases	13.7
Digestive tract diseases	12.3
Senility and ill-defined causes	4.2
Diseases of the genitourinary tract	3.7
Allergies, endocrine disorders, metabolic disorders, and diseases of the blood	3.2
Circulatory system disorders	3.2
Diseases of the joints and locomotion	1.6
Cancer and other tumors	1.4
Diseases of the first year of life	1.4
Disorders of pregnancy and childbirth	1.1
Diseases of the skin and subcutaneous tissue	1.1
Nervous system and sense organ diseases	0.9
Congenital malformations	0.9
Accidents	0.9
Mental disorders	0.4
All causes	100.0

Further reflection of the nature of the health problems in the demonstration area is given by a tabulation of deaths in Quezaltepeque by age. (See table III.4.) It is apparent that more than half of all deaths strike children four years of age or under, a further confirmation of the enormous importance in the area of the various infectious diseases.

A few other basic rates reflect the nature of the problem in the demonstration area. They are presented with approximate United States comparisons, as of 1949, in table III.5.

It is apparent that, despite the extremely high infant mortality rate and general death rate in the demonstration area, the population continues to grow because of an enormously high birth rate. The com-

Table III.4

Deaths in Quezaltepeque by age groups: 1949, by percentage distribution

Age group	Percentage
6 days or less	7.0
7-28 days	6.0
29-364 days	20.0
1-4 years	33.1
5-9	3.9
10-14	2.8
15-19	0.9
20-24	2.1
25-34	1.6
35-44	2.8
45-54	4.2
55-64	5.3
65-74	2.5
75-84	4.4
85 and over	2.8
All ages	100.0

dren under two years of age and for pulmonary tuberculosis there is no consistent relationship to season.

SPECIAL MORBIDITY STUDIES.

Deaths are an extreme manifestation of health problems, but they give a misleading picture of the day-to-day burdens of disease and disability faced by the population. Certain data on specific illnesses are available to help round out the picture.

Whatever may be its true impact on total deaths, there is no doubt that malaria is an enormous cause of disability during life, in the demonstration area. Studies have been made of children in each of the twelve municipalities and at five of the rural settlements or *caserios*. The findings are shown in table III.6.

Inspection of the data indicates an average splenic index of about fifty percent, reflecting past exposure to malaria and an average parasitic index of about ten percent, reflecting current active infection. Although it is not entirely clear from these data, the rate of infection tends to be higher at low altitudes and in the more rural sections. A great variety of anopheline vectors have been identified in El Salvador and in the demonstration area, but the most common species are *A. albimanus*, which tends to breed more abundantly in the rainy season, and *A. pseudopunctipennis*, which breeds mostly in the dry season. Both varieties are rarely found at elevations over 2,900 feet (about 1,000 meters), but the entire demonstration area is below this level. There has been a great deal of investigation of mosquito vectors in El Salvador and no attempt will be made to review it here.[3] With the modern approach of house spraying with DDT, the importance of species analysis of the malaria vectors has somewhat diminished.

Related to the problem of malaria is the potential hazard of yellow fever, which is not now found in El Salvador but which might come in from Panama or South America. In this connection, studies have been made of the *Aedes egypti* mosquitoes in the demonstration area, and about ten percent of houses were found to harbor these vectors. The percentages in different municipalities were as follows: Opico, 4.7; Apopa, 27.7; Quezaltepeque, 12.3; Guazapa, 2.5; Najapa, 3.7; Aguilares, 16.8; and El Paisnal, 5.7.

Undoubtedly of greater importance than suggested by the national death rate data is the problem of tuberculosis. Evidence for this is found in an analysis of deaths in the city of San Salvador for 1943, where medical attendance and reporting are more complete than anywhere else in the nation. There are two hospitals in San Salvador that receive tuber-

bination of high birth rate and high infant mortality represents a vast "pregnancy wastage" which must be a continual drain on the human vitality and economic resources of the people.

Seasonal death rates are not available for the demonstration area but some figures on deaths by month for the entire country have been prepared at the Sanidad. Reviewing six-year averages for 1944-1949 for some of the major diseases shows certain seasonal tendencies, if the year is divided into the six months of wet season (April to September) and the six months of dry season (October to March). On this basis, it is found that in the wet months there tends to be the peak in deaths from diarrhea and enteritis in persons over two years of age, typhoid fever, pertussis, diphtheria, and measles. In the dry months, the peak in deaths occurs for malaria, influenza, and respiratory tract disease. The peaks for all deaths of children under one year, for stillbirths, and for total deaths also occur in the dry months. These curves are by no means clear-cut and there are numerous exceptions in the individual years; moreover, the general unreliability of reporting of causes of death must be kept in mind. Nevertheless, these findings may provide some small basis for concentrating efforts at specific disease control in certain months of the year. Within the dry season, the concentration of malaria deaths in the first three months and an equally high number of respiratory disease deaths in the next three months suggests some possible causal relationship. For diarrhea and enteritis deaths of chil-

Table III.5

Vital Statistics: 1949, U.S.A., El Salvador, Quezaltepeque

	U.S.A.	El Salvador	Quezaltepeque
Birth Rate (per 1,000 population)	22	38.9	52.0
Infant Mortality (per 1,000 live births)	35	92.7	127.3
Stillbirths (per 1,000 births)	—	10.3	12.4
Death Rate (per 1,000 population)	10	13.0	19.9

Table III.6

Diagnosed malaria in demonstration area children: 1950

Location	Altitude Meters above sea level	Number Examined	Splenic Index	Parasitic Index
Tacachico	495	—	82	14
San Matias	460	—	19	7.1
Opico	530	300	33	2.7
Ciudad Arce	650	371	30.2	1.6
Colon	650	—	22	11.1
Quezaltepeque	475	375	37	5.4
Najapa	500	—	29	15
Apopa	500	—	20	3.1
Tonacatepeque	550	—	20	11.4
Guazapa	—	—	28	10
Aguilares	350	166	73	10.3
El Paisnal	330	211	40.8	7.9
Chanmico	—	484	32	3.7
Ateos	315	64	70	17.2
Zapotitan	350	424	76.6	6.3
San Andres	370	100	65	15
La Cabana	—	136	64.6	5.2

culosis cases from throughout the country, but even after full correction of tuberculosis deaths was made by place of residence, Dr. Martinez, Director of the Division of Tuberculosis, estimated that the death rate for the city was 202 per 100,000—vastly higher than the generally reported rate. Whether there has been a rise or decline in the rate since 1943 is quite unknown, but this figure may be compared with a rate in the United States of about thirty per 100,000.

Chest x-ray studies also suggest a high rate of tuberculosis in El Salvador. A study in San Salvador found 1.8 percent with "active disease" in 1948 (examinations of 38,027 persons). A study in Santa Ana (6,610 persons) in 1948 discovered 1.55 percent with active disease by x-ray. A study in Santa Tecla, on the border of the demonstration area (1,380 adults), in 1948 yielded 3.7 percent with active disease by x-ray. In 1950, the World Health Organization team in San Miguel has found even higher rates of positives by x-ray examination. Examination of the first 11,000 persons yielded 564 with lesions classified as positive (minimal, moderate, or advanced), primary infection, or suspicious. Sputum examinations were done on about half the cases, and making allowances for cases which were finally determined to be negative, the proportion of proven tuberculosis cases is probably in excess of three percent. Tuberculin tests among these persons yielded forty-three percent positive, with the percentage rising, of course, at the older age levels.

With these high findings of tuberculous infection or morbidity in various parts of the Republic, it is certain that the problem is a large one in the demonstration area. Although the studies cited are predominantly of urban groups, there is great mobility among the urban and rural population, promoting the spread of bacilli. Living conditions are probably worse in the demonstration area. It is altogether likely that a large share of deaths reported as due to bronchitis, bronchopneumonia, pneumonia, and influenza are actually due to pulmonary tuberculosis. It is only slightly less likely that a major share of the deaths attributed to malaria are really tuberculosis, especially in the far advanced stage when the patient is too debilitated to cough much.

There is limited evidence of high prevalence of syphilis in the demonstration area. A study was made of 200 persons fifteen to forty years of age at Talcualuya, a rural settlement near Opico. Blood serological tests on these persons yielded eighteen percent positive results, of which nearly three-fourths were early cases according to histories obtained. These blood examinations were done with the VDRL (Venereal Disease Research Laboratory) antigen developed in the United States and are believed to yield few false positives, even in the presence of malaria infestation. Even though physicians report that they see relatively little evidence of advanced clinical syphilis in El Salvador, the director of the nation's one mental hospital stated that about seven percent of the admissions were cases of general paresis. Moreover, it will be recalled that, despite the poor reporting, syphilis is listed as one of the major causes of death in the Republic.

Intestinal parasite infestation is another enormous problem in the demonstration area, and throughout El Salvador. A study made in 1950 in Sonsonate, not far from the demonstration area, by the Institute of Nutrition of Central America and Panama (INCAP) showed nearly all children to be infested. In this study of stool specimens from seven- to thirteen-year-old children, the results were as shown in table III.7.

Table III.7

Diagnosed intestinal parasite infestation in Sonsonate area children: 1950

Parasite	Percentage Positive
Ascaris lumbricoides (roundworm)	84
Necatur americanus (hookworm)	36
Trichiuris trichiura (pinworm)	48
Multiple positives	40
Entirely negative	4

Since the demonstration area is more completely rural than Sonsonate and excreta disposal is even more primitive, the proportions of infestation are, if anything, even higher than these figures. A physician attending a clinic at Chanmico, a hacienda in the area, reported that he gave antihelminthics routinely to all children coming to the clinic and asked them to report on the number of worms excreted; he said he had never yet received a negative response.

Accurate information on nutritional status in the demonstration area must await further studies. Superficial inspection of the population in the area, however, suggests great nutritional deficiency among both children and adults. Average body height is short, perhaps sixty-three or sixty-four inches for males, and the typical child or adult is thin. Blood examinations by INCAP in different cities found an average red blood cell count of only 4.2 million cells per cubic millimeter in males. Nearly all small children have the thin legs and large potbellies associated with flabby abdominal musculature from undernutrition. Physicians report many cases of edema due to protein deficiency. Dental disease in the area may only be surmised, but examinations by the Sanidad of schoolchildren in San Salvador found practically 100 percent to have caries.

Finally, a word should be said about the tremendous number of deaths reported as "diarrhea and enteritis" and the morbidity associated with them. The exact etiology of these cases is by no means clear. Many are undoubtedly bacillary dysentery, due to various organisms. Others are amoebic dysentery, due to *endamoeba histolytica*. Still others are probably typhoid or paratyphoid fever (a handful of cases of typhoid fever are actually reported from the demonstration area each year). Other causes of diarrhea in infants, according to local physicians, may not be due to microorganisms at all, but are related to protein starvation. It is claimed that the intestinal mucosa, like the subcutaneous tissue, becomes edematous and loses its ability to absorb nutrients, with diarrhea resulting. Further study of this large disease problem is required if effective control is to be launched. While environmental sanitation is obviously essential, the specific measures vary, and the problem must be broken down into its component parts.

Data on the general incidence of all illness are, of course difficult to obtain even in highly developed health service jurisdictions. At best, one must rely on local studies where medical records have been kept on a population group or house-to-house canvasses have been made. Two such sets of data happen to be available for the demonstration area, and, while they give crude measurements, they may give some idea of day-to-day problems of morbidity. (It need hardly be added that, even for communicable diseases, there has been no system of legally required morbidity reporting operating in the demonstration area in the past).

One source of information is a physician's summary of cases attended at the hacienda, Chanmico, in the demonstration area during 1950. The figures in table III.8 simply refer to the number of initial patient visits to the clinic for specified causes during the year. This clinic serves a population of about 2,500 persons.

Table III.8	
Causes of illness attended at Chanmico medical clinic: 1950	
Diagnosis	*Number of New Cases*
Respiratory tract infections	718
Malaria	541
Intestinal parasites	380
Acute gastroenteritis	289
Other diseases of the skin	142
Scabies	117
Extreme malnutrition	113
Rheumatic disorders	110
Other diseases of the digestive system	109
Trauma	105
Other genitourinary diseases	94
Pregnancy	65
Gonorrhea	13
Syphilis	11
All other causes	350

The physician in charge of this particular clinic is well-trained and conscientious, so that considerable credence may be given to these data as a reflection of major causes of day-to-day morbidity in the demonstration area. A breakdown of the diagnoses encompassed under "all other causes" was made unfortunately only for the last three months of the year, but in this period there were eleven cases of tuberculosis, twenty cases of whooping cough, and fourteen work accidents. One of the striking revelations of these data is that respiratory tract infections led the list of causes of illness, just as they usually do in colder climates. These data are also available by month, and the cases of respiratory disease show a decided peak for the months of July, August, and September—the height of the rainy season when the adobe huts are cold and damp.

This tabulation does not give information on the

duration of disability, but another study sheds some light on this for part of the demonstration area. In 1945, Dr. Victor Arnold Sutter, former National Director of Health of El Salvador, made a study of health and living conditions among workers on several of the properties of one of the nation's leading commercial families.[4] It contains much enlightening data on living conditions, family status, mobility, illiteracy, clothing, sanitation, and other features of the population on the De Sola lands. One of the properties investigated was La Cabana, a sugar hacienda within the demonstration area, with a population at the time of 470 persons. Data on incidence and duration of illness were obtained simply by questioning families on their disease experience during the previous year. The great independability of memory and other pitfalls of this technique are well recognized, and yet the results, shown in table III.9, are of some value.

The enormous importance of malaria in this study, compared with its lesser relative importance in the Chanmico report, reflects perhaps the comparison between medical and lay judgment; undoubtedly the people attribute to malaria many ailments caused by respiratory tract infection, virus disease, or other causes. On the basis of the total population at La Cabana of 470 persons, it may be noted that illnesses were reported at a rate of 415 cases per 1,000 persons per year (195/470), for an average duration of disability of twenty-four days per case (4,694/195), and an average experience among the entire group of about ten days of disability per person per year (4,694/470). Comparison of these findings with studies of sickness absenteeism and general illness in the United States suggests that these rates greatly understate the probable burden of sickness in the demonstration area. Separate analysis by age groups indicates that in the age group over forty-five years the attacks of illness are less frequent, but they last longer— similar to findings in the United States. There also tends to be more illness in women than in men.

The Sutter study should be consulted for a wealth of information beyond that cited here. A few other findings, relevant to the health of rural people in El Salvador may be mentioned: (1) the mobility of the rural population is reflected by the fact that only seventeen percent of persons on the De Sola properties were born there and most of the others migrated from urban centers; (2) relative to hookworm disease, fifty-eight percent of the population did not wear shoes; (3) forty percent had not been vaccinated against smallpox; (4) toilets for the use of a particular family were available to only eight percent of the families; (5) seventy-nine percent of the families lived in dwellings consisting of one room, and

Table III.9

Number and duration of illnesses among 470 persons at La Cabana hacienda: 1944, by cause

Cause	Number of Cases	Percent Distribution	Duration (days)	Percent Distribution
Work accidents	7	4	212	5
Other accidents	3	2	125	3
Respiratory	20	10	249	5
Digestive	10	5	243	5
Malaria	110	56	2,868	60
Pregnancy	11	5	72	2
Other defined illnesses	23	12	564	12
Ill-defined or unknown	11	5	361	8
All causes	195	100	4,694	100

twenty percent had only one bed for three or four persons. Finally a fact which underscores the general severity of problems in the demonstration area emerges from Sutter's comparison of illness data between agricultural workers and a group of urban industrial workers in the same study; he finds that agricultural workers tend to have more severe illness, being in bed for an average of eighteen days per illness, compared with eight days for industrial workers. This may well be related to less adequate medical care in the rural sections.

A final word about insects and rodents in relation to disease in the demonstration area. Although El Salvador is a semitropical country, insects other than mosquitoes and the common housefly are not a major factor in disease transmission. The mosquito in relation to malaria and yellow fever has been discussed, and the common fly is doubtless an agent in the contamination of foods leading to various dysenteries. Lice and fleas are found, but typhus fever has not been reported in several years (although there are cases in neighboring Guatemala), and plague is unknown. Ticks are prevalent in the cattle region, but spotted fever cases have not been reported. Rats and mice are abundant, but they have not been indicted significantly in disease transmission. Cases of yaws, trypanosomiasis, trachoma, and other diseases that may be transmitted by insects are only very rarely encountered. A useful listing of the principal insects related to disease in El Salvador is given in the U.S. Army report cited above.[5]

In summary, taking into account the burden of both mortality and morbidity, the major health problems of the demonstration area may be listed. The individual diseases, listed in table III.10, are purposely not numbered because it is foolish to argue about which problem is "number one" and which is "number two." A general order of priority is indicated only as "major," "significant," and "other"—

but even these weightings would vary with one's point of view. The proportionate emphasis in the demonstration program will depend only partly on statistical records of incidence or prevalence or death rates. It will depend also on the practicability of achieving certain objectives in the shortest time and at the least expense, and it will depend also on the wishes and responses of the people in the area.

Table III.10

Health problems in the demonstration area: 1951

Major
    Dysenteries and other gastrointestinal infections
    Pulmonary tuberculosis
    Malaria
    Malnutrition
    Respiratory tract infections
    Intestinal parasite infestation
Significant
    Cardiovascular disease
    Accidents
    Syphilis and gonorrhea
    Problems of pregnancy and childbirth
    Whooping cough
    Dental caries
Other
    Rheumatic disorders
    Cancer
    Measles
    Mental disease

NOTES

[1] Trends in mortality and much other useful data on El Salvador carried up to 1942 are given in a publication prepared by the United States Department of Commerce, in cooperation with the Coordinator of Inter-American Affairs: *El Salvador: Summary of Biostatistics.* Washington, D.C.: 1944.

2 U.S. Public Health Service, *Summary of International Vital Statistics 1937-44*. Washington, D.C.: 1947, p. 178.

3 A bibliography and an excellent summary are given in a report prepared by the Preventive Medicine Division, Office of the Surgeon General, U.S. Army, entitled, *Medical and Sanitary Data on the Republic of El Salvador*. Washington, D.C.: 1943. In addition, the section on malariology in the Sanidad has a great deal of data on the demonstration area, including spot maps, showing the particular vectors in each section.

4 Victor A. Sutter, *Informe de Estudio Sobre Algunas Condiciones de Vida de los Trabajadores, Agricoloas e Industriales de la Casa H. De Sola & Hijos en El Salvador*. San Salvador: 1945.

5 See note 3.

Chapter IV
General Living Conditions and Basic Social Programs in a Former British Colony: Ceylon

Health status is enormously influenced by general social and economic conditions, which are obviously far less favorable in the developing than in the industrialized countries. By the same token, general social programs, through affecting the standard of living, have an impact on morbidity and mortality that may be more basic and enduring than the benefits of health services as such.

As part of a planning survey for a comprehensive "health demonstration area" in Ceylon, carried out for the World Health Organization in 1951, general living conditions and overall social programs were briefly described. With the years and the intervention of various foreign assistance programs, multilateral (United Nations) and bilateral, the number and variety of these social programs have increased. The district of this recently emancipated British colony where the study was focused is named, in Singhalese, Devamedi Hathpattu—a rural region of about 60,000 people. This chapter is excerpted from A Health Demonstration Area in Ceylon, *an unpublished World Health Organization document produced for the Regional Office for South East Asia (New Delhi, India, 1951, pp. 18-28), and reprinted here by permission.*

SOCIAL AND ECONOMIC CONDITIONS

The people in Devamedi Hathpattu (D.H.) depend almost entirely on agriculture for their living. There are about 50,000 acres in coconut and 22,000 in rice paddy. There are small acreages in tobacco and *chena* (jungle land cleared about once in ten years for vegetables). There is no industrial production except a small number of village carpentry or weaving shops. In almost every village is a boutique or small store for general supplies. There are about 23,000 agricultural workers in the area, of whom roughly 17,000 work predominantly in paddy fields and 6,000 in coconuts.

Although I made numerous inquiries, I was unable to obtain accurate data on the conditions of land

tenure in D.H., a matter of great importance for the economic status of the average person. The best estimate of the divisional agricultural officer was that seventy-five percent of the coconut land was in large estates, owned by absentee landlords, and the rest in small holdings. Of the paddy land, he estimated that two-thirds was owned in small lots by the peasants themselves and one-third was rented, usually on a sharecropping basis. The person working the paddy land, if he is a tenant, seldom gets more than half of the produce and usually less than half. There are usually two rice crops a year and in between sowing and harvesting, the peasant—whether an owner or a tenant—will often seek employment on a coconut estate or in other types of work like road construction. Some idea of the economic level of the area is given by the wages paid for a day's labor—usually nine or ten hours—on a coconut estate. This wage rate is fixed by law and in June 1951 it was 1.84 rupees for a male, 1.42 rupees for a female, and 1.25 rupees for a child. (The value of the Ceylon rupee in American currency is twenty-one U.S. cents.) The yield of the paddy crops in Ceylon is notoriously low, claimed in fact to be the lowest in the world. In relation to the seed sown, the harvest is only a fraction—about one-fourth or less—of the harvest yielded in Burma or Italy or other countries. Land holdings of the peasants who own land are usually only one or two acres, ranging between one-half an acre and five acres.

There is little if any migrant labor coming into D.H., all the labor needs being met from the local population. It is commonplace for families to own a cow, which is allowed to stray about without any fixed pasture, but little milk is produced. There is one small mill in the area, manufacturing fiber from coconut husks and employing about fifty workers. There are no trade unions of any type in the area.

While accurate income data for the families in D.H. were not obtainable, it is obvious that with this type of agricultural economy, average earnings from all sources must be very low. Undoubtedly the family average is below that of ninety-three rupees per month, found for Ceylon as a whole. Moreover, it is highly variable from year to year, for if the rains fail the paddy crops may be a complete loss. It is estimated that the crop fails for the average family about twenty percent of the time. While a middle class of tradesmen, professional people, civil servants, and growers is developing rapidly in Ceylon as a whole, within D.H. it is undoubtedly less than five percent of the population. At least ninety-five percent of the people are impoverished peasants, tenants, or laborers living a hand-to-mouth existence.

The heart of life in the area is the village which is little more than a grouping of families in a small settlement. There are about 14,000 dwelling units in the area so that each of the 672 villages contains an average of about twenty-one houses. On the basis of the population estimate of 66,000 there are thus about 4.7 persons per dwelling unit. People in the villages are bound together by strong racial and ethnic bonds and generations of living together through thick and thin. Blood ties among the villagers are close because there is much intermarriage. The family is closely knit and, whatever little resources there are will be used to sustain the aged or the disabled or the unemployed—including not only the immediate members (parents and children) but also the children or parents of brothers and sisters. The story of family and village life is complex and

requires careful study if a health education program in the demonstration area is to be effective.[1]

If there is any question about the poverty of the people in the demonstration area, one has only to go into the villages and see how they live. The typical house is made of mud supported by bamboo and topped with a thatched roof of palm leaves, called locally a structure of "wattle and daub" (timber and mud). There is no floor inside except packed earth. There are usually no windows, because the family fears theft, and the unit consists usually of two small rooms in one of which is a small clump of stones used as a fireplace for cooking, while the other is used for sleeping. It is no exaggeration to say that most houses contain no furniture whatever. In the corner will be a few rolls of thin straw mats, which are opened onto the floor for sleeping at night. A more prosperous home may contain a small table and a few wooden chairs. Variously sized jugs used for cooking and eating will be seen lying about. There is no need perhaps for furniture to hold clothing, because the average man, woman, or child will possess only one or two outfits. These consist of cotton pieces for above and below waist, both the men and women wearing skirts or "sarongs." Shoes are virtually unknown.

The great majority of households in D.H. have no toilet facilities at all. Defecation and urination are done on the surface of the ground near the house, usually by a clump of vegetation, but small children will release excreta almost anywhere. Occasionally a pit latrine will be seen near a house but as often as not it is in disrepair and not used. With no shoes being worn, conditions for transmission of hookworms are ideal.

There are occasional open wells (no pumps are used) in the area, but the great majority of families depend for their water on the tanks. From these, they carry in jugs or pails of water for drinking, cooking, and home washing. How often it is boiled before consumption cannot be stated. Laundry and bathing are usually done directly in the tanks or in small streams.

The diet of the people is woefully inadequate by any standard. It is based almost entirely on rice and a few cooked vegetables flavored with curry. A little dried fish is often added, but meat is practically unknown. Tropical fruits like manioc, *kurrakkan*, *jak*, and breadfruit are sometimes consumed. Milk, milk products, and eggs are rarely taken. Food is seldom provided to workers on the estates, and when some rice is occasionally given by the larger coconut growers a deduction is made from the wages. There can be no doubt that the small stature and slight frames of most of the village people, men and women, are related in large part to the deficient diets. It cannot be entirely racial because other Ceylonese people of the middle classes in the cities, descended from the same races and ethnic groups, are considerably larger and more robust.

The educational level of the people of Ceylon is undoubtedly high in relation to other nations of Southeast Asia, but it cannot be compared with the level in the industrialized nations of either the East or West. The 1946 census found fifty-eight percent of the population of Ceylon over age five to be literate and forty-two percent illiterate, defining literacy as the ability to both read and write a language. Data are not available specifically for D.H., but for the whole Kurunegala district, the figure on illiteracy is about like the national average, 42.5 percent. That there has been real improvement in the last twenty-five years, however, is indicated by the following data for the Kurunegala district on percentage of illiteracy:

Year	Persons	Males	Females
1921	60.6%	39.7%	88.0%
1946	42.5%	27.5%	60.1%

Not only are females found to be less literate than males, but in general the more isolated rural residents are less literate than those in the towns. Exactly what this literacy means is difficult to say, because after schooling, although a mechanical ability to read and write may be retained, it may deteriorate badly from disuse. In the several hospitals I visited in Ceylon, although hundreds of adult patients, in convalescent stages, were well enough to be out of bed and walking about, I failed to see a single piece of reading matter. It should be clarified that literacy does not, of course, call for knowledge of English, although this was the official language of the government and the upper classes for 150 years of British rule (now being changed). The primary language of the great majority of people in D.H. is Singhalese and for nearly all the remainder it is Tamil. Obviously any health work in the area calls for use of these languages.

Paths of travel within D.H. are reasonably good, with paved roads suitable for automobiles available to all principal points. There is a very good road between Wariyapola, the chief center, and Kurunegala. As is generally the case, however, there are scores of isolated villages connected with the main roads only by narrow unpaved roads or beaten paths which could not be negotiated by a car. The sanitary inspectors, as we shall see, have bicycles for getting about on, but there are many places which can be approached only on foot. There are buses that travel along the main roads, but the chief mode of transportation for the average family is the bullock cart. There are no railroad connections in the area, but there are stations at Kurunegala, twelve miles from Wariyapola, and at Ganewatte, nine miles away.

ORGANIZED SOCIAL PROGRAMS

While the basic conditions of life in Devamedi Hathpattu are as described, the situation is by no means static because for several years, especially since the Donoughmore Constitution granted adult suffrage in 1931 and more intensively since Independence in 1947, improvements have been underway. It is not possible here to describe the details of all organized social services in the area, but the highlights will be mentioned, insofar as they have a bearing on the health demonstration program.

To help improve agricultural output, there is a staff of technical agricultural personnel working in the area under the direction of the Ministry of Agriculture and Lands. There are two agricultural instructors in the area, each responsible for four korales, and attached to each instructor are two food production overseers to help in working with the peasants. Advice is given on improved methods of paddy and chena cultivation, and on methods of conserving the limited supply of water. There are intensive efforts to introduce certain types of seed, through private seed farms, which give a higher yield of rice, known as Pureline Paddy. Work is done to encourage vegetable gardens, which have value for nutrition, but there are no personnel analogous to the American "home demonstration agents" for work with the peasant woman. The major need expressed by agricultural officials for the D.H. area is for an agricultural engineering program to provide a better system of year-round irrigation.

Through the Ministry of Agriculture and Lands there has been a moderate program of land reform in Ceylon, under which undeveloped Crown Lands (government property) have been distributed to landless peasants.[2] This is administered locally by the divisional revenue officer (DRO), and in D.H., the DRO estimates that since 1938, when the program started, land plots have been distributed to about 2,500 families. The plots are small, usually one to three acres each. The peasants are given assistance in building houses, through the provision of timber. The DRO estimates that about 5,000 to 6,000 families in D.H. still possess no land.

An important background to the whole question of agriculture and land development in the health demonstration area is the national plan of Ceylon for attaining self-sufficiency in its food supply. Despite the fact that Ceylon's largest product for home consumption is rice, it must still import more rice than it now produces to meet the needs of the population. Actually about seventy percent of Ceylon's total food supply must be imported. To reduce this dependence on outside sources, the government is using a variety of measures which will increase agricultural productivity, and, if successful, these should have an effect on the entire economy of Devamedi Hathpattu.[3]

To improve education, there is a network of schools in D.H. which is in many ways remarkable, relative to other underdeveloped regions. There are forty-eight schools in the area with an enrollment of about 10,600 students. The buildings seem to be well located and most of them are attractive structures. They provide instruction for the first five standards (grades) in each school. Separate classrooms, however, are not provided and the pupils in each standard simply sit in groups next to each other in one large room. Even though the government has put a great deal into school construction in the rural sections, it has been hard to keep up with the rapid growth of population and the schools are obviously crowded. With an average of about 220 students per school in D.H., there are several teachers in each, under a head teacher. Some health education is included in the curriculum and a good many posters on health subjects are seen around the school walls. Each school has a garden, where the students learn some principles of agriculture.

Some of the schools in D.H. give instruction beyond the primary five grades for one or two years, but none gives a complete secondary school education, to lead to the "Senior Secondary Certificate." It is estimated by the divisional educational officer that between eighty and ninety percent of the children attend school, but only about sixty percent continue through the fifth standard. Very few go beyond this to secondary school. Most of the rural teachers have had a full secondary school education, but very few have had university training. All the schools are supervised by a district educational officer stationed at Kurunegala, including eight temple schools or *pirivenas* which give instruction to both children and priests. Sanitation facilities at the schools are, in general, deplorable. The larger schools have latrines at the inadequate rate of about one pit per 100 pupils but most of them have nothing. Likewise the larger schools are provided with wells, but most have no protected water supply. In their lessons the children are taught to boil all water before drinking, but at one school which I visited this had not been done in the school itself for some time.

An important service in the school, or at least potentially important, is the so-called "midday meal." This is financed wholly by the Ministry of Education but only six cents is available per pupil per day. With this small amount, it is not even possible to afford the provision of milk, and the money is used for a bun and tea—a meal with little nutritive value.

The divisional revenue officer, mentioned earlier, has many functions in addition to land assignments which are related to health and well-being. He is also the local administrative officer for public assistance, under a national system which provides grants to certain categories of destitute persons. For single persons the grant is ten rupees (about $2.10) per month and for persons with dependents it is twenty rupees per month. At present those receiving assistance in the D.H. area are as shown in table IV.1.

In addition financial relief is given to persons struck by disaster, such as widespread distress due to drought, flood or fire, or other emergency.[4] In the last year, however, no such relief was granted in D.H. The funds for this public assistance are obviously limited and cannot meet the full need, but this type of program is still far in advance of other underdeveloped nations. Some indication of the unmet need is the fact that during the period January-May 1951, there were 118 applications for help in D.H. and there are currently fifty-eight applications on the waiting list in this area.

There are a number of homes for the aged in Ceylon operated mainly by voluntary agencies, and most of them receive special grants from the Department of Social Services. No such home exists in D.H., however, nor in the Kurunegala district. It is contemplated by the department that a home for the aged to accommodate initially about twenty-five persons may be constructed by the government in D.H., if a voluntary agency, like the Social Service League, can be organized to operate it. A per capita grant would then be paid to finance its operation. Likewise a crèche might be supported along similar lines, to take care of the children of working mothers. Workmen's compensation for industrial injuries is also administered by this department, but the kind of work done in D.H. is not covered by it at present.[5]

Other functions coming under the divisional revenue officer which indirectly affect health are the supervision of irrigation channels, the promotion of the National Savings Campaign, and the issuance of ration books (since rice is now rationed.) A function quite directly related to health is his supervision, through another full-time officer, of the rural development societies.

The rural development society movement was started in 1948 as an approach to the vast problem of

Table IV.1
Assistance grants to persons in the demonstration area

Category	Number
Aged persons without dependents	195
Aged persons with dependents	42
Invalids without dependents	61
Invalids with dependents	36
Widows	47
Women deprived of the help of their husbands	5
Total	386

community improvement in the villages. Even though there were village councils, constituting local governmental bodies throughout the Island, it was felt that these were not effective for work on a self-help basis in the villages. Moreover, the village council or committee usually represented a large number of villages, too large a group to make possible intimate participation of the average villager. In D.H., the four village committees, for example, each represent an average of about 167 villages. Therefore, through the Ministry of Home Affairs, these small societies were developed on a truly local basis all over the Island, so that today there are about 5,000 of them. In D.H., there are 116 rural development societies organized. In each society there are forty to fifty households represented, coming usually from two to three villages.

The functions of the societies are described as (1) health, (2) economic, and (3) social. In the field of health they attempt to promote the construction of latrines, the provision of wells, use of compost pits, and other features of the health unit program. In economic matters, they promote better agricultural methods, savings, and village industries. Under social objectives, they promote religious teaching in Sunday schools, adult education, and women's clubs. Thus their activities help to promote, through community educational backing, the objectives of the Ministry of Health as well as other ministries. Not all the societies in D.H. do all the things theoretically included in their program, but they are still young and just learning new methods of group work. There is a rural development officer for D.H. who works with them, advising on techniques. The societies are organized into eight larger groups, sending representatives to meetings of these groups monthly, while the eight groups form a Union of

Rural Development Societies for the entire area which meets twice yearly. In this way, experiences are exchanged and a healthy competition is promoted. Up to the present, no direct subsidy has been provided for any of the societies in D.H., but for the coming year the sum of 40,000 rupees has been requested from the Ministry of Home Affairs and Rural Development, with which to launch an extensive program of latrine construction. I visited one of the better rural development societies in the area (village of Hamillakotuwa) and was much impressed with work they had done in building with their own hands a new rural school, in road construction, and in developing the use of compost pits near the homes of the villagers. The opportunities for working with these societies in the development of the entire program in the health demonstration area are enormous.

The Department of Labour in the Ministry of Labour and Social Services carries out certain functions in Devamedi Hathpattu, which will have an impact on the health of the people of the demonstration area. While concerned mainly with conditions in urban industry, the department maintains wage boards which fix minimum wages and maximum hours on the coconut estates in the area. It also enforces the payment of maternity benefits to women employed on coconut estates which employ a force of ten or more workers. These consist of six weeks of leave with a grant of forty-two rupees (one rupee per day). The Coconut Wage Board also covers the fifty workers employed in the single mill in D.H., where fiber is produced. There is no restriction on labor performed by non-school-going children and women. Department officials are concerned with enforcement of ordinances on health and safety in factories, but these do not apply at present in D.H. They help to settle labor disputes, such as might occur on a coconut estate, although such disputes are nearly all confined to the larger tea and rubber estates. They help to deal with unemployment by directing unemployed workers to other areas where they may be needed, but no significant unemployment has been reported in D.H. in the last year.

Another highly important activity for the social well-being of the people in the demonstration area is the cooperative movement for distribution of both consumer's and producer's goods. Starting in 1911, the cooperatives in Ceylon early came under the supervision of the central government and in 1942, during the war, they enjoyed rapid expansion. There are today 6,634 societies organized in Ceylon, of which the chief types are cooperative stores for consumer goods and credit cooperatives, mainly for providing credit for small cultivators on reasonable terms. In a given area cooperatives are organized into "circles," which come under the supervision of a circle inspector. Such an officer is stationed at Wariyapola in the demonstration area. One circle includes the cooperatives in D.H. and just one *korale* in a neighboring district. Within this circle there are now eighty-six cooperative societies, including: twenty-seven cooperative stores for sale of food, textiles, and other supplies; forty-one credit societies of different types giving loans; eight school societies for teaching schoolchildren cooperative principles; six agricultural production and sales societies; and one each for coconut sales, pottery sales, tobacco marketing, and for wholesale services to the retail stores ("store union cooperative"). Cooperatives are encouraged and supported by the government and they even perform official functions, like retention of rice ration books for the people. This form of community organization should provide numerous opportunities for promotion of health objectives in the demonstration area program.[6]

A parallel development of economic importance in Ceylon is the promotion of cottage industries—small village enterprises through which useful products are manufactured on a small scale from locally available materials. In the absence of large-scale industrialization, these small industries can do much to improve the economic well-being and hence the health of the people. This program comes under the supervision of the Department of Cottage Industries in the Ministry of Industries. According to the records of that office, little is now done in this field in D.H. Within the general Kurunegala district there are *coir* centers (for making rope from coconut fiber), pottery centers, textile units, and cooperative carpenters' societies (for making furniture). Within D.H., the only activity seems to be a pottery center at Galwewa, near Katupotha. This program certainly deserves expansion in the demonstration area.

The development of roads in Ceylon is a responsibility of the Ministry of Transport and Public Works. At present there is no new road building activity going on in D.H., since the main channels are well provided. The ministry indicates, however, that if there are any special requests for paving of rural roads in the demonstration area, they will be given special consideration. To pave a one-lane country road in this area costs an average of 15,000 rupees per mile.

All of the above forms of organized social programs in the demonstration area are sponsored by branches of the central government. Finally, we may consider the activities of the only units of local government in the area, the four village councils. As mentioned earlier, those are elected bodies with members representing all the villages in the area. Several small villages may have a joint representative in the village council (sometimes also called village committee) so that while each village council in the demonstration area represents an average of 168 villages, they contain only twenty-four to thirty members each. The council has minor taxing powers (licenses, fines, small property taxes, etc.) with which it raises funds, but in D.H. the bulk of its funds come from the central government, through annual grants. It has legislative powers and can pass bylaws with respect to use of roads, public places, sanitation, and other local matters. (The Department of Medical and Sanitary Services sends out model sets of bylaws on sanitation in public eating places, markets, scavenging and conservancy, dangerous trades, food and drugs, etc., which are usually adopted by the village council, with supplements to most local conditions.) It may develop various public works and welfare programs for its area, maintain markets or fairs, provide housing, and other direct civic services. It is in this sphere that the village council does work of special importance for the demonstration area.

The village councils administer funds for providing milk (dried milk powder) at the maternal and child welfare centers in their jurisdictions, for helping to maintain the buildings in which dispensaries are located, for constructing walls, for conservancy services (removal of excreta from bucket latrines), and for scavenging (garbage disposal). The information in table IV.2, obtained from the assistant commissioner for local government for the Kurunegala district, gives some idea of the recent functions of village councils in D.H., relating to health and sanitation.

When it is realized that the construction of a well costs about 1,800 rupees, the meager quantities involved in these expenditures can be appreciated. Nevertheless, the nucleus of a body of participating local government is provided by the village councils and it may be hoped that they will develop further, to assume larger roles in local health service. Another activity of the village council that might have indirect bearing on health, is its development of community centers, which are primarily places of recreation for young people. The four village councils in D.H. have organized twenty-eight such centers of which about sixteen are currently described as being active, the others being inactive. It may be possible to use these centers in health education activities. In the launching of the entire demonstration area program, much is to be gained by having the support and understanding of the four village councils.

This, then, summarizes the organized social programs in D.H., all of which have some bearing on the

Table IV.2
Funds spent by village councils for health and sanitation: 1950-1951, in rupees

Function	Wariyapola	Kalugamuwa	Hettipola	Kanogama
Milk at child centers	800	1,000	500	300
Dispensary maintenance	—	2,500 (1947-48)	—	—
Construction of wells	3,600	1,500	3,600	3,600
Conservancy Service	100	—	—	—
Scavenging Service	60	—	—	—

health of the people. It may be observed that all these activities are governmental, either directly or by inspiration, as in the case of the rural development societies. There are some voluntary agencies in Ceylon, working in health and welfare services but so far as I could tell none of them is operating in D.H. As in other countries, there is heavy emphasis on maternal and child health services by the voluntary groups, which work chiefly in the larger cities. It may be possible to promote activity by such societies in the health demonstration area, to help reach specific objectives.

Despite all the organized social programs, as stated earlier, the life of the people in Ceylon generally and in D.H. particularly is, on the whole, dull and primitive. The day's activities are an endless struggle for survival, nearly all efforts being directed toward meeting the simplest needs of food, shelter, and family life. The result is inevitably a high volume of disease and death. Relative to other underdeveloped agricultural nations, Ceylon's health record is outstandingly good, but compared with the achievements technically possible in the modern world there is a long way to go.

NOTES

[1] A brief summary of "The Social Context" of Ceylon's culture is given in *Report of the Commission on Social Services*. Ceylon Government Press, February 1947. A series of important sociological studies of village life, directed by Professor Bryce Ryan, Head of the Department of Sociology at the University of Ceylon, is soon to be published. While these studies do not include a village within D.H. they do include a village in the northwestern province just to the north of D.H., near Nikaweratiya. This village is called Ellagamillawa, containing about fifty households.

[2] This program is reported in S.F. Amerasinghe, *Administration Report of the Land Commissioner for 1949*. Ceylon Government Press, 1950.

[3] See Department of Information, *Ceylon Food Plan*. 1950.

[4] More details on the operation are available in a publication of the Department of Social Services, *Public Assistance Orders and Procedure*. Ceylon Government Press, 1951.

[5] The general program of social services in Ceylon is described in A.T. Grandison, *Administration Report of the Director of Social Services for 1949*. Ceylon Government Press, 1950.

[6] For a general account of the Ceylon cooperative movement see the report. *The All-Ceylon Co-operative Congress Souvenir*. Ceylon Government Press, 1950. More detailed information on the operations of the societies is given in S.C. Fernando, *Administration Report on the Working of Co-operative Societies from May 1, 1948 to April 30, 1950*. Ceylon Government Press, December 1950.

Chapter V
The Development and Current Spectrum of Organized Health Services in a New Asian Country: Malaysia

The characteristics of health service organization in many newly independent nations of Asia and Africa have been heavily influenced by their past, as colonies, and before that as indigenous tribal cultures. This is well illustrated in Malaysia, which took shape as an independent nation in 1957. In its current health service patterns is seen the impact of not only the British Colonial Service of the past century, but also of the older Malay and Chinese practices and the planning of the new Malaysian leadership.

In 1968, an evaluation was made of a special Rural Health Services Scheme, which had been started with the assistance of the World Health Organization and UNICEF in 1953. This chapter consists of two sections of that report providing general background information, before examination of the rural scheme itself, with its network of health centers and midwife stations. It is drawn from Rural Health Services Scheme of Malaysia, *an unpublished World Health Organization document produced for the Regional Office of the Western Pacific (Manila, the Philippines, 1969, pp. 5-36), and reprinted here by permission.*

HISTORICAL DEVELOPMENT OF OVERALL HEALTH SERVICES IN MALAYSIA

As in any country, the current picture of overall health services in Malaysia is a product of several separate and distinct streams of historical development, all of which, as we will see, have a definite bearing on the Rural Health Services Scheme (RHSS). These overall services, including those for both preventive (defined in Malaysia usually as "health") and curative (defined usually as "medical") purposes, have taken shape through the influence of several historical periods.

Early Local Culture and Initial Colonization (1511-1880)

Five hundred years ago the Malay Peninsula was peopled by rural tribes, whose healing arts were believed to be influenced by the ancient medical lore of the great Asian continent. Malay traditional medicine, according to Dr. J. W. Field, was a blend of local folklore, Hindu mythology, Moslem orthodoxy, and Arabic pharmacopoeia.[1] This stream of development, despite the enormous influences of the West, is still very much alive in the work of *bomohs* and other traditional healers in the several thousand villages or *kampongs* of modern Malaysia.

The impact of the West started with the Portuguese settlement in what is now Malacca in 1511. In 1641 the Portuguese were succeeded by the Dutch in Malacca and in 1786 the British came to the island of Penang, followed in 1795 by their replacement of the Dutch in Malacca. A generation later, in

1819, the British acquired control of the island of Singapore by purchase from a local ruler. In all three of these early trading stations, the Dutch and then the British probably established small garrison hospitals or infirmaries for the care of European officials and their families. Perhaps local persons were occasionally treated at these infirmaries, but there was no significant spread of Western medicine inland until about 1873, when the British intervened among the warring Malay state sultanates. The civil administration of the three coastal cities—Malacca, Penang, and Singapore—was strengthened by the formation of the Straits Settlements Authority under the British Colonial Office in 1867, including responsibility to some extent for health protection.

Hospital Development (1880-1910)

In the early nineteenth century, tin had been discovered in Malaya, and Chinese settlers came to extract it. With them, they brought Chinese traditional medicine, and in 1880 they built a small hospital of twenty-eight beds for their countrymen in Kuala Lumpur.[2] In 1883, the British Resident established a "general hospital" also in Kuala Lumpur—the first of what now constitute a network of general hospitals in each of the state capitals of the eleven states of West Malaysia. As the Chinese continued to come to Malaya in the later nineteenth century, Chinese herbalists, with hundreds of remedies from plants and animal organs, settled in the slowly growing towns.

In 1896, the Federation of Malay States was formed by agreement between the British and the sultans of the four states of Selangor, Perak, Negri Sembilan, and Pahang. In these "federated states," the advice of the British Resident was followed on all matters (including health), except religious and Malay customs. A few years later, the northern states of Perlis, Kedah, Kelantan, and Trengganu passed from Thai (Siam) to British protection in foreign relations. Along with the southern state of Johore, these came to be the "nonfederated states," with greater autonomy in the management of their internal affairs.[3] Thus by about 1910 an administrative structure, under differing forms of authority, had been established in the three straits settlements, the four federated states, and the five nonfederated states of the Malay Peninsula.

With this extension of European influence, between 1883 and 1910, general hospitals were established in the capital cities of each of the states. In 1907, for example, in the nonfederated state of Kelantan, a small hospital was built (probably nine beds) at the town of Kota Bharu.[4] The emphasis of this period was obviously curative medicine and the hospital treatment of the desperately sick. There was, however, a dawn of sensitivity to preventive health needs in the main cities. Kuala Lumpur, in fact, set up among the British governmental personnel a sanitary board concerned with cleaning of the streets, maintenance of public markets, and so on.

The challenge of research into the causes and control of infectious, tropical diseases was met by the establishement by the British of the Institute for Medical Research in 1900. This important center in Kuala Lumpur, tied originally to universities in London and Liverpool, now plays a key role in the health services of all Malaysia. The Singapore Medical College was founded in 1905, evolving later into the faculty of medicine of the University of Malaya.

The British Colonial Medical Service and Public Health (1910-1942)

In 1910 an organized health department was established on a permanent basis in Kuala Lumpur. It was staffed by colonial government medical officers, qualified in public health, and its functions were chiefly related to environmental sanitation in Kuala Lumpur and the surrounding areas. By 1920, the staff had expanded to thirty-one medical officers and eight sanitary inspectors.

Meanwhile in the early twentieth century, rubber estates had begun to take form (after the first introduction of the trees in Singapore in 1877). By 1920 there were 1,200 such estates, and a labor code—including provisions for health and sanitation—had been enacted. Outside the main cities, it was on the rubber estates (rather than in rural areas generally) that public health efforts were concentrated. Swamp drainage and mosquito larvacidal work to control malaria in these locations, along with smallpox vaccination and some quarantine, were the chief activities.

In the decades between 1910 and 1940, medical officers of health (MOHs) were appointed in the capital cities of each of the Malay states. In some, their functions were confined to the interior of those cities and in others they extended to enforcement of sanitary conditions at the rubber estates and tin mines. In a few cities, maternal and child health clinics were established and some examinations were done on schoolchildren. In each of the federated, as well as the nonfederated states, there was a public health "adviser" who was assigned by the Colonial Medical Service. In 1948, however, the Federation of Malaya Agreement decentralized control to some extent to the several states.

Quite separate from the public health work, general hospitals were also expanded in the state capitals during this period and some small "district hospitals" were built in other towns. As satellites of some of the hospitals, small "town dispensaries" were established in a few cities, staffed mainly by hospital assistants. These were male dressers or medical auxiliaries who learned their skills by apprenticeships in the hospitals.

Thus, there took shape two sides to the health services: a "public health" side and a "hospital" side. After 1948, both came under the control of the state governments. At the federal level in Kuala Lumpur, health authority was limited to enforcement of quarantine and the control of epidemics, the allocation of personnel, the operation of certain federal hospitals (mental, military, etc.), and general advisory services. It was not until 1958 that the national government of the then independent Federation took over control of both public health and hospital functions in the states.

From 1930 to 1942, the colonial public health and medical services were faced by the setbacks of the worldwide economic depression and made little further progress. Outside the estates and mines, the only services for rural areas were a few travelling dispensaries emanating from the hospitals. In 1942, the country was conquered and occupied by the Japanese army.

The War and Postwar Period (1942-1952)

During the Japanese occupation (1942-1945), health services were severely impaired. The infant mortality rate in Kuala Lumpur, for example, leaped from ninety-seven per 1,000 live births in 1940 to 156 per 1,000 in 1943.

With the end of the war and the formation of the Malayan Federation in 1948, civil government became more systematized throughout the twelve states. Among other things, this meant the establishment of "administrative districts" as smaller units of political jurisdiction within the states. Their authorities involved land control, tax collection, road maintenance, and related functions. In current Malaysia, these administrative districts now number seventy, and they constitute—either singly or in combinations of two or three—the underlying framework of public health services (both urban and rural) in the nation. As of the present time, the seventy administrative districts are clustered into forty-seven health districts, which will have an important part in the discussion below.

In the postwar period there was also a large expansion of "district hospitals" reaching fifty, in addition to ten "general hospitals," by 1956. Emanating from most of the general and district hospitals, located usually in the headquarters town of an administrative district, were various static dispensaries in the towns. Some additional travelling dispensaries to rural locations were also organized.

Maternal and child health clinics were established in scores of cities and towns in the postwar period. In the state of Pahang, for example, eight such clinics had been established in the state capital (then Kuala Lipis) and seven district towns by 1956. These preventively oriented clinics came under the administration of the health district MOH and they have often formed the nucleus of what later took shape as health centers within the RHSS.

Origin of the Rural Health Service Scheme (1953-1956)

The "Emergency" had its onset around 1948. Since the Communist guerillas derived much of their sustenance from Chinese settlers, wresting a living at the edge of the Malayan jungles, a major counterinsurgency program consisted in resettlement of about a half million of these people into "new villages"—some 500 of these throughout the country. This was done between 1950 and 1953. While curfews were imposed and movements restricted, the inhabitants of the new villages were often provided with midwife clinics or small first-aid facilities.

The Emergency, therefore, not only contributed to the belated recognition of rural needs, but it also highlighted the special deficiencies in the hundreds of *kampongs* peopled by Malays who had taken no part in the guerilla movement. With all the attention given to the Chinese in new villages, it was argued in Parliament, what about the social needs of the greater number of rural Malays?[5] Thus a series of national programs were started, focusing attention on improving conditions in rural areas: the Rural and Industrial Development Authority (RIDA, 1951), the Federal Land Development Authority (FLDA, 1956), and the Ministry for Rural Development (1959), now functioning as the Ministry of National and Rural Development.

It was part of this swelling tide of concern for rural welfare that led to the formulation of the RHSS. The first seeds of the idea were planted with the design of a model "rural health center" at Jitra, Kedah, in 1953.[6] This center was established in 1954 to provide both a broad scope of preventive and curative service to a surrounding rural population and a training program for the staffs to be placed eventually in other rural health centers.

The First Development Plan of the then Federation of Malaya was scheduled for 1954-1956 and it contained the prospectus of the RHSS. In this initial period it was contemplated that twenty-five rural health centers would be built, more or less on the Jitra model. Around each of these would eventually be four "subdistrict health centers" and around each of these would be five "trained rural midwives"—the whole constellation serving about 50,000 rural people. With the pressures of the Emergency, only eight "district health centers" were built in this first period. The details of the whole development are presented in an excellent publication by Dr. L. W. Jayesuria appearing in 1967.[7] The step-by-step progress of the RHSS to the current day need not be repeated here, but its general movement will be reviewed below.

The Five-Year Plans (1956-1970)

Even before Independence (1957), planning on a national level had begun. The first Five-Year Plan was scheduled for the period 1956-1960. The construction of numerous components of the RHSS was part of the plan. A further boost was given to planning in the health sector by transfer of all responsibilities for public health and hospitals from the states to the federal government in 1953.[8] Henceforward, both financial support and general direction (both technical and administrative) came from a unified national "Medical Department"—later, a Ministry of Health. This permitted greater coordination of the RHSS planning with the planning schedule of other ministries.

By the end of the first Five-Year Plan in 1960, construction in the RHSS had been completed as follows:

District health centers	8
Health subcenters	8
Midwife clinics cum quarters	26

Staffing of these facilities, however, was far from adequate, since training programs take longer than putting up buildings.

It was in the Second Five-Year Plan, 1961-1965, that the concept of the RHSS became better crystallized, in relation to the overall process of "rural development planning" and the administrative structure of the Ministry of Health. In this period, it became clarified that the "medical and health officer" in charge of each "main health center" would be responsible to the MOH of the health district. The district MOH in turn is responsible to the chief medical and health officer of the state—an official appointed by the central ministry and responsible for all activities in the state, both preventive and curative (i.e., hospitals). The state chief medical and health officer would meet with the state rural development committee, the health district MOH with the district rural development committee (or committees) in his territory, and the rural medical and health officer with any *kampong* development committees that were formed.

By the end of the Second Five-Year Plan in 1965, further construction had achieved thirty-nine main health centers, 122 subhealth centers, and 643 midwife clinics cum quarters. This was obviously a period of rapid progress, even though staffing of the rural health units could not keep up with the pace of construction. The very completion of buildings, however, provided an inducement toward the recruitment and training of personnel. Perhaps the most serious deficiency was in doctors; most of the main health centers were without a medical and health officer, theoretically the team leader. This critical gap was not filled until a decision was made in 1965 to import doctors for these posts from overseas.

The third Five-Year Plan (1966-1970) became known as the "First Malaysia Plan" since the new country had taken shape in 1963. It did not contemplate construction of further main centers, but did aim at completion of sixty more subhealth centers and 450 more midwife clinics. The relatively slower pace of construction was due to channelling of funds toward urgently needed improvement of general and district hospitals, and it permitted consolidation of staffing of the various components of existing rural health units. As of December 1967, some seventeen additional subcenters had been built, plus sixty midwife clinics, bringing the total network to:[9]

Main health centers	39
Subhealth centers	139
Midwife clinics cum quarters	703

A drop in the world price of rubber has caused a decline in revenue for Malaysia so that, as of this writing (August 1968) it seems unlikely that the construction goals of the RHSS in the First Malaysia Plan will be met. Nevertheless, it is obvious that, since its beginnings in 1954, the Scheme has made enormous progress in improving health services for rural people. As noted earlier, WHO has been involved in an advisory capacity at three stages (1954-1959, 1959-1963, and 1964-1968) which happen to overlap with the Five-Year Plans.

In the whole sequence of Five-Year Plans, an active program of training has also proceeded within the RHSS at the rural health training centers at Jitra, Kedah and Rembau, Negri Sembilan. These will be discussed below, along with the other basic health training programs in Malaysia which indirectly contribute to RHSS staffing.

THE CURRENT SPECTRUM OF PUBLIC AND PRIVATE HEALTH SERVICES

With this historical development, containing as always several concurrent streams, the resultant picture of health services today is naturally complex. It is important, however, to draw its lines because there is no part of the broad picture—a dynamic moving picture, as it is—that does not affect the operations of the RHSS. If the RHSS is to be evaluated, the full spectrum of public and private health services in Malaysia must be seen.

As new cultural forms of health care or new organized patterns of service have entered the scene, the older forms have not died out, but have continued to operate. Thus the ancient forms of Malay healing and of Chinese herbalism continue to exist even after Western medicine and public health have arisen and flourished. Likewise within organized scientific health service, many older patterns continue alongside the newer ones. There is a common tendency in official health circles to overlook the whole private sector of medical care, but it must be understood if some of the problems of manpower and of service utilization in the public sector are to be appreciated.

Traditional Healing (and Drugs)

Semisubmerged under the RHSS and, indeed, the entire structure of modern health services in Malaysia, is a vast layer of traditional, nonscientific healing, the ancient origins of which were briefly noted above. Over the years, the practices of the traditional healers have changed, as new influences have impinged on them, but—in spite of their widespread operation and even some limited effectiveness (either psychological or empirical)—their overall impact today on the health of the people must be considered negative. It is perhaps less important that their ministrations are usually medically worthless (if not sometimes harmful) than that they have the effect of misleading sick people and delaying the procurement of sound medical care.

The historic streams have yielded several types of traditional healer in the current period. Most important are the Malay *bomohs* (sometimes spelled *bomors*) who abound in the villages or *kampongs*. Along with them are the *kampong bidans* or midwives. Their work is built on three pillars: (a) magic, (b) religion, and (c) empiricism. With magic they perform rites intended to exorcise evil spirits or counteract evil influences of other persons. They also win the confidence of the patient by invoking Divine aid and performing certain rituals of the Muslim faith. (Sometimes they are minor lay officers of the mosque.) Finally they use a vast variety of external and internal drugs made from local plants or animal organs. There are hundreds of these, ranging in complexity from single ingredients to a concoction of twenty-nine items for external treatment of smallpox.[10] For mild complaints, the *bomoh* tends to use a simple herbal, while for more serious illness he makes greater use of incantations and more complex regimes of drugs designed to restore the balance among the four basic properties of nature: heat, cold, dryness, and moisture.[11]

It is difficult to determine the extent of the bomohs in rural Malaysia, but everyone seems to agree that they are ubiquitous and frequently used. The commonest opinion is that every *kampong* (of perhaps 300 people or more) has at least one *bomoh* and sometimes two. Most of them, however, are not full-time, but are men engaged in agriculture who practice the healing arts on the side, when called upon. A frequent estimate is that about twenty percent are full-time. Accurate data on the numbers and rate of utilization of *bomohs* have not been collected, and questions about them frequently seem to cause embarrassment, as though the subject itself were somewhat improper. Yet, there is no question about the importance of this healing practice (found, incidentally, in some form in all countries) if rural health services are to be properly understood.

It is common practice for sick villagers to consult the *bomoh* first, and only if satisfactory improvement does not occur to seek help from a government facility. In any village, however, the older persons are more likely to use *bomohs* and the younger ones, with more education, less likely. But distance from a health center or hospital is also a factor; more isolated *kampongs* naturally depend more on healers who are on the spot. As roads and transportation improve, as education extends, and as scientific medical resources are established in rural areas, the use of *bomohs* is bound to decline.

More openly recognized than the *bomohs* are the *kampong bidans* who, from all the evidence, still deliver about half the babies in West Malaysia and probably over half in the rural areas. Their extent will be discussed below, but here it may simply be noted that their practices also represent a blend of magico-religious and empirical principles. As an older woman, who has had several children herself, the *kampong bidan* usually has the confidence of the village people and she is the authority on ancient Malay customs, such as the dietary taboos for the mother after childbirth and the prohibition on her or the infant leaving the house for forty-four days.[12] Irrational as some of these practices may seem, it should be realized that they contain an internal logic — if the premises on disease etiology are accepted. Thus, the *kampong bidan* applies certain herbs to the abdomen in the first three postpartum days, because this is a time when evil spirits are considered strong and the mother is weak and susceptible to their invasion; the herbs are designed to protect her against such invasion—essentially a form of preventive medicine.[13] The reduction of deliveries by these nontrained midwives, therefore, probably cannot be achieved by arguments or propaganda, but only by replacement with an obstetrical service that to the village people seems better.

Beyond the *bomohs* and *bidans* in the villages, there is the occasional drugseller, the *jual obat* who applies no spiritual devices but simply sells various concoctions in bottles. These are allegedly tonics, designed to give general strength and not related to a specific diagnosis. Because their work is not based on any theory, ancient or modern, these rural practitioners are usually simply referred to as "quacks."

In the small towns, as well as the cities, throughout West Malaysia is a very different form of traditional healer on whom rural people also depend for much of their medical care. This is the Chinese herbalist or *sin seh* who sells an enormous variety of drugs prepared from plants—some recipes derived from writings of Chinese physicians 3,000 years ago and others from the commonplace herbs and roots in the local region.[14] The *sin seh* has his shop on the town's main street and is not the least surreptitious. Sometimes he operates a "medical hall" with a large impressive sign. Indeed, these practitioners are registered with the national government, not as health professionals but as businesses coming under the authority of the Registry of Business in the Ministry of Commerce and Industry. The herbalist makes no use of spiritual procedures nor does he lay hands on the patient or make any examination. On hearing of the patient's complaint, he simply dispenses a remedy.

At the Department of Statistics, a compilation has been underway on the businesses registered in Malaysia in 1963 (registration is required annually). While the classification problem is formidable and the actual registrations are believed to be far from complete, the writer's own count of "businesses" which were classified as "medical and health services" (nonprofessional) or as "drug stores" (not qualified pharmacists) yielded 909 such places.[15] The general opinion is that these herbalists exceed the number of doctors in private medical practice. A recent study of *sin sehs* in Taiwan (where there is a relatively high supply also of scientifically trained physicians) reported that they saw, on the average, thirty patients per day—approximately the same number as doctors.[16] If this relationship applies in Malaysia, it would appear that the Chinese herbalists offer as much medical care outside of hospitals as doctors. Since the prices are much lower than medical fees, it may be assumed that low income rural people who come to town (rather than to a government facility) for medical care are more likely to see herbalists than doctors. The national *Household Budget Survey* of 1957-1958 (discussed more below) found, of course, a much greater expenditure for "internal Eastern drugs" among Chinese than among other racial groups, but even among rural Malays the expenditure for "Eastern" drugs was nearly as high as for "Western" (eighteen cents per month compared with twenty-two cents) despite the higher price per item of the latter.

Beyond the officially registered Chinese drugsellers, almost every provision shop in the small rural towns sells some Chinese herbals and also Western-type drugs that are dispensed without a doctor's prescription. These usually consist of vitamin pills, aspirin, or cough remedies, but sometimes even antibiotics that are marked for veterinary use. There is a national Ordinance on Sales of Food and Drugs which does not attempt to cope with the Chinese herbals but rather with officially "scheduled" pharmaceutical products. The Pharmaceutical Chemist in the State Medical and Health Office, who is expected to enforce this law, however, is usually busy with other matters (especially maintaining drug supplies in government health facilities), so that surveillance of these over-the-counter drug sales is weak.

Beyond all these nonscientific healers, there are a few Ayurvedic or homeopathic practitioners from India in the towns and a few acupuncturists. Like the herbalists, these are not prohibited, so long as they do not hold themselves out to be qualified doctors of medicine. There are also frankly religious healers, known as *tang-ki* (spirit-medium) in the Chinese urban communities.[17]

All this traditional healing in Malaysia has a distinct influence on rural health services and it must be understood if these services are to be improved. In a sense, the continued use of traditional healing can be taken as a barometer of the effectiveness of the RHSS or vice versa. The general opinion seems to be that the use of traditional healers, especially *bomohs*, has been declining as the RHSS has expanded. Firm data on this are lacking, except with respect to the use of *kampong bidans*, which will be discussed further below. It is easy enough to understand why isolated rural people will continue to use village healers, who are close at hand, inexpensive, and spiritually comforting, so long as scientific medicine is distant, sometimes hasty and impersonal, and always hard to comprehend.

Private Medical Practice and Medical Manpower

Medical care is perhaps the only major governmental function in which access to manpower resources is restricted by competition from a significant private sector. In recruiting policemen or soldiers, governments do not have to face competition, as it were, from private police squads or private armies. In a developing country, private schools do not offer any significant competition to government in the acquisition of teachers. But governmental responsibilities for medical care, and especially services in rural areas, are seriously affected by the operation of a robust sector of private medical practice in most countries.

In December 1967, the Registry of Medical Practitioners of Malaysia (maintained in the Ministry of Health) contained the names of 1,759 doctors.[18] Since registration is done only once and some of these doctors may have moved away, without notifying the registry, this number may be inflated by an estimated five to ten percent so that a more reliable figure would be about 1,600, yielding a ratio (for a population in West Malaysia of 8,500,000) of one doctor to 5,300 persons. This is much poorer, of course, than the industrialized countries of Europe but much better than many developing countries, such as Indonesia to the south. As in nearly all countries, there is a marked maldistribution among the states, ranging from a ratio (in 1964) of 1:2,630 in Selangor to 1:18,730 in Kelantan. Within all states, the available doctors are heavily concentrated in the cities.

Of the 1,600 or 1,700 scientifically trained doctors in Malaysia, 713 were attached in December 1967 to government services. Thus a balance of nearly 1,000 or about sixty percent are in private medical practice. There is almost no part-time employment in government in Malaysia (in contrast to most countries of Latin America, Africa, or elsewhere), so that the majority of medical manpower in the country is totally outside the orbit of the public programs which are subject to planning, especially for meeting rural needs.

Private doctors in Malaysia are almost entirely in general practice. They are almost exclusively in the main cities and in solo arrangements. Conversations with several practitioners and with knowledgeable observers from the University and government suggest that the qualitative level of work is not very high. Typically they do very little laboratory or other diagnostic work-up on patients. They have virtually no relationship to hospitals. If a patient requires specialist consultation, he may be sent to a hospital, but this is rarely done. It is estimated that the private practitioner sees an average of fifty to seventy-five patients a day, and the attention to each is relatively perfunctory.

In spite of this, the earnings of private doctors are relatively high. There are many quips among government doctors about how much more private doctors earn, even without any specialty training. A common estimate is that private medical net incomes are three times the level of governmental medical salaries, on the average. (The level of governmental salaries must be adjusted, however, for certain perquisites like allowances for quarters, transportation, and retirement.) Especially successful private practitioners may earn five or six times the level of government doctors. It is easy to understand, therefore, why the majority of doctors in the country are in private practice and why the turnover of doctors in government service is high—about forty or fifty leaving each year. Between 1958 and 1966, there were 480 doctors recruited into the government health and medical services, but 327 (seventy-five percent) left—nearly all for the more lucrative prospects of private practice.

The realities of private medical practice in Malaysia have a strong bearing on the operations of the RHSS. Because of its financial and other attractions, the Ministry of Health has, up to now, found it almost impossible to recruit Malaysian doctors for posts in the rural health units. As a result, nearly all the positions for medical and health officers in the thirty-nine main health centers have had to be filled by foreign doctors (mostly from South Korea and the Philippines) hired on temporary contracts. These doctors are often very well trained (with graduate degrees in public health), but they usually do not speak Malay (the language of the village people) and their time in the rural areas, being transitory, is of no permanent qualitative value to the nation's manpower. Indeed, many of the posts in district hospitals serving rural populations have likewise had to be filled by foreign doctors.

Yet, it may be noted that the total number of new doctors placed in the Medical Registry each year is relatively large and rising; in 1966 it was 166 doctors and in 1967 it was 200. The great majority of these are Malaysian who have studied medicine in Singapore or elsewhere abroad. (The University of Malaya Medical School will turn out its first graduates in 1969—the implications of which will be discussed below.) If all these doctors were to join the government service, the medical posts in the RHSS could be filled with Malaysian personnel overnight. It is the lucrativeness of private practice, of course, that makes this an idle thought.

The earnings of private doctors, one must sometimes be reminded, come from the pockets of patients. In 1957–1958, a national household survey was made by the Department of Statistics, to explore the incomes and spending patterns of rural and urban people.[19] Among other things, this survey found that people were spending between one and two percent of their total outlays on medical care. This does not seem very high, but it must be borne in mind that in developing countries the total expenditure for health services from all sources is usually less than three percent, and the Malaysian finding applies only to personal expenditures—that is, exclusive of governmental and all other organized programs. Most of the people in the household survey, moreover, were entitled to free medical services from governmental facilities. As one repeatedly hears in Malaysia, it is the crowded conditions and long waiting time in hospital outpatient departments that lead sick people, even of very low incomes, to spend the money for private medical care. In general, however, persons of lower income probably receive less total medical care of all types (public and private), if Malaysia is like other developing countries where this has been carefully studied (e.g., Colombia or Taiwan).[20]

Thus, we see in Malaysia—as in so many other countries—a sort of vicious circle in the relationships of private medical practice to the governmental program, both urban and rural. Because of higher earnings in private practice, the governmental medical services are understaffed; therefore patients are dissatisfied and seek care privately, contributing further to the disparity in earnings and the shortages of governmental medical manpower. It is the patients who are the ultimate losers, since they are paying twice—once through taxes (direct or indirect) and again through private medical fees. The challenge is to channel the money now already being spent on personal medical care into an organized public service, so that its adequacy can be upgraded.

Within very recent months, it has been claimed that private practice in Malaysia has become "saturated," that the market of private patients has been exhausted. For the first time, it is said by the medical officer of health of the municipal health department of Kuala Lumpur, there is a waiting list of doctors for public employment in the capital city. It is by no means certain, however, that this applies to medical posts in the RHSS.

The private sector of dental care bears quite a different relationship to governmental programs, but this will be discussed below.

Hospital Services

For the care of serious illness, hospitals are a necessary component of a program of rural health service, so that their current status must be examined. As we noted in the historical review, hospital care developed long before the public health services, but insofar as some critically sick rural people have been able to get to the cities for treatment, urban hospitals have always played some part in rural health service. The adequacy of hospitals, therefore, especially in the smaller towns, has a distinct bearing on the current operations of the RHSS.

Fortunately for planning purposes, the vast majority of hospital beds in Malaysia are under governmental sponsorship and control. The hospitals, built often by state governments since the 1880s in state capitals and district headquarter towns, are now all under the jurisdiction of the Division of Hospitals in the federal Ministry of Health. In addition there are a relatively large number of small hospitals operated by estates and mines, as required by the Labour Laws, and others under purely private auspices (either charitable or proprietary), but their aggregate bed supply is relatively small. Based on an estimated population in West Malaysia of 8,500,000, the aggregate ratio of hospital beds in late 1967 was 3.9 per 1,000 population—a supply much higher, for example, than in India. This figure includes, however, a relatively large proportion of beds (about forty percent of the governmental bed supply) for mental disease and leprosy, and still other beds in nearly every general hospital must be reserved for long-term cases of tuberculosis. The ratio of beds available for general, short-term illness, therefore, is approximately 2.0 per 1,000. The distribution of these beds, by sponsorship, is shown in table V.1.[21]

From the viewpoint of the RHSS, the most important hospitals are those under government, classified as "general hospitals" and "district hospitals." There are nine general hospitals, in each of the state capitals except two, and forty-five district hospitals (two of which serve the state capitals in Perlis and Pahang). Also serving rural populations, however, are the smaller and less well-developed estate hospi-

Table V.1
Distribution of hospital beds in Malaysia: 1967, by sponsorship

	Hospitals	Beds	Percentage (beds)
Governmental	66	27,579	83
Estate and mines	88	3,943	12
Other nongovernment	73	1,733	5
Total	227	33,255	100

tals, most of which serve groups of small rubber estates and, therefore, being known as "group hospitals." A special Aborigine Hospital of about 450 beds is also operated separately by the Ministry of Land and Mines to serve some 45,000 scattered isolated rural aborigines (the data on which are not included in the Ministry of Health tabulations).

Impressive progress has been made in recent years in the physical facilities and staffing of the government hospitals, especially in the state capitals. These are very important as places for theoretical referral of patients from the rural health units requiring specialist attention, particularly for major surgery. The standards for staffing and operation of all these hospitals are laid down by the central Ministry. Among these is a standard that one doctor should be on the staff (fulltime) for each fifty beds, plus one doctor for each seventy-five outpatients seen per day, on the average. (Thus a 100 bed hospital, having 150 outpatients per day should have a complement of four doctors.) According to the Ministry official responsible for hospitals, this standard has been achieved now to a level of about sixty percent. Field observation suggests that the shortcomings are most serious in the district hospitals.

From a general scanning of the map, it would appear that the geographic coverage of the fifty-four general and district hospitals in West Malaysia is quite good, in relation to the distribution of both urban and rural population. Over the last fifteen years (coincident with operation of the RHSS but not solely due to it) utilization of the hospitals has steadily increased. This pressure has been met entirely by expansion of the bed capacity, including the setting up of temporary beds, in existing facilities (usually building of new pavilions), rather than by establishment of totally new hospitals. In fact, there were sixty general and district hospitals in 1956—six more than there are today.[22] The catchment areas of the government hospitals are roughly, but not exactly, coterminous with the approximately forty-seven health districts, supervised by medical officers of health, but the latter officers have no official connec-

tion with the hospitals. Both hospital director (medical officer-in-charge or medical superintendent) and medical officer of health are responsible directly to the office of the state chief medical and health officer.

Hospital care, it should be noted, is available to the rural and urban population almost free. In the district hospitals, most relevant to the RHSS, ninety percent of the beds are in third class open wards, for which there are no charges. (The other ten percent of beds are divided between second and first class for which there are small charges, but these beds are seldom accessible to rural people.) Of the total ministry budget for hospital operation, less than ten percent is recovered in collection from patients, this coming mainly from first and second class cases. The use of hospitals by rural people is not impeded, therefore, by financial barriers, but rather by handicaps of transportation and attitude.

The question of geographic congruence of the rural health units with the district hospital catchment areas is complex. The planning of the units was evidently not done in any deliberate relationships to the hospitals, but the distribution of the hospitals is such that there is one within reasonable travelling distance (by automobile) from virtually every main health center and subhealth center. This has an important bearing on certain recommendations to be offered below.

In this evaluative study, visits were made to four general hospitals and five district hospitals. It would be tedious to read all the observations in each hospital but certain general findings relevant to the RHSS should be recorded.

In the general hospitals, there is a certain uniformity of staffing, by reason of national standards, but variations inevitably develop as vacancies occur, not promptly refilled. Differences in the availability of medical and surgical specialists are especially striking, and every hospital visited revealed gaps in one field or another. The overall complement of personnel (including professional, auxiliary, attendants, and all) comes to about 1.0 employee per bed (in contrast, for example to about 2.0 per bed in the larger hospitals of the United Kingdom and about 3.0 per bed in the United States). The commonest problem identified by the medical superintendent was the need for additional staff in nearly all categories, but especially nursing. More variation characterizes the physical plant of the general hospitals, which depends markedly on the time of construction. The older structures follow the nineteenth century European pavilion design, with numerous separate single story buildings, while the newer ones are more unified multistoried buildings. These more compact structures tend to be more efficient for both staff and patients.

The typical ward is large, containing about twenty-four to thirty beds. Occupancy levels are generally high, at eighty or ninety percent, with numerous wards containing extra beds in the middle corridor. There are the usual subdivisions by sex and medical, surgical, maternity, and sometimes other departments—always with a separate ward for tuberculosis. The operating theaters seem impressively new and well maintained, and some hospitals have developed "intensive care units" with ample staffs. On the other hand, x-ray and laboratory facilities seem usually to be quite modest, especially the latter. Trained laboratory technicians are obviously very scarce, and much of the work is done by hospital assistants, who have learned to do the simpler procedures on-the-job.

The number of admissions in all general hospitals has been steadily increasing over recent years. This has been accommodated by addition of new pavilions as well as temporary beds and by some shortening of the average length of stay. Exact data on average stay are not available in the hospitals, but national compilations for 1965 showed it to average around ten days in most of the general hospitals. There are long delays if a pathological specimen has to be sent to the Institute for Medical Research at Kuala Lumpur for analysis. The most painstaking utilization statistics seem to be kept according to racial groups, with daily admissions and patient census classified by Malays, Chinese, Indians, and others.

Quite relevant to the rural health situation is the fact that among the three main categories, the greatest proportion of inpatients tend to be Chinese and the smallest proportion Malays. At the general hospital of one state, for example, the patient census on July 29, 1968 was: Chinese, 293; Indians, 168; Malays, 108; and others, 4. Yet in this state, as in nearly all the other states of West Malaysia, the greatest share of the general population consists of Malays, followed by Chinese and Indians in that

order. An examination of national hospital admission data for 1965, for all government hospitals, shows there were 185,000 Chinese patients, followed by 127,000 Malays, 105,000 Indians, and 6,000 others.[23] Since the vast majority of the rural population is Malay, while persons of Chinese and Indian background are concentrated in urban areas, there is no doubt that these figures reflect much lower hospital utilization by the rural population.

As for diagnosis in the general hospitals, a few observations may be made. Maternity cases are admitted only if the patient is primiparous or is gravid VII or higher or if there are complications. Many patients are said to be anemic. The surgical wards have a high proportion of trauma cases, often from road accidents. On the medical wards there seem to be many cases of unexplained fever and of respiratory tract disease. On the pediatric wards, respiratory disease and gastroenteritis seem to predominate. A few cases of malaria are seen, mostly in young males, but they only stay two or three days. On the medical wards one sees a surprising number of senile men, with low-grade chronic illness, often kept for long periods because they have no home to which to go. Tuberculosis patients are also predominantly in the older age groups. Infectious cases, like typhoid fever or meningitis, are sometimes kept in open wards, isolated only by screens.

As for specific use of the general hospitals by rural people, no hospital official could give data on places of patient origin, but the general impression was that they are predominantly urban. Referrals from district hospitals are mainly surgical cases, but the vast majority of patients enter through the outpatient department, to which they have come on their own. Very few cases could be identified as having been referred from any of the rural health units. Likewise, very few patients were known to be referred from private doctors. In one general hospital, the obstetrical specialist made weekly visits to an antenatal clinic at a main health center, but this was exceptional. In another, visits of surgeons to district hospitals had formerly been made, but not in the last two years. Ambulance service is offered by all general hospitals at all times, and this is extremely important for rural people.

The outpatient departments, to which rural patients would initially come, are typically crowded. Because of the pressures, there are usually long waiting periods and each patient sees the doctor for only a few minutes. If the doctor is not available or is called away, a hospital assistant sees the patient and prescribes medication. The doctors are so busy that it is seldom possible to send reports back to an outside doctor (private or governmental) when referrals have been made—a point on which one hears complaints from RHSS doctors.

In training programs for various types of personnel, the general hospitals do very important work. For staffing of the RHSS especially, their basic training of professional nurses, assistant nurses, midwives, and hospital assistants is invaluable. Except for professional nurses, however, this training has been rather lacking in preventive or public health principles.

Preventive medicine generally was not in evidence within the four general hospitals visited. One exception was the routine practice of giving BCG vaccination to newborns. Children, however, were not being checked for immunization status and, on asking about this, one is told that "that is the responsibility of the public health staff." Case-finding laboratory tests for anemia, intestinal parasites, diabetes, tuberculosis, cervical cancer, syphilis, or other hidden diseases on which screening procedures are possible, were not being routinely or systematically conducted. Health education (which can be especially effective at times of sickness) seems to be totally lacking.

The district hospitals are, on the whole, much more modestly staffed and equipped than the general hospitals. Their medical staffs consist typically of two or three general practitioners, one of whom is medical officer-in-charge. Their overall staffing ratios are about 0.75 personnel per bed, and vacancies are frequent. Nevertheless, there has been a marked improvement in the resources of these hospitals in recent years and their utilization by rural and urban people has steadily increased.

Visits were made to five district hospitals in three states, with special attention being given to their articulation with the RHSS. The capacities of four were between 100 and 150 beds, but one was 300 beds. Their mixture of patients is somewhat similar to those in the general hospitals, with the exception of few surgical cases (although the 300 bed facility had a substantial surgical ward, with several complicated cases). Perhaps relatively more of the patients were long-stay cases—either aged chronic cases, tuberculosis, or convalescent fracture patients sent back from a general hospital. One might expect the average length of stay in district hospitals to be shorter than in general hospitals, reflecting less grave diagnoses, but this is by no means uniformly found. The explanation is probably the relatively high proportion of beds for tuberculosis and chronic patients.

Among the staff of the district hospitals, the hospital assistant plays an especially important part. Since these hospitals often lack laboratory technicians, radiographers, pharmacists, administrative personnel, dieticians, and other trained personnel, hospital assistants may be assigned to any of these roles. They are usually middle-aged men with a long and varied experience, and doubtless they make a positive contribution in the absence of specially trained staff. Still, their assumption of the doctor's role in the outpatient department—a common practice in district hospitals—is surely questionable.

As in general hospitals, the most frequent complaint of the medical officer-in-charge was the need for more staff in all professional categories. It is difficult to understand how a hospital with 125 inpatients or thereabouts, *plus* over 100 outpatients per day can be adequately served by two young doctors—the typical situation. The nurses and assistant nurses must obviously work very hard to carry the load expected. Another complaint is on the slowness of procurement of supplies, which are issued from central stores in each state.

The comments offered above on general hospitals with regard to outside relationships apply with extra force to the district hospitals. If patients are referred from a rural health unit, reports are seldom sent back (the hospital doctor is too busy for this). If a patient is referred from a rural health unit to the district hospital, he may be seen only by a hospital assistant, since the outpatient department is usually covered fifty percent (or sometimes 100 percent) by this type of health worker. Hospital doctors, furthermore, are far too busy to make any peripheral visits to the RHSS health centers. The "travelling dispensaries" which in former years emanated from many district hospitals have now been transferred to the jurisdiction of the district medical officer of health. This officer, it will be recalled, has no responsibility for district hospitals.

Several district MOHs remarked to the writer that they were seldom even notified of cases of communicable disease, including cholera or typhoid fever, admitted to the hospital. Since laboratory facilities and staffing are generally weak, the district hospital is seldom expected to do any diagnostic examinations for the RHSS. As for a preventive orientation, it is quite lacking in the district hospitals, and we could hardly expect otherwise with the pressures on the staff. Aside from the lost opportunities in communicable disease control, the lack of any efforts at health education among either inpatients or outpatients is noticeable. The weak laboratory facilities rule out the possibility of any systematic case-finding procedures. One district hospital doctor encountered made occasional visits to an antenatal clinic a few miles away, but such clinics are not held at the hospital itself.

The difficulties in the district hospitals may be partly attributed to their pattern of administration. In the general hospitals, there is a full-time medical superintendent, often assisted by a trained hospital administrator, but in the district hospitals the medical officer-in-charge is expected to carry a heavy load of clinical responsibility while, at the same time, serving as the hospital's top executive. These men estimated that their administrative work required on the average about two hours (ranging from one to three hours) per day, their assistance coming from clerks rather than trained hospital administrators. This work involves personnel management, authorization of supply procurement, public relations, responses to complaints of patients, financial matters, and the preparation of a variety of returns and reports to higher authorities. When questioned about these administrative responsibilities, the medical officers-in-charge invariably replied that they looked upon these duties as a chore, from which they would like to be relieved.

In spite of their problems, the quality of care in the district hospitals has undoubtedly improved over recent years (several with two doctors now had only one a few years ago), and their utilization by the population has steadily risen. While the proportion of Malay admissions still tends to be lower than that of Chinese, it is apparently rising. In one district hospital the Malay maternity admissions (presumably from the *kampongs*) rose between 1965 and 1967 from 194 to 221, while the Indian admissions declined from 237 to 154 (allegedly due to family planning practices). The rising trend in outpatient utilization is especially striking, and it is a sign of progress that patients are increasingly asking to see the doctor, rather than a hospital assistant. Yet, when one inquires about the source of patients, the response is usually in terms of "the towns, the estates, private doctors, and FLDA schemes or new villages" with little mention made of the *kampongs*. Perhaps the *kampong* patients are not readily identifiable, and this is a question—important for evaluation of the RHSS—that probably warrants research.

Among the five district hospitals visited, one stood out for its exceptional sanitary maintenance, its active tone and cheerful atmosphere. Its staff complement was evidently not greater than in other district facilities, but there was some evidence of greater local pride in its operation. The local visiting committee (theoretically visiting committees are attached to *all* government hospitals) is evidently quite active and the top personnel—medical officer-in-charge and matron—were residents of the local area and had a long period of tenure. Perhaps this

observation holds some lessons for hospital policy in general.

Other types of hospital in Malaysia may be mentioned briefly. Distinctly relevant to the RHSS are the estate or mine hospitals (group or single) serving mainly rubber or tin workers and their families. Their average size is small, at forty-five beds, and their occupancy rates have been low. Their staffs are meager, with one doctor sometimes covering two or three hospitals, the main responsibilities being borne by hospital assistants. Often private doctors in the main cities are engaged part-time by the estate groups to do this work. Rarely do these hospitals offer surgical facilities, and surgical cases are usually referred to a government hospital. Yet, for the population they are intended to serve (about 320,000 in West Malaysia) their relative bed supply is remarkably high at twelve beds per 1,000. Their occupancy rates are, however, very low and their staffs very sparse. Their trend has been toward declining importance, especially with the growing "fragmentation" of the rubber estates into multiple small holdings.

One group estate hospital visited was exceptionally large with 115 beds (occupancy only forty percent) to serve about 16,000 persons distributed among 320 small estates. This hospital was staffed by only one part-time doctor, one professional nurse, one midwife, and nine hospital assistants (mainly untrained). The state government subsidizes the operating costs, but each estate must pay a small amount for each day of care (ninety cents in 1968) to one of its workers. Even this cost is said to inhibit admissions. The patients in this particular hospital were overwhelmingly Indians. The commonest diagnoses were respiratory tract disease, malaria, malnutrition, and maternity. Peripheral to the hospital on the larger estates were ten hospital assistant stations, as required by the Labour Law.

As rubber prices have declined and as the government hospitals have improved, the estate hospitals have lesser importance and it has been commonly suggested that they be absorbed into the governmental system. At the moment, they meet a partial need for a section of the rural population. Their relationships to the district MOH and the RHSS, however, are virtually nil.

Another type of hospital, under purely private or charitable sponsorship, is found in the main cities, and has very little significance for the rural population. These seventy-three facilities average only twenty-four beds each and the great majority are limited to maternity cases. Most important among them are several "Chinese maternity hospitals" established by wealthy benefactors and other donors for the confinement of Chinese mothers whose urban housing is typically extremely cramped. One of these maternity hospitals was visited, and its maintenance showed obvious diligence by the small but highly devoted staff.[24] In its twenty-five beds, 1,480 maternity cases had been accommodated in the last year, or about four deliveries per day. Most of the costs are met by patient fees ($3.50 per day), but about twenty percent are met by grants from the state and federal governments. Only normal maternity cases are accepted (complicated ones being sent to government hospitals), so that the mortality record is very low. Perhaps the chief meaning of these private hospitals for the RHSS is that they take a small amount of pressure off the government hospitals.

A visit was also made to the Aborigine Hospital, mentioned earlier, where a remarkable compromise is presented between the requirements of modern medical care and the cultural habits of these jungle people. This hospital, and its satellite field stations throughout the entire country, are obviously playing a distinct role in the rural health services of the nation, in spite of complete separation from the RHSS.[25] Starting as a twelve bed unit in 1957, with about twelve first aid stations in the jungle attached to police posts, it has grown steadily to accommodation for 450 persons and to sixty-six manned field posts, plus another sixty-four nonmanned sites (where helicopters may land and provisions may be dropped). Not all the 450 "persons" accommodated in the hospital are "patients," since admissions often consist of whole families, but seventy-five percent of the beds are occupied by sick people. Tuberculosis is highly prevalent, so that every new patient gets a chest x-ray (by daily van transport to the National Tuberculosis Centre in Kuala Lumpur) soon after admission. Most of the food preparation is done by the families themselves (cooking areas are provided near the wards), but medical care is provided by a staff of thirteen professionals (mainly from overseas) plus ninety "medical assistants" manning the field posts. A system of rotation is followed, at three-month intervals, between the field posts and the hospitals, so that each person acquires both types of experience. The three doctors currently on the staff, furthermore, make periodic visits by helicopter (this air transport is provided by the Ministry of Defense) to the field posts. There is also an impressive system of daily radio communication between the hospital at Gombak (near Kuala Lumpur) and the field posts.

The auxiliary health personnel for this program have all been trained by the small professional staff at the hospital in courses of six months' duration. The prior education of the aborigines, of course, is quite

deficient, so that few of them would meet the requirements for health personnel in the regular Ministry of Health service. Many gifts of equipment and supplies have been provided by charitable international agencies (British Commonwealth and American), but the bulk of costs are met by the Ministry of Land and Mines, Department of Aborigine Affairs. Only the medical director is in the budget of the Ministry of Health. Proposals to integrate this entire program with the overall resources of the RHSS have been made, but so far without fruition.

This somewhat detailed discussion of hospitals is offered in order to emphasize the relevance of hospitals to any rural health service administration. The reasons for this emphasis will, it is hoped, become evident below.

The Public Health Administrative Structure

The RHSS is administratively a responsibility of the Ministry of Health, which, as noted earlier, took shape as the central government health authority in 1958. Its scope of responsibilites is very broad and these have been well summarized in a brochure issued in July 1968.[26] The range of functions is reflected in the list of ten divisions in the "Technical Department," which follows:

(1) Hospital Division
(2) Health Division (with six public health subdivisions)
(3) Dental Division (both preventive and curative)
(4) Tuberculosis Division
(5) Medical Research Division (the Institute for Medical Research)
(6) Development Division (new construction)
(7) Training Division
(8) Pharmaceutical Division
(9) Medical Records and Health Statistics Division
(10) Nursing Division (both for hospitals and public health)

The organization chart of the ministry is much more complex than this, but one does not see in it any unit earmarked for the RHSS. The reason is perfectly sound—namely, that the RHSS is part and parcel of the responsibilities of *several* divisions, including those for health (i.e., public health), dental, development, training, and nursing. The principal leadership and responsibility, however, fall to the Health Division, under which are included also functions of control of communicable diseases, environmental sanitation, health education, maternal and child health, malaria, leprosy, and nutrition. Even this division does not contain an earmarked unit on the RHSS, but rather fulfills its responsibilities largely through coordination by the top officer (deputy director of medical services) and by delegation of responsibilities to the state chief medical and health officers. Since the state chief medical and health officer is appointed by the central ministry, uniformity in policy implementation is achieved.

Because of their key role in the administration of the RHSS, visits were made to the chief medical and health officer offices of five of the eleven states of West Malaysia. Since their separate historical backgrounds might be expected to generate different current characteristics, these were chosen to represent former federated states (3), nonfederated states (1), and straits settlements (1).

In general, the state chief medical and health officer offices are busy places, in which the RHSS is obviously a prominent subject of interest. The walls are covered with charts showing the progress of the Scheme, with respect to the geographic location of current and planned facilities, the staffing, and the health activities. The top staff beyond the chief medical and health officers consists of two deputies (one for hospitals and one for public health), two matrons (also for hospitals and for public health), a principal dental officer, and a senior public health inspector. Frequently, however, there seems to be a vacancy in one of the two medical deputies positions. It is of interest that between these two deputies, the senior rank is always assigned to the officer on the curative side, and the same applies to the two matrons. In four of the five states visited, the chief medical and health officer office was located in a general administration building of the state government, but in one it was on the grounds of the general hospital (which would seem to have certain advantages).

Thus, the chief medical and health officer has overall responsibility for both the hospitals (general and district) and the public health programs. The top official of each hospital reports to this office, as does the medical officer of health in charge of each health district. Any coordination must occur at this state level. While the planning of the RHSS is done largely at the state level, the responsibility for each of the rural health units lies with the district medical officers of health. Ordinarily all local public health facilities that may not yet be included within rural health units (such as separate static dispensaries or separate maternal and child health clinics) also come under the district medical officer of health. The definition of boundaries for each of these health districts, composed from all or part of one or more administrative districts, are drawn by the state chief medical and health officer office. Since there are frequent vacancies in these medical officer of health

positions, reassignment of responsibilities must often be made, and sometimes the state chief medical and health officer himself or his deputy for health (senior medical officer of health) must take on the task.

The state chief medical and health officer's office is also responsible for selecting field personnel for various training programs, such as auxiliary health workers to be sent to the rural health training centers at Jitra or Rembau. Central stores for medical supplies for both the hospitals and health centers are maintained at this level. The state chief medical and health officer participates regularly in the planning meetings of the state rural development committee. He collects information periodically from all hospitals and health districts, on the basis of which annual reports are submitted to the Ministry of Health.[27]

There are other official health programs in the states which, it should be noted, are carried out more or less independently of the chief medical and health officer office. These are principally the malaria eradication program (operating now in several northern states) and the tuberculosis program, both of which are directed straight from the central Ministry of Health. There is also the program of the National Family Planning Board, which emanates directly from the national office of the Prime Minister. More will be said about this later.

It is at the health district level that direct administrative responsibility is carried for the operations of the RHSS. While the overall staffing of these important positions changes almost from day to day, there are forty-seven health district offices established as of March 1968 to cover all seventy administrative districts in West Malaysia. As of that date, however, there were fourteen vacancies in these posts, leaving thirty-three medical officers of health to cover the field.[28] Of these thirty-three officers, twenty-one had graduate degrees in public health, but several were foreign doctors in Malaysia on temporary contracts. It is evident, therefore, that much remains to be done to achieve proper coverage of the country with public health executives even in the forty-seven health districts established, let alone the full seventy administrative districts through which other governmental services are administered.

Visits were made to five health district offices in three states. The offices were relatively humble and crowded, and only one of the five was close to a district hospital. Associated with the district medical officer of health are a public health sister and a public health inspector, plus limited clerical staff. A major responsibility of these personnel is to supervise the rural health units within their borders, but in instances where the position of medical and health officer in a unit is vacant, the medical officer of health may also have to play this role. Numerous statutory duties fall upon the medical officer of health, especially for environmental sanitation and control of communicable diseases. Within towns, governed by town councils, the role of the district medical officer of health is theoretically only "advisory," but since those towns have no personnel except environmental sanitarians, activities relevant to maternal and child health and communicable disease control are essentially the obligation of the health district staff.

As observed earlier, most health districts are composed of more than one administrative district. In the state of Kedah, for example, there are ten administrative districts, plus the capital city of Alor Star. These eleven jurisdictions come under the wing of five district medical officers of health (although in early 1968 two of these positions were vacant). The North Kedah health district includes three of the administrative districts plus the capital city, with a combined population of 317,000. In this health district there are two main health centers, four subhealth centers, and twenty-seven midwife clinics under the RHSS. In addition, there are four static dispensaries for general outpatient medical care unattached to rural health units. The overall staff coming under the direction of this office is large, as shown in table V.2.[29]

Table V.2
Staff of North Kedah health district

District health office (including clerks)	9
Medical and health offices (RHSS)	2
Sanitation (P.H. inspectors and overseers)	29
Nursing personnel (all levels)	20
Midwives	42
Female attendants	11
Male attendants	8
Laborers and others	104
Total	235

For another example, the Central Pahang health district in the state of Pahang includes two main health centers, six subhealth centers and forty-two midwife clinics, with a total of 219 persons. This staff includes some antimalaria inspectors, in contrast to the North Kedah staff, where the malaria eradication program maintains a completely separate staff.

The work of the district medical officer of health varies to some extent among the states but, in a word, it includes responsibility for general public health

activities outside of hospitals and exclusive of two disease campaigns which are centrally controlled: tuberculosis control and malaria eradication. The general public health activities, however, include both preventive and curative personal health services as well as environmental sanitation. His specific role is both administrative or supervisory and clinical. Thus, in the North Kedah health district, the medical officer of health follows a monthly schedule of activities in which each of twenty-four days has an assigned task. The breakdown of these activities, shown in table V.3, provides an interesting analysis of his time allocations.

Table V.3
Monthly activities of district medical officer of health, North Kedah health district, by days

	Days
Environmental sanitation	5
Rural projects	2
Town duties	3
Administrative work	9
Town council meetings	2
Rural development meetings	2
Office work	4
Staff meeting	1
Clinical functions	9
Antenatal clinics	3
Well-baby clinics	2
School health services	2
Outpatient clinics	2

Thus nine out of the twenty-four days or thirty-seven percent of the time, the medical officer of health is engaged in purely clinical functions. Some medical officers of health evidently do less clinical work than this, and others more, depending on the availability of medical and health officers in the rural health units to carry this load, which is intended to be mainly theirs. The medical officer of health and his staff may also give some assistance in other fields for which they do not have statutory responsibility, such as tuberculosis case follow-up, family planning activity, or general health education.

The immediate responsibility of subhealth center staffs, it will be recalled, is to the medical and health officer and his colleagues in the main health centers. There are in nearly all states, however, some subhealth centers established without a parent main health center, so that these centers come under the direct supervision of the district medical officer of health.

Another level in the public health administrative structure of Malaysia is the local health authority in urban places. The municipalities of Kuala Lumpur, Georgetown (Penang), Ipoh, and Malacca engage their own medical officers of health and associated public health staff.[30] In all other urban places, however, the town councils or town boards engage personnel only in the field of environmental sanitation, looking to the state or district public health officials for advice or supervision on technical matters. Visits were made to the local public health offices in one municpality and one town, where it was evident that the predominant activities concerned maintenance of a sanitary environment. The operation of hospitals and static dispensaries in the cities remains a state and federal responsibility, although the largest municipal health departments do operate their own maternal and child health clinics. The main relevance of these activities to the rural health services is the tendency of "squatter areas" to develop in the fringes of towns as rural people come in search of work. These areas of very poor housing are often just outside the town boundaries, and they present serious hazards of communicable disease with which the district health office must cope.

Finally in the structure of public health administration are the various components of the RHSS itself.[31] Before proceeding to this discussion, however, brief attention must be given to certain other special programs coming under the Ministry of Health, not already discussed, and to other organized health programs outside the framework of this ministry.

Special Health Programs in the Ministry of Health

Because of the historical developments reviewed earlier, certain organized health activities have a distinct impact on the rural health services, although they are not specifically under the administration of the RHSS. The process of integration is usually a slow one, and all of these services are partially or even predominantly included within the RHSS, but here we will mention those activities which are currently separate.

Static dispensaries, it will be recalled, started as satellites of the hospitals and only about ten years ago most of them were placed under the supervision of the district health offices. In many instances, they have become the sites of health centers in the RHSS, but in March 1967 there were still eighty of these that operated separately. Three of these were visited, two being in very small towns that must be considered rural.

The urban static dispensaries are busy places, which have obviously been serving the ambulatory

sick for many years. One in Alor Star is in the center of the town, but it sees many patients who come in from the surrounding rural area. It is staffed by two hospital assistants but there is no physician. Difficult cases are referred to the general hospital outpatient department about a mile away, but this is done only rarely. In the month of June 1968, there were 2,875 new cases seen, of whom 2,040 were Malays. The ten commonest diagnoses made by the hospital assistants were:

Coryza	561
Diseases of larynx, trachea, and bronchitis	482
Intestinal worms	386
Boils, carbuncles, and other skin sepsis	312
Pyrexia of unknown origin	261
Ringworms and other skin diseases	137
"Clinical" malaria	121
Anemia	96
Scabies	91
Dyspepsia	84

In another city, Seremban, the static dispensary was unusual in being still attached administratively to the general hospital, although located about a mile away from it. This was actually a polyclinic, staffed by four full-time doctors, with a laboratory, x-ray equipment, and a pharmacy. Even an ophthalmologist and a psychiatrist had periodic sessions.

At Nenasi, a very small town in the state of Pahang, the static dispensary serves an estimated 5,000 rural population. It is staffed by a hospital assistant and an attendant. The building is small, but very well maintained with good water and toilet facilities. In June 1968, there were 357 new cases seen (plus 197 repeat visits), among which the commonest diagnoses were skin disorders (69), bronchitis (34), influenza and coryza (27), gastroenteritis (13), and other stomach disorders (12). In addition, the hospital assistant made monthly visits to ten other sites ("travelling dispensaries"), seeing 272 other patients in June. It is obvious that this type of clinic is meeting a medical care need for rural people. Eventually, it is expected to integrate it into the RHSS, with expansion to a subhealth center.

Maternal and child health clinics have likewise been largely incorporated into the RHSS, but some are still operating as separate entities. In 1967 there were forty-one of these and, while some are in state capital cities, most are in very small towns, undoubtedly serving nearby rural people.[32] They all come under the district medical officer of health, though not within the rural health units. In one of these visited, the attendance in May 1968 had been 582 antenatal women and 1,243 infants and children—obviously a busy place. The staff consisted of two staff nurses, three assistant nurses, and two midwives.

Dental clinics for children are part of the standard plan of the RHSS main health centers but many dental clinics still operate separately from these centers, as well as outside hospitals. Most of these clinics are located in urban schools, but there are forty-nine located elsewhere in the towns to which children from some rural schools are transported for dental care. These are staffed both by dental officers and dental nurses. The latter are young women trained and authorized to do not only cleansings but also restorative dentistry (i.e., fillings) and extractions on children up to twelve years of age. Two of these separate dental clinics were visited and the dental nurses appeared to be working very efficiently. It was estimated that each would complete treatment (usually several visits per case) on 700 to 1,000 children per year. The chief dental officer in one state estimated that the overall dental service reached about twenty to thirty percent of all school-age children, this figure being higher in the towns and lower in the rural areas. Of special interest is a "floating dental clinic" on a boat which travels up the Pahang River twice a week, treating about thirty persons per day.

Tuberculosis control is a special program in the Ministry of Health which obviously affects rural people but is carried out quite separately from the RHSS. Emanating from the central ministry as a separate division, this program fans out to all parts of the country with an impressive balance of case finding, immunizing, and treatment activities. The National Tuberculosis Centre, as it is called, operates directly a fleet of fourteen mobile units (large vans) for miniature chest x-rays; these stop periodically at general and district hospitals and occasionally at main health centers for filming anyone who comes. Routine chest x-rays, however, are not done as a permanent routine on all hospital admissions in any of the hospitals visited.

For prevention, BCG vaccine is supplied by the National Tuberculosis Centre to all hospitals throughout the country, where it is administered to newborns. It is also provided to the rural health units for administration to infants as well as entering schoolchildren (who have been previously missed). There are two hospitals exclusively for tuberculosis and other chest diseases in the national capital, but virtually every general and district hospital in the country has special wards for tuberculosis, adding up to nearly 4,000 beds (including a 219 bed nongovernmental institution, the Lady Templer Hospital) in 1968. The hospitalized cases, based on observations in the wards of several hospitals, are predominantly aged or middle-aged patients (mostly male) with far advanced disease that cannot be treated at home. The majority of patients, however, are treated at home through a regime of drugs (streptomycin, isoniazid, and P.A.S.) which are dispensed mainly through a network of special tuberculosis clinics.

The tuberculosis clinics are located at the established hospitals and also at static dispensaries throughout the country, but they are administered entirely by the National Tuberculosis Centre (that is, they are not delegated to the control of the state or district public health officials). None of these clinics currently is within the rural health units. Follow-up of positive cases detected through the chest x-ray surveys and other methods is done by these clinics, as well as epidemiological tracing of contacts. A commonly discussed problem, however, is the failure to reach positive x-ray cases which is variously estimated at twenty to forty percent; another problem is the dropout of cases under home therapy (intended for about two years) before complete cure. These problems are especially serious in the rural population who are more distant from the established tuberculosis clinics.

The provision of a monthly supply of antituberculosis drugs to selected rural patients has been delegated to a few of the rural health units (main centers or subhealth centers), but this is not routinely done. As expressed at one of the special tuberculosis clinics in a general hospital, the preference is to have the patient return to that clinic for his drugs, so that he can be seen by the specialized staff. Evidently, it is only certain "defaulters" from the rural areas who are reluctantly referred for follow-up or continuing therapy by the staff of the RHSS.

The record of achievement of the tuberculosis control program is impressive. From a death rate of sixty-five per 100,000 in 1949, it declined to seventeen per 100,000 in 1959, and to about fourteen per 100,000 in 1966.[33] It may well be that this progress has been due in part to the strong, centralized direction of the program. There are doubtless organizational advantages in this approach as a strategy for launching a *new* service. Still, problems have emerged with respect to case follow-up, especially in rural areas. A WHO consultant has also suggested greater emphasis on sputum examination to identify infectious cases, as against reliance on the chest films. Training on tuberculosis problems is currently not included in the courses for rural health personnel at Jitra and Rembau, but is confined to special courses for its own staff conducted by the National Tuberculosis Centre. Some limited integration with the RHSS has been developing in recent years, but perhaps more could be promoted for the mutual benefit of the RHSS and the tuberculosis control program.

Malaria is another important disease, now predominantly in rural areas, for which action in Malaysia is being taken largely through a centralized strategy. A distinction must be made between "malaria control" efforts, which are largely decentralized to the cities and towns, and the "malaria eradication program," which is the major current emphasis in rural areas and is heavily centralized in its administration.

The older "malaria control" efforts have long consisted of larvacidal work in and around the urban centers, carried out under the direction of the health districts or the local authorities. The clearing and maintenance of open drains along the streets of all the towns and cities are designed to prevent mosquito breeding. In all the outpatient clinics of the country—in hospitals, health centers of the RHSS, and static or travelling dispensaries—suspected malaria cases are, of course, treated with chloroquine, which eliminates foci of spread as well as helping the individual. In certain *kampongs*, moreover, where many malaria cases have been identified, chemoprophylactic drugs are sometimes given to all residents by the district medical officer of health to halt the spread of the disease.

In 1967, however, the national government of Malaysia, with the advice of WHO, decided to embark on an extensive malaria eradication program (MEP). This was based on estimates, from blood film surveys, of an endemic rate in rural areas of about five percent nationally, with higher rates in the northern and hillier regions and lower rates in the southern and coastal regions.[34] With the clearing of jungle to open up new areas for land development, the rural incidence of the disease had recently been increasing. Preparatory work for the MEP actually started in 1966, and through its four phases— preparatory phase, attack phase, consolidation phase, and maintenance phase—it is scheduled to operate for ten more years, until 1978. The work will proceed in geographic stages from the northern to the southern states. In each area, teams of trained personnel will systematically attempt to do internal residual DDT spraying of all houses in all the *kampongs* and rural areas.

The complex problems of malaria eradication need not be discussed here, but the relationship of the program to the RHSS is important. In each state where the MEP sets up its operations, they are carried out more or less independently of the basic state public health administrative structure. While liaison is, of course, maintained with the state chief medical and health officer, the direction of the program both technically and administratively stays with the national division in the ministry. At the district medical officer of health and the RHSS levels, there are no responsibilities delegated from the MEP. It is expected only that after the consolidation phase has been completed, the local public health staff will continue with the maintenance phase by detecting any new malaria cases occurring and subjecting them to prompt chemotherapy.

In one respect the MEP has had a direct impact on the RHSS which has generated many critical comments from the personnel of the Scheme. The MEP is expensive—estimated at about M$10,000,000 per year over the next eight years—and, in order to economize, a large share of the environmental health personnel required are being withdrawn for special training and assignment to the MEP in each state during the attack and consolidation phases. (In Kedah, where the MEP is now in its attack phase the medical and health officer of one important rural health unit complained that three of the four public health overseers on the staff had been withdrawn recently.) Eventually these personnel will return to their former posts, with increased knowledge, but in the meantime the regular environmental sanitation work in the *kampongs* (latrine construction, improved water supplies, etc.) is suffering a setback. It is also no secret that several distinguished malariologists question the wisdom, in terms of cost-benefit analysis, of the whole MEP concept. Two leading authorities in Malaysia expressed this view to the writer, explaining that the great cost of eliminating the last few cases in an area might not be worth the investment—especially compared with the relatively large achievements possible from a much less costly "control" program based on selective spraying, larvacidal work, and chemotherapy in sites of known high endemicity. They also point out the recent sharp rise of malaria in Ceylon some years after an allegedly successful eradication program.

The whole problem of malaria illustrates the consequences of a public health administrative structure which is relatively weak at the local level. (The same applies perhaps to tuberculosis.) In the absence of a firm local structure, the tendency is to launch national campaigns in a highly centralized manner with personnel stationed locally, of course, but responsible "vertically" to a national office. In the short run, this may well achieve results more rapidly, but it does nothing to build up the local organizational competence and is probably more expensive. If campaigns against specific diseases can be delegated to local public health organizations—like the district health offices and RHSS in Malaysia—with technical advice from a central office, then a more balanced local health program can develop. Emphasis can be focussed on the problems which are greatest in each local area, rather than with a broadside stroke. In the long run, the local public health organization is built up, so that it can be effectively applied to new problems as they arise.

In contrast to malaria eradication strategy, one may take note of activities in Malaysia on filariasis control. While this is also a mosquito-borne disease, attacked both by antivector work and by chemotherapy, the approach has been a highly focussed one, even for rural areas. In Penang Island, for example, where the disease has high prevalence in certain *kampongs*, the direction of the control program has been delegated, with advice from national experts, to the state chief medical and health officer.[35]

Other Governmental and Voluntary Health Programs

While the overwhelming bulk of governmental responsibilities for both preventive and curative health services rest with the Ministry of Health, certain functions come under other ministries in Malaysia. There are also certain nongovernmental or voluntary health agencies. Insofar as these activities affect the operations of the RHSS, a few words must be said about them.

Occupational health services are partially a responsibility of the Ministry of Labour, although the Ministry of Health is also involved. Inspection of rubber estates and mines in rural areas, to assure compliance with regulations on housing, sanitation, and medical services, is a responsibility of the Ministry of Labour. This ministry also supervises a Workmen's Compensation Ordinance, under which injured workers may receive financial awards from their employers (but without provision for medical care). In 1966, the greatest share of "industrial accidents" reported under this law were in agricultural occupations and mining (9,000 out of a total for all occupations of 15,000), so that the rural population is obviously affected. The district medical officer of health, on the other hand, is expected to look after the health conditions on estates and mines, and may make recommendations to the labor authorities for correction of defects. In November 1967, for example, a medical officer of health recommended (and the Labour Inspectorate required) that action be taken at a tin mine to halt the breeding of mosquitoes for prevention of malaria.[36]

Quite recently, Malaysia has undertaken steps toward development of a social security program which would eventually provide medical care to selected groups of workers and their families. Planning has been done by the Ministry of Labour, with international technical advice. While the proposed program will start only in the four largest cities for workers in establishments of five or more, it is to be extended eventually to rural estates and mines. Medical care would be financed both through fees to private doctors and payment to government hospitals. From the viewpoint of rural health services, this program may have the effect of partially lightening the financial burden on the Ministry of Health for services to some of the urban population, thereby permitting more resources to be devoted to the rural population.

Family planning is another function with obvious implications for rural health but carried out under the wing of other agencies. The program started in 1953 under the aegis of voluntary agencies in the states which have now formed the Malaysian Federation of Family Planning Associations. There is no religious objection to contraception in Malaysia, and the program grew rapidly. In 1966 official action was taken by government, with the formation of the National Family Planning Board, responsible directly to the Prime Minister.[37] While the work of the associations is principally in the larger towns and cities, the goal of the governmental board is to reach the rural population as well. Its program has proceeded in four phases: first, to establish clinics in all general hospitals; second, in all district hospitals; third, in the health centers of the RHSS and in the rubber estates; and fourth, in the remainder of the rural areas. A family planning clinic is typically a session that meets once a week, staffed usually by a professional nurse. The commonest method used, by far, is oral steroid pills, although obstetricians in the general hospitals also do insertion of intrauterine devices in selected cases.

At present the National Family Planning Board is in the third phase of its programs, and the impact was quite evident in the various health centers of the RHSS. The maternal and child health staff of the RHSS do not currently engage in family planning, but they refer mothers, on request, to the weekly clinics, held in the same buildings. This has been described as "physical integration," as distinguished from "functional integration."[38] Steps are now starting, however, toward training of RHSS nursing personnel in family planning practices, so that functional integration may perhaps also be expected eventually. In looking to the fourth phase of the work, the board is also starting a program of training for *kampong* midwives, with the intention of paying them fees for every woman who is enabled to become an "acceptor" of the techniques.[39] Since the birth rate in rural areas is higher than in cities and since rural families are likewise of lower income levels, it is likely that this program will have a long-term beneficial effect on the health of the rural population.

Other organized voluntary health programs are not highly developed in Malaysia, but there are a few that complement the activities of government. The Malaysian Association for the Prevention of Tuberculosis assists families with a sick breadwinner through small financial grants. There is an Association of the Blind and an Association of the Deaf, which conduct education programs for children with these handicaps. Emergency services are also provided to some extent by the Red Cross and the St. John's Ambulance Service.

One other government program has an indirect bearing on health services. The national Department of Social Welfare operates a number of small institutions for aged and homeless persons. It will be recalled that many beds in district hospitals are occupied by aged patients not truly in need of active hospital care, so that the capacity of these welfare facilities will indirectly influence the availability of hospital beds for acutely ill patients. The welfare department also gives small cash grants for food to destitute individuals. Finally, note must be taken of the important Ministry of National and Rural Development, mentioned earlier, which is responsible for coordinating all rural development activities, including the RHSS. In the famous "Red Book" used for planning at the local level by the district rural development committees, section VII includes the mapping out of health centers and related facilities.[40]

NOTES

[1] J. W. Field, "The Historical, Racial and Cultural Background of Western Medicine in Malaya." In (various authors) *Institute for Medical Research 1900-1950*. Kuala Lumpur: Government Press, 1951.

[2] E. M. B. Wylde, "Short Outline of Growth of Public Health in Kuala Lumpur and Malaya." *The Medical Journal of Malaya*, Vol. 13, June 1959, pp. 316-321.

[3] Gayl D. Ness, *Bureaucracy and Rural Development in Malaysia*. Los Angeles: University of California Press, 1967, p. 26.

[4] R. E. Anderson, "Half a Century of Medicine in Kelantan." *The Medical Journal of Malaya*, Vol. 5, June 1951, pp. 265-284.

[5] Ness, *Bureaucracy and Rural Development*, p. 99.

[6] Colony of Singapore, *Report of the Committee of Enquiry on Medical Education in Malaya November-*

December 1953. Singapore: Government Printing Office, 1954. p. 12.

[7] L. W. Jayesuria, *A Review of the Rural Health Services in West Malaysia*. Kuala Lumpur: Ministry of Health, 1967.

[8] Federation of Malaya, *Report of the Medical Department for the Year 1958*. Kuala Lumpur: Government Press, 1961.

[9] Ministry of Health, "Rural Health Scheme: Lists of Main Centres, Sub-Centres and Midwives' Quarters cum Clinics Completed Since 1956 to 1967." Processed report, 1968.

[10] J. D. Gimlette and I. H. Burkill, *The Medical Book of Malayan Medicine*. (*The Gardens' Bulletin-Straits Settlements*, Vol. VI, Part 3), October 1930.

[11] Richard Winstedt, *Malaya and Its History*. London: Hutchinson's University Library, undated c. 1950.

[12] Ali Bin Sheikh Alhady, *Malay Customs and Traditions*. Singapore: Eastern Universities Press, 1962.

[13] I. H. Burkill and Mohamed Haniff, *Malay Village Medicine*. (*The Gardens' Bulletin-Straits Settlements*, Vol. VI, Part 2), April 1930.

[14] David Hooper, *On Chinese Medicine: Drugs of Chinese Pharmacies in Malaya*. (*The Gardens' Bulletin-Straits Settlement*, Vol. VI, Part 1), December 1929.

[15] Based on unpublished listing of the Department of Statistics, Distributive Trades Section, 1968.

[16] Alan J. A. Elliot, *Chinese Spirit-Medium Cults in Singapore*. Singapore: Donald Moore Books, 1964.

[17] *Ibid.*

[18] Ministry of Health, "Registered Medical Practitioners in the States of Malaya as on 31 December 1967." Processed document.

[19] Department of Statistics, *Household Budget Survey of the Federation of Malaya 1957-58*. Kuala Lumpur.

[20] Timothy I. Baker and Mark Perlman, *Health Manpower in a Developing Economy: Taiwan, A Case Study in Planning*. Baltimore: Johns Hopkins Press, 1967.

[21] Based upon tabulations of "Governmental Bed Distribution . . . as on 1 January 1968," "Estate and Mine Hospitals . . . 1967," and "Non-Government Hospitals . . . 1967," provided by E. J. Martinez, Senior Medical Records Officer, Ministry of Health.

[22] Ministry of Health, "Statistics on Health Matters, Report No. 1, October 1966." This useful compilation was produced by E. J. Martinez, Senior Medical Records Officer, and provides data on numerous subjects discussed in this chapter.

[23] *Ibid.*, p. 10.

[24] Negri Sembilan Chinese Maternity Association, *32nd Annual Report*. December 1967.

[25] J. M. Bolton, "Medical Services to the Aborigines in West Malaysia." *British Medical Journal*, No. 5608, June 29, 1968, pp. 818-823.

[26] *Organization and Function of the Ministry of Health in Brief*. Kuala Lumpur: processed document, July 25, 1968.

[27] A. S. Sandhu, *Annual Report, Medical and Health Department, Negri Sembilan for the Year 1967*. Processed document, April 1968.

[28] Ministry of Health, "Medical Officers of Health as of 1 March 1968." Processed document.

[29] Health Office, North Kedah, *Annual Report–1967.* Alor Star: processed document, 1968.

[30] See, for example, *Annual Report–Municipal Health Department.* Kuala Lumpur: 1965.

[31] See orginal WHO report for this discussion.

[32] E. J. Martinez, Memorandum on "Maternal and Child Health Clinics." Ministry of Health, September 21, 1967.

[33] Based on figures from two sources: Federation of Malaya, *Report of the Medical Department for the Year 1959.* Kuala Lumpur: 1962; and Department of Statistics, *Vital Statistics–West Malaysia 1966.* Kuala Lumpur: 1968.

[34] Based on numerous processed documents provided by Dr. Rosman Kass, Assistant Director of Medical Services (Malaysia), Ministry of Health.

[35] Chee Chin Seang, "A Short Review of Filariasis Control Work in Penang and Province Wellesley 1933-1967." Penang: processed document, November 1967.

[36] Ministry of Labour (Malaysia), Monthly Report, November 1967, p. 6.

[37] Ariffin Marzuki, "Malaysia: The Family Planning Program, 1967." *Studies in Family Planning* (The Population Council), No. 26, January 1968, pp. 12-15.

[38] Raja Ahmad Noordin, "Integration of Family Planning Services in Health Services." Proceedings of the Family Planning Seminar, Kuala Lumpar, June 1968.

[39] National Family Planning Board, Malaysia, *Annual Report 1967.* Kuala Lumpur: 1968.

[40] Ministry of Rural Development, District Rural Development Plan. Kuala Lumpur: undated c. 1965.

Chapter VI
Health Resources and Planning
in an African Kingdom: Ethiopia

In sub-Sahara or Negro Africa, health services are generally less well developed than in Asia or Latin America. In Ethiopia, one of the few lands not colonized by a European power (except for a brief period under Italian rule), conditions are especially primitive and health resources are especially sparse.

The prominent and overwhelming health need of Ethiopia is to build up its supply of personnel and facilities for modern health service. The U.S. Peace Corps has made a small contribution to that end, along with other bilateral and international health agencies. In 1963 a brief inspection was made in Ethiopia in preparation for a Peace Corps project bringing two teams of medical and allied health personnel to staff two provincial hospital-health centers—at Makelle in Tigre province and Dessei in Wollo province. To give an appreciation of the problems of staffing such combined facilities, the full complement of personnel at one of them is listed. This chapter is drawn from a document prepared for orientation of the Peace Corps volunteers, Peace Corps Health Service Project in Ethiopia *(Los Angeles: University of California, 1963, pp. 1-10), and reprinted here by permission.*

GENERAL SETTING

A few points of Ethiopian geography, political structure, and culture relevant to health services are in order. Since the nation is an Empire with governmental power lodged in the central government, virtually all planning for health services is done at the national level. The intention is to establish provincial public health organizations, under the governor of each of the fourteen provinces, but at present the leadership is all coming essentially from Addis Ababa. From the point of view of long-term planning, this has certain advantages, and it helps to assure a significant role for the Peace Corps projects.

The great poverty and overwhelming rurality of the population mean, of course, that health needs are very great and that any effective action in this field can have a great social and political impact on the country. The enormous social problems also mean that striking health improvements will probably not be seen rapidly, unless the health services go hand-in-hand with basic measures of agricultural, technological, and educational development.

A cultural feature of importance in the health projects is that one of them, at Dessei, is in a province near Addis (Wollo) where the language is Amharic. The other, at Makelle, is in the province of Tigre, where the language is Tigrinya.

DISEASES

Basic information like the death rates, crude or disease-specific, is not available for Ethiopia, but a good deal is known from local studies that have been made. The best information has been published in the *Ethiopian Medical Journal* which began to appear in 1962. The principal problems are, of course, the communicable diseases, most of which are preventable. High causes of mortality and morbidity are: tuberculosis, gastrointestinal infections due to both bacteria and parasites, malaria, typhus fever, syphilis, and leprosy. The hospitals and ambulatory care clinics also receive a heavy load of less exotic afflictions found in temperate zones like accidents, respiratory tract disease, complications of pregnancy, and even diabetes, heart disease, and cancer. There is also much goiter (nontoxic), cirrhosis of the liver, and skin disease. The people are generally very thin, but specific diseases of malnutrition have not been commonly reported. In 1958, a severe epidemic of malaria (falciparum) took a high toll, but it has been under control since then. The exceptionally high rate of typhus fever (louse-borne) may be valid or may represent faulty diagnoses.

GENERAL HEALTH SERVICE RESOURCES

Realistically, the principal resources for meeting health needs of most of Ethiopia's 20,000,000 people are probably the indigenous healers, of which there are three types: (1) *wageshos*, who offer physical measures—including such techniques as cutting out a child's uvula as a treatment for fever; (2) *qualichas*, who engage in magical rites; and (3) *debteras*, who are priests and offer religious help.

Scientific medicine was brought to Ethiopia for the first time about 1920, through religious missions from Europe. During the Italian occupation, 1935-1941, some hospitals were established. Both the religious groups and the Italian authorities trained "dressers" as the main auxiliary health workers, although no Ethiopians were trained in medicine or other fields of major responsibility until very recently. After the Second World War, several Western European nations offered assistance in establishing hospitals and clinics, as well as did India and Soviet Russia. The United States assistance program began about 1952.

In 1947, the Ethiopian Ministry of Health was established. The policy of the ministry is to accept help from many different sources and try to weave it together into a system. Thus, it now regards the health personnel and facilities of the nation as consisting of two principal components: (1) governmental, including resources provided by foreign nations as well as by the Ethiopian government, and (2) religious missions. Most of the mission activities consist of ambulatory care clinics, without hospital beds.

There are about 6,200 hospital beds in Ethiopia now, of which 300 are for military personnel and about 2,000 are for leprosy cases (largely custodial). Of the remaining 3,900 beds, 650 are in mission-operated facilities and 3,250 in governmental hospitals. The overall ratio of 0.3 hospital beds per 1,000

people is one-thirtieth of the U.S. supply (nine beds per 1,000).

About half the hospital beds are in Addis, where only a very small percentage of the population lives. The great majority of hospital beds, moreover, require the patient to pay something for admission. Only one hospital (St. Paul's) in Addis is completely free, and only about ten to twenty-five percent of the beds in all the other hospitals in the nation are without charge. There is, however, at least one hospital located in each of the provincial capitals.

The vast majority of the approximately 200 physicians in the country are located in the national capital. At an overall ratio of one doctor per 100,000 population, Ethiopia has one of the poorest supplies in the world. (U.S. ratio is one doctor per 750 people).

A major resource for medical care throughout Ethiopia, although on a very primitive level, are the "dresser stations"—more recently called "health stations." These are simply one-man units in a small hut, staffed by a dresser, who has typically had about a one-year course of training in a hospital, following six grades of elementary school. There are probably about 150 to 200 of these stations around the country. The dresser is expected to treat common ailments with drugs, which he obtains (a) from the hospital in the provincial capital, or (b) from the central stores of the Ministry of Health in Addis. Some dressers have been authorized to sell "common household remedies," thus constituting private druggists. The great majority of the 1,300 dressers in Ethiopia, however, are engaged in hospitals and clinics as the rank-and-file staff, in the absence of trained nurses. (The formal training of dressers is only recently being standardized—see below.)

The newest type of health resource in Ethiopia is the "health center," of which there are now fifty in all. Thirteen of these are "major" centers in each of the provincial capitals (except Asmara—the most "Europeanized" city in the country) and thirty-seven are peripheral or "minor" centers in more rural districts. These urban and rural centers, for provision of general preventive and curative health service on an ambulatory basis, have been established largely with the aid of the United States, WHO, UNICEF, and other international agencies. They are key elements in the long-term planning of Ethiopian health services, and will be further considered below.

PERSONNEL TRAINING

The critical need of the Ethiopian health services is for an enormous expansion of trained personnel, and several important actions are being taken toward this end:

1. There are nine schools for training dressers, located at hospitals in nine cities around the country. Five of them train "elementary dressers" (one year), two train "advanced dressers" (two years), and two train both types. The principal school (Menelik Hospital, Addis) is establishing curriculum standards for dresser training to be used throughout the country. About 175 dressers are currently enrolled in these schools.

2. There are five schools, also located in hospitals, for training of professional nurses, with a total enrollment of about 200. Two-thirds of the students are women; one-third are men.

3. A school for training pharmacists, laboratory technicians, and x-ray technicians—the Medical Auxiliary Training School (MATS)—is located in Addis (Menelik Hospital).

4. Plans are being made for developing a medical school in Addis. In the meantime, about sixty Ethiopians are being trained in medicine in several countries abroad, the largest number being at the American University in Beirut. Of the current supply of 200 doctors in the country, thirty are Ethiopian and twenty-five of these are located in Addis; none has yet entered the field of public health. (The Ministry of Health officials are trained in health education, chemistry, and related fields.)

5. The most significant training program is at Gondar, where a remarkable Public Health College and Training Center has been established through the joint effort of the World Health Organization, UNICEF, and the United States. This institution, staffed with a large teaching team of foreign physicians, nurses, and others, is turning out personnel to man the health centers. These consist of "community health officers" (three years of study after twelfth grade), "community nurses" (two years of study after eighth grade), and "community sanitarians" (one year of study after sixth to eighth grade). All three have a year of "internship" at a peripheral health center near Gondar. The latter two types of personnel play roles similar to those in other countries, but the health officers have a scope of duties very similar to that of physicians in more developed countries. They are authorized to diagnose and treat disease (including almost everything except major elective surgery), as well as to direct a generalized public health program in the area served by the health center.

LONG-TERM HEALTH SERVICE PLANNING

In the last few years, with technical advice from WHO, the United States, and the West German government, Ethiopia has clarified its long-term plans for health service. It is intended that each province will have a provincial health department, directed by a medical officer of health. There will be a provincial advisory health council, elected from municipal and district jurisdictions in the province, but the provincial medical officer of health (PMOH) will report directly to the national ministry.

This centralized authority is justified partly by the fact that nearly all the funds for operating the program will come from the central government. A major source of these funds is the special health tax on land, imposed by the Emperor in 1960. The overall budget of the Ministry of Health for 1963-1964 is 16,000,000 Ethiopian dollars (about U.S. $6,400,000), of which about 1,000,000 Ethiopian dollars are derived from patient fees and the balance from various taxes.

The provincial medical officer of health is to be responsible for all health activities in his province, including public health campaigns (such as the malaria control program via spraying of houses with DDT), all ambulatory services at health centers and dresser stations, as well as all hospitals. This wide scope of authority is remarkable, compared with the great fragmentation of services in the more industrialized countries. (Certain health service responsibilities are vested in the Ministry of Education for schoolchildren, and also in a special "community development program" for services in selected villages, but I was unable to get clear information on these programs.)

Within each province, the health services are conceived as a network starting from the provincial hospital in the capital city, and branching out to several peripheral hospitals in the other main towns. Parallel with the hospitals would be health centers, to offer ambulatory medical care as well as preventive services (immunizations, health examinations, health education, etc.) and a home base for community nurses and sanitarians. In smaller towns there would be health centers, without hospitals. Peripheral to the hospitals and health centers would be the health stations (dresser stations) to meet day-to-day needs in the villages. The functions of health centers have been outlined in a number of documents issued by the Ministry of Health.

The key positions of PMOH are now all theoretically filled by physicians located in the main provincial hospitals. Actually these men are all clinicians practicing surgery or medicine within the hospital walls, and none of them is really functioning in the broad administrative capacity visualized. All of these doctors are foreign employees of the ministry, most being expatriates but some being "on loan" from the official health agencies of their own country. One of the key tasks lying ahead is eventually to staff these key PMOH positions with Ethiopian doctors trained in public health work.

For the present, the supervision of the network of fifty health centers throughout the country is being provided by a skilled team composed of a Chinese physician, a Finnish nurse, and an Indian sanitary engineer, on loan to the Ministry of Health from the World Health Organization. This team is stationed in Addis but travels a great deal throughout the provinces. The establishment, construction, and equipping of the health centers themselves is one of the major activities of the USAID mission in Ethiopia.

A closely related undertaking of the USAID mission is the "Demonstration and Evaluation" project on the benefits of overall public health and curative medical services. A well-staffed research team is gathering detailed data on the health status and practices of a sample of families in eight communities; then a comprehensive health center program will be introduced in four of these, the other four being left alone. After two or three years, detailed measurements will again be made, comparing the two sets of villages with the hope of determining the exact consequences of the health program. This "field experiment" is being watched with great interest by the World Health Organization.

THE MAKELLE AND DESSEI PROJECTS

Against this background, one can understand better the objectives of the health projects at Makelle and Dessei, in which the Peace Corps is playing the key role. In a word, these two places are intended to serve as "model" demonstrations of the operation of hospital-health center units, such as are to be at the hub of each provincial health program in the long-term planning of Ethiopia.

These two provincial capital cities were carefully chosen for this demonstration purpose. Dessei, capital of Wollo province, is about a one-day drive south of Asmara—Ethiopia's second main city. Both cities have important ties to the family of His Imperial Majesty Haile Selassie I, which helps to assure a stability in their role. Dessei has a population of about 40,000 and Makelle about 24,000—each serving as the cultural and trade center for a provincial population of between 1,000,000 and 2,000,000.

The hospital-health center buildings at these cities were constructed with United States funds and designed by a U.S. architect. They are simple, functional, and admirably suited to a conception of integrated preventive and curative health service. But it is important to understand that they are not United

States operations; the physical structures have been turned over completely to the Ethiopian Ministry of Health.

The obvious gap has been the professional staffing of these physical units, and this is where the Peace Corps comes in. Consultation between the Ministry of Health, the USAID public health consultants, and the Peace Corps Medical Division yielded a roster of eighteen medical, nursing, and related health personnel needed to supplement the currently available staffs in each health unit. The composition of these two health teams has been outlined in a Peace Corps document. Their pattern of work will be discussed below.

The projects are conceived as being province-wide and not simply confined to the capital cities. In Wollo province (Dessei) there are now other facilities as follows: a second hospital in Dessei operated by a religious mission, a leprosarium operated by the Sudan Interior Mission (with 250 beds and 8,000 registered outpatients!) not far from Dessei, three peripheral health centers staffed with Gondar graduates, a small mission clinic, and fourteen dresser stations in villages.

In Tigre province (Makelle), aside from the central facilities, there are three peripheral governmental hospitals (at Aksum—where the Queen of Sheba was supposed to have reigned at the time of King Solomon, at Adua, and at Adigrat). There are four peripheral health centers, staffed with Gondar graduates, two small mission clinics, and about eighteen dresser stations.

Transportation is very difficult throughout both provinces, and some of these units can only be finally reached from the provincial capital by mule or on foot (part of the way being done by car on the few main roads). Nevertheless, the conception of the projects at Dessei and Makelle is to serve as the central directorates for these province-wide services, and to weave them all into an integrated system.

THE PEACE CORPS ROLE

At both Makelle and Dessei there are medical and public health staffs now at work, and the infusion of Peace Corps manpower will obviously add great strength, while presenting a challenge in effecting smooth integration. The usual conception, in international health agencies, of having a national "counterpart" for each foreign professional worker may not be so easy to apply. It will require great flexibility.

The problem of integration to be faced may be better clarified by a listing of the personnel currently on the job at Makelle. While the hospital and health center are physically united and work closely together, their staffs are paid from different budgets, and they are conventionally listed separately.

The hospital staff consists of:

- ADMINISTRATOR—an Ethiopian high school graduate who received one year of training at the American University in Beirut.
- MEDICAL DIRECTOR AND ACTING PMOH—a Polish expatriated physician, mature and agreeable.
- REGISTERED NURSE—a male nurse trained at the hospital school (staffed by Swedish personnel) in Lekempte.
- NONGRADUATE NURSES (3)—young men who started training at the U.S.-operated nursing school in Asmara, but who were dismissed before completion of their studies for disciplinary reasons (they were involved in a student riot). They are evidently working very well in Makelle.
- PHARMACIST-TECHNICIAN—trained for two years at the Medical Auxiliary Training School in Addis.
- LABORATORY TECHNICIAN—trained for two years at the Gondar Public Health College.
- ADVANCED DRESSER—female (though these are usually males).
- ELEMENTARY DRESSERS (3)—males, trained in an Italian occupation hospital.
- STOREKEEPER
- ACCOUNTANT-SECRETARY.
- REGISTRAR—an admissions clerk who collects payments from patients.
- ARCHIVES LIBRARIAN—records-keeper.
- TYPIST—who serves also as interpreter.
- HELPERS (5)—males, who work like elementary dressers, but have had no training.
- CLEANERS (7)—village women.
- CASHIER—works for both hospital and health center, handling money.
- CARPENTER
- MECHANIC
- AMBULANCE DRIVER
- KITCHEN STAFF (4)—one chief and three assistants.
- GARDENERS (2)
- LAUNDRY WORKERS (4)
- GENERATOR ENGINEER
- GUARDS (5)
- PRIEST—on the regular hospital staff.

This aggregates to a staff of fifty hospital personnel to serve about sixty beds. This ratio of 0.83 personnel per bed is relatively good, compared with the usual level of underdeveloped countries—although an American hospital of sixty beds would be staffed by an average of about 120 personnel.

The health center staff, in addition, consists of the following persons:

- HEALTH OFFICERS (2)—Gondar-trained for four years.
- COMMUNITY NURSES (2)—Gondar-trained for three years (one may leave soon).
- COMMUNITY SANITARIANS (3)—Gondar-trained for two years (one is expected to leave).
- REGISTRAR
- ACCOUNTANT
- ELEMENTARY DRESSERS (2)
- HELPER—office boy.
- DRIVER—general truck (not ambulance).
- GUARD
- MULEKEEPER (to be discontinued).

These fifteen health center personnel work in the ambulatory care services as well as out in the surrounding community.

Finally, there are two Peace Corps volunteer physicians, who have been stationed at Makelle for the last year. They work very hard in both the hospital and the health center, with an extremely wide range of duties. When the new Peace Corps health teams arrive, these men may both remain at Makelle or one may move to Dessei or they both may leave for another post; this is not yet decided. They have been doing an excellent job under great difficulties. A surgeon visits periodically from Asmara for elective operations, such as excision of large goiters.

It can be seen from this roster of personnel that there are potential "counterparts" for many but not all of the Peace Corps volunteers scheduled to come to Makelle. The present staff at Dessei is not quite so large, but is of the same general composition. Obviously it will take a few months to work out the relationships of the new volunteers to the current staffs.

There is certainly freedom to make technical arrangements in whatever pattern seems best. In Dessei, for example, the work flow in the health center is handled very differently from the scheme in Makelle. There are differing arrangements for general medical clinic sessions, specialty clinic sessions (e.g., tuberculosis, child health, or leprosy), and for distribution of outpatients as between the physician and health officer. Likewise there are different systems for dispensing drugs to bed-patients, for maintaining records, for operating the food service, and so on. There are plenty of problems and endless room for administrative imagination.

Some of the most vexing problems concern the operation of technical equipment. All the basic diagnostic, sterilizing, refrigeration, plumbing, and related equipment at both Makelle and Dessei is modern, but much of it is not in good operating order. For certain items—like expensive x-ray machines— there are servicing agents in Addis, but for most of the items, great skill and resourcefulness will be necessary to keep things operating and to repair them when they break down. This will be a task for everyone, as well as the electrical repairmen on the Peace Corps team.

Supplies are provided by the central medical stores of the Ministry of Health in Addis. It will be helpful if several members of each Peace Corps health team can become acquainted with the scheme of operation of this agency before leaving Addis for their posts. Ethiopia gets supplies from many different countries, and problems of terminology— especially for drugs—can be confusing.

Modern reference books in all aspects of clinical medicine and public health have been assembled in Makelle by the two Peace Corps doctors there. It is urgently recommended that the same be done for the Dessei unit at the very outset; perhaps it would be wise for each volunteer to bring a few basic books in his own field of work for ready reference.

The tasks for the "community health workers" in the Peace Corps teams will be particularly challenging because this type of community organization for health purposes has not yet been developed as part of the program at Makelle or Dessei. Their work will include assistance in the organization of "community health councils" and carrying out various educational programs through these. They can work on selection and training of "peripheral health workers" out in the villages, for assistance in sanitation, education, and vaccination efforts. Such young village workers have been organized around the health centers near Gondar, but this is yet to be done around Dessei and Makelle.

A critical problem for the success of the whole demonstration program at Makelle and Dessei is the appointment of properly qualified provincial medical officers of health. As noted earlier, these positions are now held by clinical physicians who really confine their work to the hospital, where the demands are great enough. With the current lack of qualified Ethiopians for these major positions, foreign aid must be sought, and it is the expectation that the USAID program will select and assign public health trained physicians from the United States for this purpose.

The basic purpose of the Makelle and Dessei projects is, in summary, to serve as demonstrations of good comprehensive health services in rural Ethiopia. A "demonstration" implies that there will be people from other provinces and from the national capital to observe it.

The Ministry of Health leadership is not yet willing to commit itself on using Makelle and Dessei as "field training centers." Their viewpoint is that the initial task is to develop a smooth and effective operation at these two hospital-health center units. Then, one can later decide if these units should serve as field centers, to which certain health personnel may be sent for brief periods of training or experience, prior to their assignment in one of the other provinces.

If such a training role is to be played eventually by the Makelle or Dessei programs, it will not apply to the graduates of the Gondar College, which has its own "training health centers." It could apply, however, to training for (a) physicians who have been educated in an urban medical school, (b) professional nurses graduated by any of the five Ethiopian schools, or (c) technicians graduated from the Medical Auxiliary Training School in Addis.[1]

With or without the training function and even short of the demonstration function, the projects at Makelle and Dessei should also be regarded as basic programs of service to people. In the areas served by these units are several hundred thousand Ethiopians, whose lives can be made happier and more productive through health service. This task alone will merit all the effort that Peace Corps volunteers can put forth.

NOTES

[1] In the late 1960s, a modern school of medicine was started at Addis Ababa.

Chapter VII
Health Service Patterns in Latin America:
Peru, Costa Rica, Mexico, Brazil, and Chile

In the health service patterns of Latin America one sees the influence of many forces: the early Indian culture, the Catholic church of Imperial Spain and Portugal, the social security concept of modern Europe, the public health ideas of North America, and of course the blend of all these entities forged in the Latin American culture of today. The resultant picture is a complex montage of many elements. Several discrete subsystems of health service–each oriented, in a sense, toward a different social class–operate side-by-side and serious problems of incoordination have resulted.

To lay the basis for improved coordination, especially between ministries of health and autonomous social security agencies, the Organization of American States (through its secretariat, the Pan American Union) sponsored a study in five countries: Peru, Costa Rica, Mexico, Brazil, and Chile. The summary chapter of that report follows, drawn from Medical Care in Latin America, *(Washington, D.C.: Pan American Union (Studies and Monographs III), 1963, pp. 246-272); it is reprinted here by permission. In the later 1960s and early 1970s, a good deal of progress was made in coordination among different autonomous social security systems (e.g., in Brazil), as well as between social security agencies and ministries of health (e.g., in Venezuela).*

From a review of the structure and function of the varied systems of medical care in five countries of Latin America, there are certain general features that can be identified. The differences between countries are great and, in this study, we have only looked at a sample of the twenty-one American republics—Peru, Chile, Brazil, Costa Rica, and Mexico. In Argentina, in Venezuela, in Cuba, in Haiti, in every other country there are unique characteristics to the social organization by which medical care is provided, and these have not been examined.

There seem to be enough similarities, however, in the approach to a population's health needs in the larger Latin American culture to permit an overview of the total situation and to allow a certain delineation of significant problems. In this chapter, we will attempt to draw, in rough lines, the shape of these main features and the disturbing problems associated with each of them. The viewpoint here will be critical, as it must be if we are to arrive at constructive proposals for the future.

INDIGENOUS MEDICINE

Millions of people in the Latin American hinterlands, especially those of pure-blood or heavily Indian background, still depend today, in 1963, on various forms of primitive nonscientific medicine for the healing of their ills. Starting from irrational or unproven concepts of the causation of disease, various systems of therapy follow logically and are applied by different types of healers or *curanderos* in the isolated villages. Their approach may be magical or it may be empirical, involving the use of certain herbs and physical measures, or it may be a combination of these approaches. In addition, while not part of the traditional culture, there may be true charlatans or "quacks" who know a little about scientific medicine and pretend to be "doctors," using or misusing some of the scientific drugs.

The use of these healers by the people is, of course, perfectly understandable, in the absence of other more effective modern resources. They are usually deeply rooted parts of the culture. They are close at hand in the village and are inexpensive; sometimes the service is just given on a neighborly basis without any economic transaction. A great deal of the service might be described, in scientific terms, as psychotherapy, and it may sometimes be effective because of the role of psychogenic factors both in disease causation and in the process of recovery. The indigenous healer understands the feelings and the fears of his patient and can, therefore, often help him.

When scientific measures of preventive medicine are first introduced into a rural area, where the population has previously depended on these primitive healers, naturally there are bound to be frictions.[1] The local people will not accept the new practices overnight. The impressive experience in Latin America, however, is how rapidly people do come to accept modern health service, when it is shown to be more effective and is physically and economically accessible to them. Rejections of scientific medicine, reported by anthropologists, can often be traced to overt causes like great physical inaccessibility (long distances to travel), fears which have not been answered in an understandable way, or a nonsensitive and condescending attitude by the practitioner. Despite these experiences, the long-term trend is clearly toward a reduction of the dependence of rural people on primitive medicine and a heightened utilization of scientific services that are offered.

In developing modern health service programs in rural areas, the governmental health authorities of Latin America have usually ignored these indigenous healers. They have been bypassed rather than being offered any training that might incorporate them into the modern system. The main exception is the local midwife (not truly a *curandero*), who is often given some education and encouraged to work under the supervision of a professional nurse. In India and China, however, governmental policy has taken the other approach—to give these village personalities some training and incorporate their services, under some supervision, in the official system. There are, of course, hazards in this approach, but on a selected basis it might be worth exploration in Latin America.

At present, the "system" of medical care available from indigenous healers can only be described as extremely deficient. It is, of course, a pattern of ambulatory care or home care, without benefit of hospitals or equipment. It permits people to suffer and die

from illnesses for which modern medicine has perfectly effective cures. It persists where there is nothing better, but it must eventually be replaced.

THE CHARITY SYSTEM

Stemming from the initiative of the Catholic church in the Spanish colonial days and later from the sense of "noblesse oblige" of the wealthier families, there has developed throughout Latin America a great network of charitable hospitals to serve the poor. Known as *santas casas* or as *beneficencias* or by other designations, these are in many countries the principal resource for medical care of the mass of the population, especially in the larger towns and cities.

While there are outpatient departments attached to most of them, the principal focus of the charity hospitals is the bed-care of the seriously sick. It is the philosophy of mercy for those in great distress, rather than the more preventively oriented approach of a modern medical center. Indeed, purely preventive services—like well-baby clinics or health education—are rarely if ever offered. Outpatient departments available are usually small and inadequate in relation to the demand. The typical charity hospital is an old building, poorly designed for current medical concepts. The wards are large and quite lacking in privacy or bedside attachments that add to patient comfort. The laboratory and x-ray equipment are usually meager. Most important, the staffing is poor both in nursing personnel and in the various forms of technician and therapist required by modern medicine. Hard-working religious sisters frequently form the basic corps of the staff, both for labor and for supervision, and one can only admire them for their patience in working against great handicaps.

Of course, not all charity hospitals fit this grim picture. In the capital cities, several of them are associated with medical schools and offer a fairly high level of technical service—if not great personal comforts for the patient. Moreover, most charity hospitals have come to make provision for private patients at various levels. For a little extra payment, the patient may be assigned to a ward with simple partitions between the beds, and his diet may contain a little more meat. The well-to-do may be served in completely private or *pensionado* rooms by private doctors of their own choice. The doctors attending the indigent patients receive only small honoraria, although in recent years these payments have been rising—in order to attract physicians in competition with other organized medical care programs.

Historically, the charity hospitals were financed

67

by bequests on the death of wealthy people, by operation of cemeteries, by lotteries, by donations, and so on. These sources of income continue, but as the costs of medical care have risen, as more technically trained personnel have become necessary, as doctors have had to be remunerated, these sources have proved less and less adequate. The adjustment everywhere has been through subsidy from government, both local and national. To enable them to survive, governmental subsidies to the charity hospitals have taken many forms—both for operating and for construction costs—and probably exceed fifty percent of total costs, on the average, rising often to ninety percent.

With these subsidies, governments have stipulated certain standards—such as requiring that over half of the patients be indigent— but the technical demands are very limited. In some ministry of health budgets, the subsidies to the charity hospital system of the nation represent the largest item of expenditure, but the controls associated with these large outlays are very weak. The immediate authority over the hospital is typically a board of leading citizens from the local city; while these men and women may be kind and public-spirited, their knowledge of modern medical requirements is usually very limited. Nor is there a trained hospital administrator, except rarely, to compensate for these deficiencies. The top direction is often in the hands of a busy doctor, who does clinical work in the hospital, maintains a private practice in the town, and can give little attention to administrative matters.

With such conditions, it can be no surprise that the medical care provided in the charity hospitals is usually of a meager quality. The time that physicians can devote to the diagnosis and treatment of indigent patients—either in the wards or in the outpatient department—is very limited. Many essential diagnostic procedures cannot be done and many needed drugs are simply not available. As a result, the average length of stay of patients is very long—usually exceeding twenty days. Death rates are often high.

The trend toward governmental intervention, which began with subsidies, has in several countries proceeded beyond this. Some of the larger and more costly *beneficencia* hospitals have been transferred to government entirely and are operated by the ministry of health. In certain countries the whole system has been transferred. In Mexico, as part of the general movement against the Church, all charity hospitals were taken over by the government—central or state—many years ago. In Costa Rica, a general transfer of ownership occurred about ten years ago, but local *beneficencia* boards still play a part in the direct management of the institutions. In

Chile, the entire charity hospital system was placed at the disposal of the central government with the inauguration of the National Health Service in 1952.

The whole charity system of medical care in Latin America, therefore, is in very active transition. It has played a major role and continues to render much service, but it has had to come under increasing influence of government to adjust to modern conditions. The medical profession is generally dissatisfied with the system, and everywhere seems to welcome a shift to direct control by government.

There are other limited programs of medical care under charitable auspices, aside from the *beneficencia* hospitals. Voluntary societies operate under religious and nonsectarian auspices for service to children, for custodial care of the aged, for campaigns against tuberculosis and other diseases. Some of these, like the cancer societies, operate hospitals mainly for private paying patients. In some countries, like Brazil, the voluntary societies receive heavy governmental subsidy and carry major responsibility for child health services. But the general importance of these bodies is declining.

MILITARY AND OTHER NATIONAL PROGRAMS

As everywhere in the world, the military forces in Latin America are a favored group and their health is well protected as a matter of high public policy. The very first hospitals constructed by the Spanish settlers were for their military men, and some of the finest facilities today are devoted to the army and navy. The medical and nursing personnel to serve these men are also abundant; in some countries they are even trained in special schools to assure a good supply of persons with high competence.

The dependents of military personnel are also often entitled to special services at military expense. In communities where the number of military personnel is too small to justify a special facility, there are often special departments reserved for them in local hospitals under other auspices.

Other national employees, necessary for the smooth operation of the government, are also generally favored in Latin America. The railroads are, in large part, owned by the central governments, and elaborate systems of medical and hospital care are found everywhere for railroad workers and their families. Likewise for the employees of nationalized industries like petroleum in Mexico. The utilization of services in these special programs tends to be much higher than among the general population.

The great bulk of other employees of the national government are also often protected by special social insurance programs, to which the employees make financial contributions but which are predominantly financed from general revenues. In Brazil and Mexico, the most elegant hospitals in the nation are reserved for these workers—who are largely white collar—and their families. While a high proportion of such beneficiaries are, of course, in the national capitals, some of them are located throughout the country. For the care of the latter, special contracts are often made with local private and public facilities. These services are typically independent of other organized programs which are similarly designated as "social security."

SOCIAL SECURITY

In terms of their rate of growth and energetic policies, the arrangements for medical care under the social security systems are perhaps the most impressive in Latin America. The concept of social security was derived from Europe and it has been applied widely to the small but growing industrial population and even to sections of the agricultural population in the Latin American countries.[2]

Social security programs have established a mechanism for raising money out of the process of economic production in a more or less automatic way. Taxes are imposed typically on the workers—deductions of a certain percentage of their wages; on employers—i.e., through deductions based on payroll costs; and thirdly on the general public treasury. The money contributed by the workers might otherwise have been paid directly to them for personal spending, so that they rightfully feel a personal sacrifice and involvement—hence an entitlement to the benefits that this money can buy. The money contributed by employers, however, is derived from payments received for the sale of their products, so that it is really contributed by the whole community (or indeed the whole world) which purchases these products. The money contributed from general governmental revenues, of course, is derived from the total population through various systems of direct and indirect taxes.

It is important to keep in mind these sources of social security funds, because insofar as less than 100 percent of the population is covered, then one must realize that money derived from the total population is being spent on the welfare of a share of it. There may well be sound reasons for such inequity, in terms of the economic or political objectives of a nation, but it is well to understand the reasoning in back of such policy decisions.

The fact is that in most Latin American countries with social security systems, despite the widespread sources of their money, only a minority of the population is protected—ranging from ten to twenty percent. Typically this population is concentrated in the main urban centers, although the prevailing policy is toward gradual extension into the outlying areas. There are great deficiencies in coverage of agricultural workers, both wage earners and small landowners or tenants.[3] Different kinds of benefits are provided in the various countries; sometimes dependents are included, sometimes not. The details of coverage, financial sources, benefits, and administrative patterns of the Latin American social security systems are well summarized in various publications of the Organization of American States.[4,5] Of twenty Latin American countries, fourteen include provisions for medical care and maternity benefits in their social security systems. These include most of the larger nations and all five of the countries examined in this study.

The money derived from various sources may, as a rule, be spent with considerable latitude by the agencies controlling social security programs. Indeed, one of the special features of social security in Latin America is the relative "autonomy" of these agencies. This is designed to protect them from some of the vicissitudes of political changes but, at the same time, it may lead to policies poorly coordinated with other governmental programs of health service. For various reasons, moreover, there may be several social security programs operating side-by-side, for different occupational and social groups, with little interconnection in the provision of medical benefits. In fact, in only a few countries is there a single, unified social insurance agency for all public and private occupational groups.

Medical care is provided to insured beneficiaries along two general lines. The older pattern, which was followed by the first program—in Chile after 1924—is to use social security money for purchase of medical, hospital, and related services from existing facilities and personnel. They are paid on the basis of contracts involving various schemes of remuneration. The later pattern, starting in Peru around 1940, is for the social security organization to establish its own facilities and engage its own personnel, paid by salaries to provide services to the designated beneficiaries. In all countries both of these mechanisms are used in varying proportions, but the trend appears to be toward more of the second pattern—that is, operation of independent hospitals and ambulatory care centers directly by the social security agencies.

The reasons for development of the latter pattern are not far to seek. The existing facilities for medical care, at the time of origin of the social security programs, were typically quite deficient. The largest resource has often been the charity hospital system, and we have noted its technical weaknesses. Rather than simply turning money over to these institutions, the social security authorities have considered it wiser to use their funds for building new facilities according to their own standards. With large sums of money available, these standards could be relatively high. Somewhat later, central governments began to build hospitals and health centers of good quality, and one may wonder if reasonable standards could not be applied by channelling social security money back to the ministries of health—as has, indeed, been done to some extent in a few countries.

In any event, the resources of medical personnel and facilities available to socially insured beneficiaries—by one device or another—are generally much more abundant than those for the noninsured population. In addition to hospitals of their own or hospitals with reserved blocs of beds, there are impressive networks of *consultorios* or medical posts. Drugs are also provided, on medical prescription, and dental care may be offered. There are often special provisions for long-term illness, including tuberculosis and mental disorder. Organized preventive services may also be promoted, including immunizations, health education, maternal and child health examinations and counselling, and routine disease-detection tests on adults.

Not that all the health needs of insured persons are being fully met; far from it. As workers and their dependents have become educated about the programs, their rates of utilization of medical and hospital service have risen. The resources, therefore, are typically under pressure, and medical examinations are often hasty. The medical departments of social security agencies are continually seeking ways to upgrade the quality of service, through surveillance, medical audits, and training programs. The pressures are greatest in those social security institutes that are devoted to manual, industrial workers or *obreros* (as distinguished from commercial or white collar employees or *empleados*)—programs in which the membership is usually greatest and the per capita financial resources lowest.

Nevertheless, the more educated and higher income employee population is enlarging throughout Latin America and, as the costs of modern medical service rise, is making increasing demands for social insurance protection. At the same time, the medical profession is resistant to the loss of these persons as private patients, when they come under a social security umbrella. The problem has been faced in a few countries by using the system of "free choice of doctor" for white collar employees (even though it is relatively costly), with reimbursement by the social security fund on the basis of fees for each service. In

some programs, the employee has still a further freedom of choice: as between a private physician and an organized facility of the social security program. The precise arrangements may differ in different cities, depending on the resources locally available. There may also be differences in benefits between private and public employees. This whole question of social security coverage of the expanding middle class is one of the most critical issues of medical care organization in Latin America. Indeed, the whole system of social security is in active flux, with a constant tendency toward wider coverage and benefits.[6]

One of the most positive influences of the social security medical care programs has been their emphasis on proper ambulatory, as distinguished from purely hospital services. In most countries, impressive polyclinics and peripheral medical stations have been developed, even when hospital care is provided in existent public institutions. While most of these ambulatory care centers are under heavy pressure, they tend to provide a much higher volume of services for insured persons than is obtained by others of the same income level. Some insured persons, to avoid long waiting periods, also avail themselves of the services of private doctors for which they pay.

The cash disability or sickness benefits in Latin American social security programs are usually administered by the medical care system. This has the great advantage of placing responsibility for certifying disability in the hands of the same doctors who can give medical care to reduce the disability; yet, the doctor has no financial interest in prolonging the sickness period—as he may in systems based predominantly on "free choice and fee payments" (as in Western Europe). The disability certification and cash benefit program, however, puts an additional administrative strain on the system.

Insurance for medical care and cash benefits in industrial injuries is handled in different ways. In several countries, it is simply part of the social security system for general medical care. In most countries, however, this workmen's compensation legislation was enacted separately, and the arrangements for medical care may be quite independent. Private insurance companies are usually involved, and the services are frequently rendered in private hospitals.

A number of significant measures of coordination have been taken by the social security programs with respect to health services. Although Brazil presents seven major, autonomous *institutos* for insurance of different categories of private and public employees, a coordinating council has achieved much uniformity among them. New hospitals are henceforth to serve the members of all the programs jointly, just as has long been true for a special network of emergency care stations. In Costa Rica, there is an interchange of hospital service between the social security agency and the Ministry of Health, to avoid duplication of facilities in the smaller towns. The greatest coordination has been achieved in Chile, where the medical care program of the social security system for manual workers (though not yet for white collar employees) has been, in effect, turned over to the Ministry of Health. These and other coordinated activities demonstrate the value of teamwork, which can be achieved in the field of health service, even though—for purposes of tax collection and for payment of monetary benefits—the social security organizations remain autonomous and independent.

The overriding question, in examining the total medical care scene in Latin America, is the effect of the social security program in each eountry on the development of an adequate system of health service for everyone. On the one hand, the financial device of earmarked contributions from workers, employers, and government has succeeded in channelling a great deal of money into health activities. Overall resources in the way of hospitals, polyclinics, and medical manpower have obviously been strengthened. Higher quality standards have also been promoted. On the other hand, the restriction of these benefits to a minority of the population creates marked inequities. By attracting personnel, usually through higher salaries and better professional conditions, into the social security sector, the task of the ministries of health to meet the needs of the great balance of the population becomes all the more difficult. In terms of long-term economic development, there may be sound reasons to give priority to the medical needs of industrial workers (and other selected occupational groups), and the question is whether this might still be done within a unified national medical care system.

GOVERNMENTAL MEDICAL CARE

While social security programs have been energetic, particularly for the benefit of urban populations, ministries of health in Latin America have also made great strides in the provision of health service—both preventive and curative—especially for the benefit of rural populations. And if the social insurance philosophy was derived largely from Europe, the more heavily preventive orientation of the ministry of health programs comes in large part from the influence of North America. The best known activities of the ministries of health have been their campaigns against the great epidemic diseases, but our focus in this study is on their role in the provision of medical care.[7]

Government operates, of course, at many levels. At the city or municipal level, there are governmental hospitals to serve the poor. One sees these facilities in Mexico, Argentina, Puerto Rico, and elsewhere—some of them having been acquired from older *beneficencias* and others having been built directly by the local government. Provincial or state governments also operate hospitals largely for the care of the poor, especially in the federated nations like Brazil or Mexico. These facilities of local government are of very uneven quality, varying with the affluence of the region; most of them are crowded and inadequate. Local governments may also contribute financially to the costs of operating charity hospitals.

The central governments exercise responsibility for medical care in many ways. There are the systems of grants to the charity hospitals, mentioned earlier, along with which may go a very limited imposition of standards. Federal grants for operating costs may also go to state-owned hospitals, as in Mexico. Hospital construction planning has also been done modestly by a number of Latin American ministries of health, with designation of technical standards to be met by all new hospitals constructed, under any organizational sponsorship.

The larger role of ministries of health is through the direct operation of networks of facilities for both ambulatory health service and hospital care of the sick. The *Servicio Cooperativo Interamericano de Salud Publica* played a large part in the development of these facilities, since about 1942. A variety of health centers, medical posts, sanitary posts, and other types of unit have been established all through Latin America, especially in the small towns and rural districts, for ambulatory care.

In the rural areas, these facilities usually offer both preventive and curative services; the latter may be quite rudimentary, depending mainly on auxiliary personnel (with periodic visits from a physician). In the larger cities, where hospitals are more accessible for referral of sick patients, the emphasis tends to be overwhelmingly preventive. Maternal and child health services get the major attention. Indeed, there are often a number of separate governmental units, especially in Brazil, for services to children. Even where the service is theoretically open to everyone, the primary users of these ambulatory health units are women and children, rather than adult males. Many of the small rural health centers contain also a few beds for maternity cases (often staffed by a midwife), emergencies, and minor illnesses.

In recent years, the ministries of health have constructed a number of large regional hospitals, located usually in the trade centers of great rural regions at a distance from the national capital. These institutions are usually well-designed and equipped, with staffing in all the medical and surgical specialties. Often their program includes responsibility for public health services as well.

In Brazil, Mexico, and elsewhere, the movement has been strong toward establishment of regional health authorities. The regional health officer is in charge of all ministry activities in his geographic area, whether they involve medical care, personal preventive service, or environmental public health campaigns. In Chile, the concept has been carried farthest with the creation of "health zones," including all the medical care activities that were previously under social security sponsorship. Regional officials everywhere in Latin America, however, are still limited in their authorities to programs controlled by the ministry of health and, even in Chile, many health service activities remain outside of that arena.

In a few places, governmental hospitals have come to acquire a very comprehensive role. Tacna, Peru is one such example, where a large Ministry of Health institution serves as the center for virtually all health services in its territory, including the care of beneficiaries of the two social security agencies in that country. A former *beneficencia* hospital was absorbed as a branch facility for the chronically ill. All the preventive and public health activities of the area are also based at this hospital. Peripheral medical and sanitary posts in the rural areas report to the hospital director. This comprehensive conception is being applied also at the new national capital of Brazil, the remarkable district of Brasilia—although it is not yet fully realized. In Costa Rica at Quepos, a hospital acquired from a private company is being converted by the Ministry of Health into such a multipurpose center for an isolated region. Here and there in several countries are examples of such truly integrated health service administration, under a ministry of health, and these may serve as models for the future.

Governmental hospitals of the newer type are not limited exclusively to the indigent, but may also contain some private beds. These may be in separate rooms, elegantly furnished, in which the patient is treated by a personal physician. In addition, patients on the regular wards, where treatment is given by governmentally salaried doctors, may have a modicum of privacy and slightly more attractive surroundings by paying a supplemental hospital fee. It is of interest to see this adjustment of governmental

hospitals to the rising expectations of the population of Latin America.

In addition to their operation of general hospitals and ambulatory service health centers, central governments throughout Latin America also operate special institutions for mental disorder, tuberculosis, leprosy, and other long-term disorders. As everywhere in the world, these institutions have a relatively low priority in the competition for limited funds. Compared with North America, the proportion of total hospital beds allocated for mental illness is very low (about one-tenth instead of one-half), which is probably quite reasonable. The condition of those beds, however, is often disgraceful—just as it commonly is in the wealthiest countries.

The persons served by governmental hospitals and health centers are, of course, primarily the low income and indigent population which still predominates in Latin America. As a rising proportion of the urban population comes to be enrolled under social security programs, the coverage of the governmental services is increasingly focused on the rural populations and low income families in the smaller towns. In most of the great capital cities of Latin America, moreover, there are slum settlements—*barrios* often making a great belt around the metropolitan center—and the families in these places must usually depend on some type of free medical care. Since these slums and "shantytowns," despite their squalor, are relatively new, they are in neighborhoods distant from the center of the city, where the old *beneficencia* hospitals tend to be located. Medical services for these slum dwellers, therefore, are provided largely by governmental facilities.

The impact of governmental medical care programs, it may be noted, tends to be somewhat complementary to that of the charity system. The patients served by the two systems are of a similar social class, but in more or less separate locations. The governmental facilities, however, are on the whole more subject to uniform technical standards at a higher level. Their personnel are more likely to meet merit requirements, rather than being appointed on the basis of local loyalties or religious preference. Their equipment is usually newer. Their philosphy is more likely to be imbued with a concept of prevention and comprehensive service, rather than a spirit of merciful relief of distress.

Governmental health services are, in a sense, the twentieth century response to the need for medical care by masses of the population, while the charity services symbolize the nineteenth century approach. Yet, the line is not really this sharp, since almost all Latin American governments have built upon the foundations laid by the older charity system. They have done this by a variety of actions, ranging from (1) simple subsidies, to (2) subsidies with technical standards, to (3) legal transfer of controls while local boards are retained, and finally to (4) complete governmental acquisition and operation. Each Latin American government, moreover, has struck a somewhat different balance in its use of governmental money, as between support of the charitable facilities and complete replacement of them by governmental units. The trend is certainly toward the latter solution.

One of the principal carry-overs of the past is seen in the arrangements for first aid and emergency medical care in many Latin American countries. Because of their origin separate from the charity system and their provision for twenty-four hour service (in contrast to the limited schedules of medical hours in hospitals), these emergency units tend to be separate administrative entities under government. While this separateness may generate a certain "esprit de corps" in the personnel, there would doubtless be great technical advantages in integration of these units with the rest of the governmental health services. Still other emergency services are operated by the Red Cross, outside of the wing of government but usually dependent for most of their money on governmental grants.

The broad, theoretical conceptions of governmental health services in Latin America are not always implemented as effectively as they appear on paper. Salaries for medical personnel, from top to bottom, are usually insufficient to provide a satisfactory livelihood, even when they are supposedly "full-time." As a result, nearly all governmental physicians engage also in private practice, which is perhaps less of a problem of compromised time than of compromised spirit. Loyalties divided between a private clientele and a public duty create a strain for both sectors. If an hour devoted to private patients yields higher earnings than an hour in a public function, it is easy to understand the temptations. There can be no real solution to this problem until the governmental agencies can pay salaries sufficient to hold the full time and full loyalties of their personnel.

Other difficulties spring from the sparsity of travel funds, which makes it hard for central ministries of health to exercise proper supervision over peripheral activities. Between regional headquarters and rural posts, also, there are elementary deficiencies in transportation. The whole field of public administration in Latin America, moreover, requires further development to grapple with the tasks of national planning and efficient program execution, and the health services are no exception.

INDUSTRIAL MEDICAL SERVICES

Private industry has filled many gaps in Latin America left by the inadequacies of charitable or public services. Especially in isolated rural areas, where medical facilities were totally lacking, mining, oil exploration, electrical power, construction, agricultural processing, and other enterprises have established some excellent hospitals and health stations. The company, of course, needs a healthy work force, but the usual program covers also the worker's family—sometimes with extra charges. Many, if not most, of these enterprises are under foreign ownership and they enjoy a high rate of profit, so that they can well afford to provide these services as a business expense. Indeed, they usually pay much higher than average salaries to medical and nursing personnel, thereby attracting an ample staff even to very isolated locations.

In many countries, laws have been passed requiring private industry to provide these services, if there are more than a certain number of workers (e.g., 100) and if the enterprise is located more than a specified distance from an urban center. With the development of social security programs, under which the same industrial workers are compulsorily covered, arrangements have been made for reimbursement of the company for these medical care expenses; these reimbursements, however, may not equal the full expenditures of the company.

The utilization of these industrial health services tends to be quite high, compared with rates in general population. Being in small tightly-knit communities, the clinic and hospital tend to be conveniently located, and are readily used. The ratios of hospital beds and of medical and nursing personnel are also usually high. There is frequently a high rate of accidents in these industries. In almost all industrial establishments of any size and location, moreover, there are usually minor first-aid services for emergencies. And in the larger cities, some companies engage physicians for doing health examinations and minor medical care in the plant for a few hours a week.

In Brazil and perhaps elsewhere, private industries have banded together to offer medical and welfare services through special associations, financed entirely by the employers. A network of *consultorios* and polyclinics is established in the main cities to serve the workers of many companies. These programs do not replace those at isolated localities, but they complement to some extent the services offered by the social security agencies in the cities.

Medical care for industrial injuries is usually provided under separate administrative arrangements in Latin America, as in most of the world. The workmen's compensation legislation often antedates that for general social security, and under it separate systems have been developed for treatment of injured workers, not to mention distribution of cash benefits. Most insurance, as noted earlier, is carried by private companies or by special agencies of government intended exclusively for this purpose. Under these systems, the injured worker is usually treated in private medical offices or hospitals, with payment made on a fee basis. In some countries, responsibility is carried under the wing of the overall social security program, and the injured worker is treated in the same facilities as he would be for nonoccupational injury or illness. Even in Chile, however, where so much integration has been achieved, arrangements for medical care of industrial injury cases are outside of the National Health Service; they involve use of special hospitals of an independent governmental insurance agency or else purely private facilities.

PRIVATE MEDICAL CARE

Despite the large and varied development of socially organized programs of medical care for diverse population groups in Latin America, an appreciable share of medical needs is still met through purely private arrangements. For a small section of the population, private medicine is the total resource for medical care, but for a large section it is a partial resource. This private world of medical care is, at the present time, in very active flux. It represents, on the one hand, a response to the inadequacies of the publically organized programs while, on the other hand, it is a response to the rising expectations of a growing middle class.

Private medical service takes many forms. As for physicians, there is a small percentage in every country—probably less than ten percent—who are exclusively in private practice. They would constitute mainly specialists in the main cities. At the other end of the scale are perhaps twenty-five percent of physicians who do no private practice at all, and are in full-time dedication to some organized program. Between these extremes are about sixty-five percent of physicians who hold part-time salaried positions, but spend part of their time in private practice, ranging perhaps from one to six hours per day. These include not only doctors in the main cities, but those in the small towns and villages as well.

In a village post, conditions are often crowded in a

morning session, and the doctor may advise an anxious patient that later in his private office there would be more time for a careful examination. This happens in the large city polyclinics as well, and it occurs under social security programs as well as governmental or charity systems. The patients who can afford private fees thereby obtain a larger share of the doctor's limited time, even though they may be theoretically entitled to proper service under the public program.

There is probably no way to correct this type of inequity until funds become adequate to pay for a full measure of the doctor's time. The priority of medical attention would then depend on medical judgment of the patient's need, rather than monetary gain. Even if a clinic session is not crowded and time is not a critical factor, however, the doctor's attitude may be condescending and insensitive simply because of the social class distinction between doctor and patient. This whole problem is being tackled in the better-financed social security *institutos* by providing more attractive physical surroundings and by education of the doctor; it is also being approached by making a fixed assignment of patients to certain doctors, so that they get to know each other.

Hospital care for private patients is provided in several ways. The private or *pensionado* beds in the governmental and charity hospitals have been mentioned. In addition, there are in all the main cities of Latin America a variety of small, relatively elegant hospitals, known as *clinicas privadas, casas de saude,* or by other names. Most of these are privately owned, often by prosperous and successful surgeons, and run for profit. Sometimes, they may be conducted by nonprofit associations or religious groups, but still restricted to private paying patients. The staffing of these small hospitals is usually abundant, especially with respect to professional nurses who look after the patient's comforts. The focus of these hospitals is on maternity cases and acute surgery, so that their average length of stay is short and their per diem costs are high.

Another type of private facility is the hospital operated by a nationality association, like the Spanish, the Portuguese, or the Germans, for the benefit of its members. These are called *beneficencias privadas,* not to be confused with the public charity hospitals operated by *juntas de beneficencia.* Membership in the association depends on annual fees and donations, and there are also charges at the time of hospitalization. In addition, a proportion of the beds may be occupied by nonmembers who can pay the full costs. There may be a few beds also for charity patients, who pay low fees but get the free attention of a doctor.

Probably the most widely used type of private health service in Latin America is the purchase of drugs. Except for narcotics in certain countries, almost all drugs can be purchased directly by anyone from a *farmacia*, without requirement of a doctor's prescription. This is a relatively cheap, if wholly inadequate, form of medical care for many indigent and uneducated people—who report their symptoms and ask advice of the proprietor (frequently not a trained pharmacist). Studies of the private expenditures of Latin American populations for health services suggest that the outlay for drugs, mainly self-prescribed, is the largest item. Medically prescribed drugs, of course, are also provided as a benefit of social security and other organized programs, but these private drug expenditures are undoubtedly wasteful and probably often harmful.

As a proportion of the total medical care in Latin America, private service is probably a contracting share. Not that it is declining absolutely, because more doctors are being trained and an enlarging middle class is using their private attention. But the relative weight of socially organized programs, especially under ministries of health and social security agencies, is increasing more rapidly. These programs can offer a secure income to the doctor, so that he is generally happy to be appointed in them, leaving less of his time for private practice. The associations of physicians in Latin America seem anxious to preserve at least a partial sector of private practice. They have no objections, however, to salaried public systems of service, so long as the scale of remuneration and the conditions of professional work are adequate.

RESOURCES IN PERSONNEL AND FACILITIES

We have discussed the many systems of organization of medical care in Latin America, and all of them depend on the mobilization of human and economic resources. In a sense, the organized programs of medical care in any country can be defined in terms of the proportionate claims that each makes on the total supply of personnel and facilities available.

With respect to personnel, the most prominent feature of these relative claims is the great disproportion between cities and rural areas. The cities attract the lion's share of physicians in all countries for many reasons. They are more pleasant and interesting places to live for the doctor and his family. The opportunity for earnings from private medical practice are much greater, because the average purchasing power of the urban population is much higher. Even the socially organized programs of medical care are more highly developed in the cities, especially under the charity system and the social security system. The ministry of health programs are exerting the chief compensatory force to attract physicians and other personnel to the rural regions. In Mexico, a system of rural "social service" for new medical graduates is a special approach to providing some medical manpower in the villages, if only for temporary periods. In every Latin American country, however, a very high proportion of doctors are concentrated not just in the cities, but in the capital city of the nation.

Maldistribution is only part of the problem, because even if health personnel were evenly distributed in relation to population, the total supply is far from adequate. In all Latin America, there were in 1960 about fifty-five physicians per 100,000 population, compared with 132 in the United States and Canada. Five countries had fewer than thirty physicians per 100,000.[8] The very shortage aggravates the urban-rural distribution, because it means that the main cities can easily absorb the limited supply (in terms of providing them a livelihood), leaving very few for rural localities. In the last ten years, however, important strides have been made in training doctors, and the ratios are generally improving in almost all countries. Nearly 100 medical schools are now producing physicians in Latin America. Most of them, however, suffer from inadequate financing and lack of full-time faculties.

The relative supply of professional nurses is much worse. If the United States and Canada are taken as a basis of comparison, there are about 290 active professional nurses per 100,000 population in those two countries, and about twenty per 100,000 in Latin America as a whole. The supply of nursing auxiliaries is better (six Latin American countries have more than fifty per 100,000), but even so it is still much lower than the ratio of 330 per 100,000 in the North American countries. The basic problem in providing nursing personnel is the relatively small proportion of young women who complete secondary education; those who do tend to come from the upper social classes and seldom wish to enter nursing service. Much greater reliance must be put, therefore, on auxiliary nurses who receive short courses of training (six to twelve months) after only an elementary school education.

More reliance is placed also on midwives in Latin America than in North America, especially in the rural districts. When properly trained, these women can effectively manage the childbirth process, but even so there were only about five per 100,000 population in 1960 in Latin America. The deficiency of dentists is also extremely serious, with only about twenty per 100,000 in 1960, compared with fifty-six in the northern countries.

More vitality seems to be going into the expansion of education of physicians in Latin America than of other classes of health personnel. Undoubtedly they have the most critical role to play, but one might like to see greater energies applied to the training of larger numbers of auxiliary personnel who could, under suitable direction, provide certain minimal health services to the mass of rural people.

The maldistribution of health personnel prevails not only between localities, but between programs. Since the social security programs tend to have more money per capita to spend than the ministries of health, and the latter agencies tend to have more resources than the charity hospitals, the attractions that can be offered to medical personnel are in corresponding order. Both in quantity and quality, the available personnel naturally depend on economic foundations, which seldom parallel the extent of health needs.

The supply and distribution of hospitals and other health facilities in Latin America also correspond to economic forces. The different systems of medical care we have reviewed are each associated with special hospitals, and the amplitude of those hospitals depends on the money available in the system. Leaving aside the private hospitals, for which it is difficult to compute a population base, the hospitals under social security auspices tend to be most generously financed, those under ministries of health next, and the charity hospitals are most frugal. The ratios of hospital personnel to bed-patients tend also to run in this order. The largest relative supplies of hospital personnel are often found in the purely private institutions.

Argentina has the highest supply of hospital beds in Latin America, at 6.4 beds per 1,000 population; Costa Rica and Chile have 5.1 and 5.0 beds per 1,000 respectively, while all the other countries have less than 4.0 per 1,000. This includes beds of all types, for which the comparable figure in the United States is 9.1 per 1,000.

The effective use of these beds, moreover, is reduced by a high average length of stay, compared with North American experience. The Latin American figures are about twelve to twenty days, compared with eight days in the United States. Each bed, in other words, accommodates fewer patients per year when the average patient stay is long. Judging from research observations made in Europe and the United States, these long average stays are probably caused by many factors. The greater poverty of the patients means that their rate of recovery from illness (due to poor nutrition) is slower, and their poor home conditions mean that they cannot be properly discharged until recovery is complete. The average severity of cases admitted moreover, is probably greater than in the United States. Another factor is probably the meager hospital staffing, which slows up the process of medical diagnosis and treatment. Increased personnel, therefore, might reduce average stays and enhance the capacity of Latin American hospitals to serve patients, without expanding their bed complements.

The usual pattern of occupancy of Latin American hospitals is great overcrowding of the large city institutions and low occupancy levels in the rural districts. This is in spite of the fact that the ratio of beds to population is nearly always lower in the rural areas. The explanation is not elusive. Rural people simply receive much less attention from doctors in the first place, and it is the doctor's decision that usually sends a patient to the hospital. The therapy of indigenous practitioners does not call for hospital admission. Transportation to the towns where doctors are available is usually difficult, and the rural patient undertakes the trip only when illness has become grave. Many hospitals, moreover, are not attractive places, and one cannot blame the patient, even with a critical illness, who might prefer to stay and even die at home.

Some of the newer hospitals built either by social security agencies or ministries of health in Latin America are very impressive structures. To some extent, it appears that hospitals have been built as monuments, designed to impress the population for various ideological reasons, rather than mainly as centers of medical care; the money invested in some palatial hospitals in a capital city could often construct double or triple the number of beds for a building of more modest design. Nevertheless, most of the new hospitals in Latin America are well planned, and they serve to inspire the people working in them to do good work. In fact, it is important to recognize that fine hospitals have been built under diverse auspices—social security, ministry of health, private, industrial, military, and so on—so long as money has been available. No one type of agency seems to have a monopoly on skilled leadership. Newer hospitals are nearly always better than old ones, and the point in history when a hospital is built seems to determine its quality almost as much as the agency sponsoring it.

The hospital, in general, is more of a center for medical care in the Latin American community than it is in the United States. This is doubtless because the relative importance of the private doctor's office in meeting the health needs of people is less. From the point of view of long-term planning this is all to the good, because much more technical service can be effectively organized in and around hospitals than in hundreds of small independent offices. In the National Health Service of Chile, the focus of *all* health activities—including ambulatory service and public health—is the hospital.

Facilities for ambulatory care take many forms in Latin America. Almost all governmental and charitable hospitals tend to have active outpatient departments. As satellites to hospitals or as independent units, various kinds of *consultorios* and polyclinics have been developed by the social security agencies. The ministries of health have organized hundreds of health centers which have a heavily preventive theme, but also offer medical care. For children and mothers there are many special units under both governmental and voluntary agency auspices. Small medical and sanitary posts, staffed mainly by auxiliary personnel, have been set up in the villages and towns. Their equipment, however, is meager and their medical supervision may be very limited. Almost all these ambulatory care facilities are open to everyone, except for the social security centers, at which eligibility is restricted to insured persons. Unfortunately, there is seldom any administrative connection between health facilities—either ambulatory or hospital—under different auspices in the same community.

The resources of personnel and facilities for medical care in Latin America, in a word, tend to function in vertical systems of sponsorship throughout the geography of a country, and these systems are each based on a certain type of authority and financing. Some facilities and personnel, of course, are purely private or local in control and not really part of any nationwide "system." Horizontal relationships among the personnel and facilities within a local community, across sponsorship lines, are relatively rare.

APPROACHES TO COORDINATION

The problems created by multiple sponsorships of medical care programs have come to be increasingly appreciated in Latin America, and numerous steps have been taken toward improved coordination.

The policy of many central governments to subsidize charity hospitals, rather than to build new ones, is in a sense a gesture of unity rather than separatism. While the technical standards tied to these subsidies have been minimal, they represent at least an approach to establishment of some uniformity in hospital service for the indigent. In most countries, moreover, certain charity hospitals have been transferred to direct governmental control. In a few countries the entire charity system has been passed over to governmental operation, although the local *juntas* may retain some minimal administrative role.

Under the ministries of health, advisory councils have been established for the purpose of planning new hospital construction and promoting minimal architectural standards. Usually these councils include representatives of other agencies of government and important professional groups as well. The authorities exercised, however, are typically advisory rather than mandatory—except as they affect the hospitals of the ministry of health itself.

Within the ministries of health, there is also a growing sensitivity to the need for unified administration of the preventive and curative services (both ambulatory and hospital), that typically fall under different divisions or bureaus. This is expressed both through reorganizations at the top, and the establishment of various forms of regional offices in the field. The legal authority of these regional offices, however, seldom extends beyond the programs under direct ministry control. Typically, the regional officials are intended to supervise the public health, ambulatory care, and hospital services of the ministry in defined geographic areas.

The social security agencies have developed their medical care programs along both independent and coordinated lines. All of them make some use of existing facilities (under governmental or private sponsorship) through contracts—in addition to establishment of their own facilities. In some countries, the social security program not only contracts with the ministry of health for certain services, but the opposite also occurs—ministries contracting with social security hospitals for services to noninsured (and usually indigent) persons. It is common also for social security agencies to follow the directives of ministries of health on technical matters, like drug standards or policies with respect to immunizations. Some social security agencies have supported preventive programs with direct grants to a ministry of health for malaria control. On the governing boards of the social security *institutos*, moreover, it is frequent to have representation from the ministry of health—which may be the minister himself.

Where more than one social security program is operating for different population groups in a country, there may be little contact between them, as in Peru or Mexico, or there may be increasing liaison, as in Brazil. The "Medical Council of Social Security" in Brazil is important in demonstrating the possibilities of developing uniform policies, and even joint use of facilities, by agencies that have been legally independent of each other. The joint operation of the emergency services (S.A.M.D.U.) by several *institutos* in that country is another demonstration of the same principle. With respect to private industrial medical services, reimbursement of private corporations by social security agencies, for medical services rendered to insured workers, is a further sensible adjustment that avoids duplication of programs.

These varied approaches to coordination of medical care in Latin America indicate a widespread realization of the problem, even though there is obviously a long way to go. In general, a coordinated approach has been more successfully achieved in the smaller towns and rural areas. In the large cities, each separate program tends to have highly specialized services, which develop independent strength. With fewer overall resources in the rural regions, the need for *joint* use of resources is all the more compelling. Some of the most impressive demonstrations of integrated medical services—involving ministries of health, social security agencies, and charitable societies—have, therefore, been developed in isolated communities. Important leadership toward this objective of coordination has come from the World Health Organization and UNICEF.[9]

The achievements of Chile in integrating several major programs of medical care must be given special attention in any review of Latin American progress toward coordination of health services. The Chilean National Health Service was built from an amalgamation of several previously independent systems, including principally (1) the *beneficencia* hospitals, (2) the social security program of medical care for *obreros*, and (3) the Ministry of Health program of preventive and curative services.

Thus, medical care systems serving the indigent of the cities, the insured manual workers, and the low income rural people were unified under one direction. The insured white collar workers, railroad workers, the noninsured well-to-do, and industrial injury cases still remain outside the National Health Service. Money is derived both from general revenue and social security sources, but in its expenditure no distinction is made among different beneficiaries. The physical and personnel assets acquired from the several health systems have been woven together into an integrated program. The preventively oriented health centers of the Ministry of Health have acquired therapeutic functions; the therapeutically oriented polyclinics of the social security agency have been enriched with preventive functions; and the old *beneficencia* hospitals have come to fill the key role of medical centers.

The Chilean hospital occupies the focal position as the center of all health services, both therapeutic and preventive, in the area it serves. All separate ambulatory care units function as satellites to a hospital. Several hospital service areas constitute a "health zone," and the director of each zone is the delegated respresentative of the central headquarters of the National Health Service. He is responsible for coordination of all the health services in his territory, as well as for planning improvements to better meet the needs in the future.

Of course the Chilean National Health Service has not yet solved all the problems. There is still a substantial minority of the population (between twenty-five and forty percent) not covered under it and, even within the Service, there are serious problems in personnel, equipment, and operating policies. The "Preventive Medicine Law," which theoretically requires periodic health examinations of all workers annually, is far from fully applied. Polyclinics are crowded, and effective personal relationships between doctor and patient are not always achieved. But these problems are being systematically tackled. Steps are being taken to increase the resources in personnel and facilities, to improve the organizational process, and to broaden the coverage more nearly toward 100 percent of the population.[10] The Chilean National Health Service doubtless has many lessons to teach both in its courageous integration of previously independent systems and its cautious preparation and step-by-step movement ahead. The leaders of this program did not try to accomplish everything at once; yet they are moving deliberately toward a goal of comprehensive health service for everyone.

THE PEOPLE SERVED

In broad perspective, enormous progress has been made in providing medical care to the population of Latin America. Hospitals, centers for ambulatory medical service, and preventive health programs have been established both in the cities and rural areas of all countries. The ratios of personnel and facilities to population have gradually improved. Death rates have declined and the access of the people to scientific medical care has, on the whole, steadily increased.

Yet, as of the present moment, grave deficiencies remain. If one takes as the standard, not the level of medical care in North America, but rather the level achieved by the more comfortable social classes of any Latin American country, then immense inequities are found. The available resources are being applied to meet health needs in an extremely uneven manner. Since separate programs are organized in most countries for different population groups, and since the per capita resources of those programs vary greatly, the medical services available through them differ widely in quantity and quality. The program with more money to spend tends to attract more and usually better trained personnel. Its buildings are more spacious, its equipment more modern, its drugs and supplies more abundant. The whole inequity is exaggerated further by the operation of a substantial private sector.

Thus, there are large numbers of impoverished rural people in any Latin American country—typically about fifty percent of the national population—who are ultimately accessible to only a small proportion of the nation's total medical resources. At the other end of the income range, there is a small number of affluent urban people who are served by a very large proportion of the nation's medical resources. Between these poles are various groupings of urban and rural workers and their families who have access to variously sized shares of the total resources, depending on their exact geographic location, their place of employment, social security coverage, and other attributes.

In this chapter, we have reviewed briefly the several systems of medical care found to operate side-by-side in most Latin American countries. As a mode of summary we can sketch the situation from the point of view of the people served. If we take another look at one of the countries analyzed—Peru—we can distinguish several different social classes in the population, each of which is served in a somewhat different way. A similar recapitulation might be done for any Latin American country, but in Peru the story would appear approximately as follows:

1. *Rural Indians.* Outside the mainstream of civilized life in Peru, the Indian population depends for its medical care mainly on the primitive, nonscientific healers reviewed earlier. These are the principal resource. If they live near a town with a *beneficencia* hospital, Indians will also get some care in the public wards of this institution. Such care is usually obtained only when illness has reached so critical a stage that life in the family setting has become impossible. Some limited ambulatory care is obtained at the outpatient departments of the *beneficencia* hospitals or at a medical or sanitary post of the ministry of health. The latter service is rendered usually by an auxiliary health worker, rather than a physician. In the towns, patent medicines for self-care are purchased in *farmacias*.

2. *Peasants and Peons.* The rural agricultural workers and their families get their principal medical care from the *beneficencia* hospitals in the small towns, and their *consultorios*. If they are fortunate

enough to live near one of the towns where a more modern Ministry of Health hospital has been built, they receive a somewhat better quality of care in the wards or outpatient clinic of this institution. *Consultorios* tend to be crowded, however, and the attention is rather perfunctory. If the family's anxiety is great, they may scrape up the money to see a private doctor. Some ambulatory care is also available from the various stations of the Ministry of Health, especially for children and mothers. The *farmacias* are a resource for self-medication. This social class, it must be realized, is the most numerous of any in Peru.

3. *Urban Manual Workers.* Those who work in some form of industrial employment are entitled to somewhat better medical care, through the social security system. If they are in or near a city, they receive care in a hospital of the *seguro obrero* or one of its associated *consultorios*. The demand for services in these ambulatory facilities is high and the time per patient is relatively brief. Nevertheless, the resources are distinctly better than in the countryside. Prescribed drugs are obtained right in the hospital. The dependents of urban manual workers, however, may not obtain services in these facilities. Instead, they must get care in the public wards of a *beneficencia* or governmental hospital in the larger towns. Their drugs, either prescribed or self-selected, must be purchased in a *farmacia*.

If the manual worker is employed at an isolated mine or oil exploration point, both he and his family may receive medical care at a hospital maintained by the company. The supply of beds and personnel in these industrial medical establishments is sometimes exceptionally high. The small urban self-employed worker not covered by social security, on the other hand, must depend for his care mainly on the *beneficencia* hospital system.

4. *Urban White Collar Workers.* These are a favored social class in Peru, entitled to care in the exceptionally well built and well staffed hospitals and polyclinics of the *seguro del empleado*. The resources available to them are relatively generous both in quantity and quality. Taking the social security population as a whole (including the *obreros*), some 620,000 persons are served by about 3,700 hospital beds—or a ratio of about 6.0 beds per 1,000. This, it must be realized, is almost three times the national average in Peru. It even understates the matter, since social security beneficiaries may also be served in Ministry of Health hospitals by contractual arrangements, or by "free choice" in private hospitals.

The dependents of white collar workers are served for maternity care in the *empleado* hospitals. For other conditions they must seek care elsewhere. Because these people are of somewhat higher income than manual workers, they often are able to afford the *pensionado* sections of *beneficencia* or Ministry of Health hospitals, paying a private physician for the service. They also get care from private physicians in the office and home.

5. *Military Personnel and Police.* These functionaries are important to the whole operation of the state, and they are in a favored class for medical care. Special hospitals and *consultorios*, with relatively abundant staffing, are available for meeting their needs. The higher officers among them receive elegant service in private rooms of the military and naval hospitals. The rank-and-file men receive care in larger wards, but the attention is active and conscientious. Relatively large numbers of physicians, dentists, nurses, and other health personnel are reserved for their exclusive service.

6. *The Social Elite.* Finally there is the small group of prosperous persons in the upper middle class or the topmost social stratum—property owners, professional persons, businessmen. These people get their medical care mainly from the private sector of medicine. If they live in a small town or rural district (for example, landowners or merchants), they usually travel to a main city (usually to Lima) for the care of any significant illness. Most of them, however, reside within the main cities, where they are served in the office, or through home calls, by private physicians. Their hospitalization is in the *clinicas privadas* or sometimes in the *pensionado* sections of a public hospital. They are the main clientele of private dentists. The drugs they purchase in pharmacies are mainly prescribed by a physician.

This may be somewhat of an oversimplification of a complex social situation, but it probably conveys the main features of the impact of diverse medical care systems on the population of Peru. The proportions of the different social classes and the precise programs, of course, differ among the Latin American countries. In some the Indian population is small, in others there are special programs for selected governmental employees, and so on. But major social class differentials and corresponding medical care variations are found everywhere. It is obvious that there are serious social inequities in the whole pattern, that the receipt of medical care of a given quantity and quality bears very little relationship to the volume of disease and the severity of human need.

From the more stern and hardheaded viewpoint of economic development, the disparities may not be so faulty. Thus, the industrial and white collar worker classes are extremely important for the economic development of a nation, and in this sense it is reasonable that they should receive attention of higher priority. Moreover, their medical demands and expectations—because of a somewhat higher educational and social level—are also likely to be somewhat greater. The ultimate question for national planning is whether account can be taken of these practical realities, while at the same time achieving a sound expansion and coordination of services, so that all resources of personnel and equipment are applied with optimal economy and effectiveness.

NOTES

[1] Benjamin D. Paul (ed.), *Health, Culture and Community: Case Studies of Public Reactions to Health Programs.* New York: Russell Sage Foundation, 1955.

[2] Beryl Frank, "Social Security in Latin America Today." *Americas*, May 1961, pp. 31-34.

[3] International Labor Office, *Social Security in Agriculture.* Prepared for the Inter-American Social Security Conference, VI Meeting, Geneva, 1961.

[4] Pan American Union, "Trends and Problems in Social Security." *Annual Survey of the Economic and Social Situation in Latin America.* Washington, D.C.: 1962.

[5] Union Panamericana, *Sintesis de la Seguridad Social Americana.* Washington, D.C.: 1961.

[6] International Social Security Association, "The Fourteenth General Meeting of the International Social Security Association" (including "General Summary of the Developments in America"). *Bulletin of the International Social Security Association* (Geneva). November-December 1961, pp. 664-670.

[7] World Health Organization, "Special Issue: The Americas." *World Health* (Geneva), September-October 1961.

[8] Pan American Health Organization, *Summary of Four-Year Reports on Health Conditions in the Americas 1957-60.* Washington, D.C.: 1962.

[9] Organization Panamericana de la Salud, *Atencion Medica: Bases para la formulacion de una politica conetenental.* Washington, D.C.: November 1962.

[10] In 1968, white collar employees were brought under coverage by the Chilean NHS, with an option of using the established facilities or choosing their own doctors and getting reimbursement of about fifty percent of the fees.

Chapter VIII
Politics and Health Services in Two Former Spanish Colonies: The Philippines and Cuba

The Revolution of 1959 in Cuba brought to Latin America its first modern socialist nation. Starting from a similar heritage of Spanish colonialism, the Philippines came under strong American influence (as did Cuba) not only after their freedom from Spain in 1900, but also after their complete independence following World War II. In the 1970s, therefore, one can see interesting contrasts in the comparative effects of socialist and capitalist ideologies on the organization of health services in these two former Spanish colonies.

In late 1971, an opportunity was presented to examine the health care systems, especially hospital services, in both of these countries, as a World Health Organization consultant. These comparative observations were published originally as an article entitled "Political Ideology and Health Care: Hospital Patterns in the Philippines and Cuba" in the International Journal of Health Services *(Vol. 3, Summer 1973, pp. 487-492, copyright Baywood Publishing Company, Inc. 1973). It is reprinted here by permission of the publisher, Baywood Publishing Company, Inc.*[1]

In late 1971 (September-December) I had the opportunity, as a World Health Organization consultant, to visit Cuba and the Philippine Islands, and to study briefly their patterns of health services organization. Both countries have a somewhat similar heritage, with an originally similar Spanish-Catholic culture superimposed on earlier primitive Indian or Polynesian societies; both were Spanish colonies until the Spanish-American War of 1898-1899. As a settlement of that conflict, the Philippines came under the direct control of the United States as a U.S. "territory" ruled by an American governor. Cuba was granted independence, but came under great American influence both politically and economically; a high proportion of its industrial and agricultural resources were owned by U.S. citizens, and its trade was mainly with the United States.

Over the next forty years or so, both countries developed economically and culturally, but Cuba more so. The Philippines, its population spread over 7,000 islands (although most of its people are concentrated on five large islands), consist of many different ethnic and tribal groups. Cuba, with a smaller homogeneous population, is essentially one island across which communication and governmental authority are more manageable. Thus, by the end of World War II, while average conditions of life in both countries were very poor and underdeveloped, they were somewhat better in Cuba than in the Philippines. According to the United Nations, the annual gross national product per capita around 1950 was about $160 in the Philippines and $320 in Cuba (as compared with a figure of $3,250 per capita in the United States at the time).

Although the Philippines were granted independence from the United States in 1946, American influence remained strong. Foreign investments were actively encouraged and much economic development occurred, especially in lumbering, mining, sugar, and other products for export. The Cuban economy, too, was tied to the United States, because it remained essentially dependent on the export of its sugar to the U.S. Its rate of development was lower than that in the Philippines, and government corruption under a military dictator, Batista, became rampant: as a result, a revolutionary movement developed, first among students and then among peasants, leading to the triumph of a socialist revolution led by Fidel Castro in January 1959. In the Philippines, a guerilla revolutionary movement by the Huks during the early 1950s had been started but was repressed.

Since 1946 there has been, in the Phillipines, a typical growth of free private enterprise (the capitalist model) with considerable American foreign aid and private investment. In Cuba, this pattern also prevailed until 1959, when there was the relatively abrupt change to the socialist model. The purpose of this chapter, then, is to examine, as of late 1971, the effects of the prevailing ideologies of the two countries on their health care systems.

PHILIPPINE HEALTH SERVICES

Ambulatory medical service in the Philippines is regarded mainly, or at least ideally, as a function for the private market. Thus, compared with other Asian countries like India or Indonesia, a relatively large number of doctors have been trained, yielding a strong ratio of about one doctor for every 1,500 people. There are eight medical schools training these doctors, one operated by the central government and seven private institutions. The medical classes are very large; the policy is to accept virtually any applicant (thereby collecting his tuition), failing the poor students after the first year or two, and graduating about one-third of those who enter. After graduation, a large proportion (perhaps as high as eighty percent) leave for hospital training in the United States; many never return. Although a law was passed some years ago requiring a six-month period of rural service of all new medical graduates, it was never implemented.

The vast majority of doctors are in private practice in the major Philippine cities. Because doctors compete for patients, their fees are very low. To meet rural needs, the government has established some 1,500 rural health centers, only two-thirds of which are staffed by a doctor. The scope of the centers' service, moreover, is restricted to prevention; for treatment, the patient is expected to see a private doctor or visit a congested hospital outpatient department. Since both of these resources are obviously limited in rural districts, there is still a heavy dependence in the villages on untrained primitive healers.

It is in the distribution and conditions of hospitals that one sees most dramatically the effects of private enterprise ideology on Philippine health services.

The basic figures for 1970, provided by the National Department of Health, are as shown in Table VIII.1. For the approximately 38,000,000 population of the Philippines in 1970, this consistutes about 1.0 hospital bed per 1,000 population. The government hospitals figure, however, includes 7,000 beds in one huge mental facility in Manila, the national capital, so that general hospital beds amount to 0.82 per 1,000 population.

More significant than this low overall ratio of hospital beds is their distribution in relation to the socioeconomic status of the population. A common estimate is that sixty percent of the people are so impoverished that they must depend entirely on government facilities for hospital care.[2] About thirty percent of the population are estimated to be able to pay some share of the costs of hospitalization, and the remaining ten percent presumably can afford the full costs. Relating these estimates to the above figures on hospital bed supply, we can conclude that about fifty percent of the beds (in proprietary facilities) are devoted to serving ten percent of the people who can pay the full costs. In actuality, some of this ten percent are also served in the fifteen percent of beds in voluntary nonprofit hospitals. Between sixty and ninety percent of the population must depend for their hospital care on the thirty-five percent of beds (really fewer, if the mental beds are excluded) in government facilities, although a small share of the voluntary nonprofit hospital beds are open to those who can pay some of the cost. In government hospitals, moreover, patients are charged for drugs and x-rays, if they can possibly afford to pay anything.

The result of these substantial inequities is apparent to any observer visiting the different types of hospitals. The proprietary and some of the nonprofit hospitals are half empty because they are competing for patients from the small private market. Impartial observers from the Philippine Department of Health have commented on unnecessary elective surgery being performed on private patients. Most of the patients are in semiprivate rooms of two or three beds, while single-bed private rooms are usually empty. Government hospitals, on the other hand, are typically jammed at over 100 percent of capacity, with beds in the corridors. Outpatient emergency units, intended to observe patients for a few hours, are filled with sick patients who are there for days. Maternity wards have two mothers in each bed. Surgical, laboratory, x-ray, and other such facilities are understaffed and poorly operated. Single-bed rooms for private paying patients are seen in some government hospitals, but they are usually empty.

The government hospitals may be operated at the national, provincial, or local level. At all three levels,

Table VIII.1
Distribution of hospital beds in the Philippines: 1970, by sponsorship

Hospital Sponsorship	Number	Beds	Percentage of Beds
Government	208	13,375	35
Voluntary nonprofit	36	5,671	15
Proprietary	423	18,879	50
Total	667	37,925	100

grants of ten pesos (U.S. $1.60) per bed per day are intended to be made by the national government, supplemented by support from provincial and local revenues. It is widely admitted, however, that political favoritism determines the extent that this support is actually received. Thus, a municipal hospital in the relatively affluent city of Manila is well financed and maintained, while a provincial hospital in a poor province functions under miserable conditions.

Within the sector of Philippine government hospitals, there is a theoretical plan of regionalization: the nation is divided into eight regions, which are subdivided into fifty-six provinces. The eight regional hospitals each average 120 beds; forty-three provincial hospitals average fifty-five beds; and 126 "emergency" rural-level hospitals each average thirty beds. This regionalization seems to apply to the standards for staffing each type of hospital, rather than to any administrative relationships within a network. All government hospitals report directly to a full-time regional health officer, but he has no influence over the much larger number of proprietary or voluntary units. Each of the fifty-six provinces is intended to have a provincial health officer, but his duties are limited to the preventively oriented health centers and do not include any responsibility for hospitals.

To cope with the obvious problems and inequities in hospital and medical care, the Philippine Republic enacted a law in 1969, entitled "Medicare" in obvious emulation of the United States plan. Yet unlike the U.S. program's focus on the aged, it establishes a social (compulsory) insurance program for all persons with steady employment, to help pay for their medical care. Theoretically, this includes between 2 and 3.4 million employees (there are different estimates quoted from different sources) of private industry and from 0.4 to 0.6 million government employees. Periodic contributions made by these persons (wage deductions) and their employers into a medical care fund form the source from which

payments are made for hospitalization and doctor's care on a fee basis (dependents are not to be covered initially). The fees paid for services are a flat amount (e.g., five pesos or U.S. $0.80 for a general practitioner's visit) beyond which the doctor or hospital can charge extra.

After nearly three years of procrastination, the Medicare law was finally implemented in April 1972. Although we do not yet know the degree of the program's success, a recent medical visitor indicated that insurance contributions were being received from only about one-fifth of the anticipated number of covered persons. In any event, the purpose of the law is to provide an underpinning for private medical practice and proprietary hospitals, to reduce the heavy load faced by government hospitals. This is explicitly stated by members of the Medical Care Commission (principally representative of the Philippine Medical Association) responsible for administration of the law. In October 1972, a state of national emergency, with martial law, was declared by President Marcos, implying that, along with other public services, the Philippine Medicare program was probably in trouble.

CUBAN HEALTH SERVICES

The approach to health services in Cuba reflects the socialist political philosophy as strikingly as Philippine services reflect private enterprise. Before the 1959 Revolution, most of the physicians were in private practice in the major cities, although about ten percent of the population were insured for medical care through mutual aid socieites (*mutualistas*). The great majority of the population, who were poor, received care through forty-six meagerly staffed government hospitals, some first-aid stations in Cuba's main cities, and eight maternal and child health stations for the national population of about 8.5 million people. The rural population had to be mainly dependent on traditional healers for ambulatory care or, if they were close enough to a town, on a crowded hospital outpatient department.

The revolution in health services was not achieved overnight, but the strategy from the outset (developed largely on advice from Czechoslovakia) was to make medical care a civic right for everyone. Great difficulties were encountered in the early years after the Revolution by the exodus from Cuba of about forty percent of its physicians and dentists. By 1970, however, through enlargement of the original single medical school in Havana and the creation of two additional schools, the deficit was more than made up, and Cuba now has a ratio of one doctor to about 1,100 population. All the medical schools are part of the government universities and are free to all students. There is also a large program of training nurses and other allied health personnel under the Ministry of Public Health.[3]

Because the government rapidly built up the public medical services, private practice steadily declined and has now almost disappeared. The basic facility for ambulatory care is the polyclinic, staffed by several salaried doctors, nurses, technicians, and others. There are 308 polyclinics, each serving about 30,000 people for the full range of preventive and treatment services reasonable for the ambulatory patient. Public health nurses and sanitarians also work out of the polyclinic. The next higher echelon in the health scheme is the "health region" (of which there are thirty-eight) and these fit into eight "health provinces." In very sparsely settled rural areas, furthermore, there are ninety-six medical posts, each staffed by one doctor for primary care. Other specialized units also exist for tuberculosis, dental care, and first-aid services.

The hospital network of Cuba displays striking contrast to that of the Philippines. In 1958 there were 4.4 beds per 1,000 population; in 1969, ten years after the Revolution and despite the growth of the population, there were 5.1 beds per 1,000 population. General hospitals account for seventy-two percent of the beds, with the remainder in special facilities for tuberculosis, mental disorders, cancer, and other special problems. More important, however, is the distribution of hospital beds by both type of structure and location. In the pre-Revolutionary period, a majority of the hospital beds (as in the Philippines) were in private units (*clinicas privadas*); there were 242 of these in 1958, mostly small with poor standards. However, by 1969, all but twelve of these had been converted to polyclinic buildings or to other purposes, and meanwhile many new hospitals had been built and some old ones enlarged. Altogether, there was a reduction over the first decade of the Revolution from 339 hospital structures, with an average capacity of eighty-three beds, to 219

structures with an average capacity of 190 beds. This meant a net increase from 28,236 to 41,706 hospital beds, with the rise in bed-population ratio noted above. All facilities are now governmental.

Cuban hospitals are administered at three levels: provincial, regional, and "health area," in descending size. The latter two types of hospital, as well as the polyclinics, come under the full-time director of each health region; the regional directors, in turn, report to the provincial health director, who reports to the national Minister of Health. In the reconstitution of the hospital system, there was a net increase in bed-population ratio of about fifty percent in all the rural provinces and a net reduction in the city and province of Havana.

To achieve medical staffing of all the polyclinics and hospitals in the rural districts, every new medical graduate is required to serve two years in a rural area; he is then offered a higher salary to stay on longer. Much use is also made of nurses and other auxiliary workers. All medical graduates now take an oath that they will not engage in private practice. Thus, when the output of doctors becomes great enough, all rural posts should eventually be filled through the dynamics of finding employment in an organized framework.

In sharp contrast to the Philippine pattern, in all hospitals as well as polyclinics, service is free. There are no class distinctions in access to private rooms or multiple-bed wards in the hospitals; the use of single-bed rooms depends solely on the patient's medical condition (though it is likely that, as in all countries, persons of high political influence probably can get private rooms). The equipment in Cuban hospitals is limited by U.S. standards, having become dependent on Soviet and Eastern European supplies after the U.S. embargo; however, it is better than that in the average Philippine hospital.

The cost of almost all these services is borne by the earnings of the central government from its control of industry and agriculture. Out-of-hospital drugs and certain dental services and eyeglasses must be paid for, although the prices are low and the pharmacies or other stores are operated by the government. Drugs for tuberculosis, venereal disease, maternity care, and certain other conditions are free. The whole system is still developing, and almost all hospitals, as well as the universities, are engaged in training additional health manpower.

DISCUSSION AND CONCLUSIONS

Although these are doubtless oversimplified descriptions of the health services of the Philippines and Cuba, quite aside from the overall supply of resources (facilities and personnel) which were greater in Cuba even before the Revolution, the striking differential between the two countries is the distribution of those resources and the access to them by different classes of the two populations. In the Philippine pattern there is not only extreme frugality in the public sector—and extravagance in the private sector, even to the point of unnecessary hospitalization and surgery for profit motives—but also the restriction of ambulatory care largely to preventive services in public health centers so as not to "compete" with a relatively large supply of private doctors. In Cuba, on the other hand, preventive and curative services are given together at the same polyclinics, which is not only more efficient, but also more convenient to the patient.

The crucial issue, illustrated by the comparison of these two countries, is whether health service is to be regarded as a social or human right, equally available to all, or whether it should be subject to a substantial determination by the commercial market (that is, the access to a limited supply of resources should depend on purchasing power). There are, of course, many gradations between these two ideologic poles, and neither Cuba nor the Philippines is totally at one extreme or the other. Yet there is manifest a preponderance of the market philosophy in the Philippines and the human right philosophy in Cuba. In government circles, moreover, one sees a spirit of frustration and pessimism in the Philippines, in striking contrast to the spirit of creativity and optimism observed in Cuba.

It is important to point out, nevertheless, that all countries seem to be moving toward the human right ideology in some degree; it is not just a phenomenon of socialist countries. The British National Health Service has surely established health care as a social right for everyone, although there are limitations in resources which lead a small percentage of affluent people to "break the queue" and pay privately for health care. The ultimate question is how much of a nation's resources will be channelled into the public sector—for health care, education, housing, or any other need—so that the service is available at a reasonable level, without regard to personal wealth or social status. There have been some steps in this direction in the Philippines, in the United States, and in all capitalist countries, as well as in socialist countries. In fact, health service has sufficient political appeal to be channelled toward a semisocialist model more rapidly than most other essentials of life.

NOTES

[1] Note added to article while in proof for *International Journal of Health Services*. Since submission of this paper in October 1972, numerous political changes have occurred in the Philippine Republic. According to certain international observers, these changes have resulted in a movement of the pattern of hospital services toward a more socially equitable model than that described in this paper.

[2] P. N. Mayuga, "Hospital Services in the Philippines." *World Hospitals*, Vol. 4, 1968, pp. 70-71.

[3] Milton I. Roemer, "Cuban Health Services and Resources—Transition to Socialism." Washington, D.C.: processed report to the Pan American Health Organization, March 1972.

Chapter IX
Principles of Health Services
in Socialist China

The Liberation of China, as the Chinese call the change of power and birth of the People's Republic in 1949, was surely one of the most far-reaching events of the twentieth century. After about twelve years of comradely ties with the Soviet Union, a break in friendly relations occurred, and the People's Republic of China demonstrated that socialism could develop in different nations along quite different paths. The Great Proletarian Cultural Revolution in China 1966-1970, involving a massive shake-up in Communist party leadership, brought further changes through a policy of "local self-reliance" and involvement of the "masses" in all social decisions.

These events naturally shaped the development of the structure and function of health services in modern China. Through the auspices of the General Evans Carlson Friends of the People's Republic of China, a visit was made to the P.R.C. for three weeks in April-May 1975. In this brief chapter, an attempt is made to summarize the main principles in back of the remarkable achievements of the health services in China, during the brief span of twenty-five years since its Liberation. This paper was published in the Public Health Newsletter *of the UCLA School of Public Health Alumni Association, (Summer 1975, pp. 8-11) and is reprinted here with permission.*

A three-week visit to the People's Republic of China is not a firm basis for understanding a nation of 800,000,000 people with a 4,000-year recorded history. Nor can a visit to seven cities and three rural sections provide an adequate sample of a nation larger than the United States, with some twenty-seven provinces or "autonomous regions," over 2,000 counties, and countless diversities in ethnicity, culture, and geography.

But ten books have already been published in English about the health services in modern China, and these, along with scores of articles on special apsects of health and medicine, and many other volumes on the overall scene, provide one with orientation that permits better interpretation of observations in the People's Republic itself and discussions with its health workers.[1]

FROM "BITTER PAST" TO HAPPY PRESENT

Regardless of one's personal philosophy, a visit to modern socialist China seems to make a profound impression on everyone—on the delegation of officials of the American Medical Association last year, no less than on our group of General Evans Carlson Friends of the People's Republic of China in April-May 1975. For almost everyone knows that until twenty-five years ago, China was probably the most destitute nation on earth—a land of massive misery, endemic malnutrition with periodic famines in which millions died, rampant infectious disease, filth, widespread opium addiction, prostitution, slavery—every suffering known to mankind. By comparison, neighboring India was well off.

Today, in China one sees a people giving every evidence of happiness, good health, unity, dignity, and a passionate sense of purpose to move forward. Hunger is gone, along with the pestilential diseases (smallpox, cholera, and plague), opium addiction and venereal disease have been wiped out, everyone is employed—or if disabled is cared for—rates of death and birth are both greatly reduced, and virtually everyone has access to medical care.

Explanation of these remarkable achievements can hardly be given in a few paragraphs, but it is not an oversimplification to say that its roots lie in the incredible dedication of the Chinese Communist party (about 20,000,000 members or 2.5 percent of the population) and its brilliant leader, Mao Tsetung. Small wonder that statues and pictures of Chairman Mao are seen everywhere, in a peasant family's small bedroom no less than in front of virtually every public building. Westerners may find it annoying to see a living man made into a god-figure, but he is no less an inspiration and the symbol of a whole system of values than the cross or the flag in our country. As Chairman Mao said to American journalist Edgar Snow, he did not like this "cult of personality," but it seemed to serve a positive purpose for the present period.

BASIC HEALTH SERVICE PRINCIPLES AND THEIR APPLICATION

The Chinese like to summarize major policies in brief slogans, and two of the most important are "Politics in Command" and "Serve the People." In the health services, evidence of these policies is apparent at every turn. Soon after Liberation, as the Chinese designate the Revolution of 1949, Mao summarized Party policy in the health sector as: (1) serve the workers, peasants, and soldiers; (2) prevention first; (3) unite traditional and Western medicine; and (4) combine health service with the mass movement. In part, these principles were probably influenced by the Soviet Union, but after the break with Soviet communism occurred (1960-1962), Mao broadcast a fifth principle in 1965: (5) in health and medical work put the stress on the rural areas. The Great Proletarian Cultural Revolution (G.P.C.R.) broke out in 1966, lasting to 1970, and added two further principles to the whole society, with special meaning in the health services: (6) fight against bureaucracy; and (7) promote local self-reliance.

In practice these seven principles have enormous implications for health, but only a few examples can be cited here. *Serving the workers, peasants, and soldiers*—or the people—has meant that there is today no private, commercial medical practice; all health workers are civil servants on modest salaries. All hospitals, pharmacies, and other facilities are public entities. Economic support of all resources is mainly through collective mechanisms (government revenues, social insurance, or cooperatives), but at this point there are still charges, though very low, for some services. The plan is to collectivize all support as soon as feasible.

Prevention first has been the principle behind mass immunization campaigns (against smallpox, poliomyelitis, diphtheria, etc.), closing down all VD-spreading brothels and rehabilitation of prostitutes, prohibition of the growing of poppies or the sale of opium, reconstruction of canals and burying of snails to tackle schistosomiasis, and awards for destruction of the "four pests:" flies, mosquitoes, bedbugs, and rats. These "patriotic health campaigns" enlist the promotional help of the masses—women's groups, young pioneer youth, workers, peasants, and soldiers of the People's Liberation Army (P.L.A.). Prevention also includes family planning, for which information, pills, and devices are distributed at all levels down to the barefoot doctor health stations; birth rates are also kept down by promotion of late marriage (twenty-eight years for males, twenty-five for females) and severe social disapproval of premarital sex. Abortion, nevertheless, is readily available.

The call to *unite traditional and Western medicine* may seem to many of us less rational than the other principles, but one must recognize that before Liberation the great majority of China's hundreds of millions of people had simply no access to modern, scientific medical care. With "politics in command," it was important for the new government to assure that everyone had access to health care. This meant that traditional doctors, with their herbals, acupuncture, and moxibustion, must be used to serve the people. By "uniting with Western medicine," the strategy has been to cull out those elements of ancient Chinese healing which are effective and discard what is not. We all know that ephedrine, the staple of sympatho-mimetic drugs in Western medicine, came from Chinese herbalism, and more recently acupuncture anesthesia has appeared like a miracle before Western observers. The whole unification process is gradual and will doubtless take many forms in the years ahead.

The fourth principle about *combining medicine with the mass movement* has already been mentioned in the preventive campaigns. It is also embodied in the implementation of the fifth principle on *stressing the rural areas*. To apply this approach, China developed a radically new conception of a health worker. In the country's 27,000 communes (20,000 to 60,000 people each), where eighty percent of the people live in agricultural pursuits, how was day-to-day primary health care to be provided? The "barefoot doctor" was the answer—a young peasant, male or female, who was given a three- to six-month training course in the rudiments of hygiene and first aid. He or she would continue to work in the fields one-third to two-thirds of the time (depending on local circumstances). The other time would be spent on health work, preventive and curative. Cases beyond his (her) skill would be sent to a health center or hospital staffed by "regular doctors." Every year additional training would be given for a week or two, either from a city-doctor coming to the village or by going to the nearest hospital. Over a million of these part-time health workers have been trained, and they serve each of the ten to twenty production brigades (of 500 to 3,000 peasants each) which make up a commune. The great majority of communes have a cooperative health fund to pay the barefoot doctors and support other expenses, like medications or the admission of someone to a hospital. Urban industrial workers are protected by a social insurance fund.

Finally, the principles of *fighting against bureaucracy* and *encouraging local self-reliance,* which gained special force after the G.P.C.R., have come markedly to distinguish the Chinese health system from its initial Soviet model. Instead of centralized planning and uniform operations through a hierarchy of authorities, the prevailing theme is decentralization. It is also egalitarianism. Just as army officers wear no insignia and all military men are dressed alike, so also in hospitals there are no symbols to distinguish doctors from nurses or other health workers. Teamwork is the rule in patient care. There are no national norms for the supply of doctors or hospital beds in an area; it is left up to each commune or urban district, as it sees its needs. To maximize the output of doctors, while also reducing elitism, training in China's eighty medical schools has been reduced from five years (after middle school) to three years—only a year longer than the training of a nurse or technician.

THE OVERALL HEALTH ADMINISTRATIVE STRUCTURE

Not that China's governmental administration lacks structure. At the central level is the Council of State, containing the Minister of Health—currently a woman, incidentally. Responsible to the Minister is the health department or bureau of each province. Each of the counties (averaging about seventy-five per province) has a health bureau, which is administratively responsible for all hospitals and health centers within it. But this responsibility, both upward and downward on the organization chart, is described as not authoritarian but advisory, and designed to be helpful in achieving local goals. Within

the county are communes and municipalities. (Three large cities—Peking, Shanghai, and Tientsin—come directly under the national government, like the provinces.) All the approximately fourteen communes per county are served by a county hospital of 200 to 300 beds—usually in the largest city. The commune itself is typically served by a health center staffed with "regular doctors" and a few short-term or transfer beds. Within the commune are the ten to twenty production brigades, noted earlier, which support the barefoot doctors in small health stations. In cities the subdivisions are districts, which in a metropolis like Shanghai (10,000,000 total population) may average 900,000 people each. Within each district are "neighborhoods" of 40,000 to 70,000, served usually by a general hospital, and equivalent, in a sense, to the rural commune. In each district are "lanes" of 1,000 to 8,000 persons each, corresponding to the rural production brigade and served by the urban equivalent of the barefoot doctor. The most local functional unit in the rural areas is the "production team" of fifty to 300 people or, in the cities, the "work group" of fifty to 150; no special health unit operates at this level.

How is this enormous pyramidal structure tied together, so that China functions as the cohesive, unified nation that everyone can observe? I am not certain that I know the full answer, but it seems to be by the Chinese Communist party, which—through literature, conferences, and periodicals—is guided by the "thoughts of Chairman Mao." These "thoughts" (note that the translation is not "directives" nor "commands" nor even "guidelines") include the seven principles explained above. The interpretation and application of these principles is left up to the leadership at each of the five levels described. This leadership, at each level (that is, central, provincial, county, brigade, and production team in rural areas, and their urban equivalents) consists of a Revolutionary committee, headed not by a chairman but by a "responsible member," as it is translated. About eighty percent of the fifteen to twenty persons on each Revolutionary committee belong to the Communist party, and the "responsible member" is invariably a dedicated Communist.

The Revolutionary committees at each level are said also to represent three groupings: the political cadres, the technically skilled workers, and the P.L.A.; at the same time they are selected to represent the young, the middle-aged, and the old. The responsible member of the Revolutionary committee of a county health bureau, for example, would not necessarily be one of the doctors who, in medical school, has had specialized training in "public health;" rather he would be the most politically reliable and respected member. Likewise, the "responsible member" of the Revoluntionary committee of a hospital might be a veteran nurse or kitchen worker as likely as a doctor. In both examples, appropriately trained doctors would always be on the committee, and decisions are reached by majority vote. There are countless meetings at which decisions are made and policies formulated. As the Chinese quip goes, "before Liberation we had oppression; since Liberation we have meetings."

This sketchy account may serve only to suggest the contours of socialist China's health service system. It is a system in which the health workers appear to be hard-working, devoted, and optimistic. Above all, they radiate—like all the people one sees in China—a certain dignity which says: "We know we are still a poor country; we have a long way to go; but we are on the road, the socialist road; and we know which way we are marching."

NOTES

[1] Joshua S. Horn, *Away with all Pests: An English Surgeon in People's China 1954-1969*. New York & London: Monthly Review Press, 1969.

Medical Workers Serving the People Wholeheartedly. Peking: Foreign Languages Press, 1971.

Population Crisis Committee, *Population and Family Planning in the People's Republic of China.* Washington, D.C.: Victor-Bostrom Fund, 1971.

Joseph R. Quinn (ed.), *Medicine and Public Health in the People's Republic of China.* Washington, D.C.: Fogarty International Center for Advanced Study in the Health Sciences, June 1972.

R. O. Whyte, *Rural Nutrition in China.* New York: Oxford University Press, 1972.

Committee on Scholarly Communications with the People's Republic of China, *Report of the Medical Delegation to the People's Republic of China.* Washington, D.C.: National Academy of Sciences, 1973.

Victor W. Sidel and Ruth Sidel, *Serve the People: Observations on Medicine in the People's Republic of China*, New York: Josiah Macy, Jr. Foundation, 1973.

Myron E. Wegman, Tsung-yi Lin, and Elizabeth F. Purcell (eds.), *Public Health in the People's Republic of China.* New York: Josiah Macy, Jr. Foundation, 1973.

Topics of Study Interest in Medicine and Public Health in the People's Republic of China. Washington, D.C.: Fogarty International Center for Advanced Studies in the Health Sciences, November 1973.

Leo A. Orleans, *Health Policies and Services in China, 1974.* Washington, D.C.: U.S. Senate Subcommittee on Health of the Committee on Labor and Public Welfare, March 1974.

Part Three

Industrialized Countries

Chapter X
Health Service Systems
in Western Europe: Great Britain, Sweden, Switzerland, and France

In Western Europe, the Industrial Revolution and the rise of a politically conscious working class led to social organization of health services much earlier than in America. Social insurance to support the cost of physician's services, public hospitals for most of the population, public health protection applied everywhere in a nation—these and other social programs have made health services available much more widely, without financial obstacles to the individual. The political and economic setting has given a different character also to professional education, medical practice, and hospital administration than characterizes these fields in the more individualistic and laissez faire American scene.

A study was made of European health service patterns in 1950 through visits to four countries. The British National Health Service was then in operation only two years, and other changes characterized the French, Swedish, and Swiss systems in the wake of World War II. In the succeeding twenty-five years, of course, further changes have occurred—such as the conversion of Swedish health insurance in 1956 from voluntary to universal coverage and the integration of the three parts of British National Health Service in 1974 through a network of local health areas. Greater regionalization of hospital facilities, widened coverage of the health insurance programs, increases in health manpower, and more systematic quality surveillance have occurred in all these countries. Yet the main organizational features evident in 1950 remain generally the same today. The American patterns, with which the European are inevitably compared, have probably changed even more than the European, becoming more like theirs—as seen, for example, in the enactment of mandatory health insurance for the aged in 1965, comprehensive health planning in 1966, and the generally expanded role of government in all health affairs. This account of health service patterns in four Western European countries was published as "Health Service Organization in Western Europe" in the Milbank Memorial Fund Quarterly *(Vol. 29, April 1951, pp. 139-164) and is reprinted here by permission.*[1]

So much of America's cultural heritage derives from Europe that it is small wonder that health workers in the United States have been interested in developments there. Social trends in the Old World have so often marked out the paths of change in the New World that a study of the organization and problems of European health services can shed much light on the meaning of events in the United States. It was with this motivation that a party of fourteen American professional people undertook a brief but intensive study of health service organization in England, Sweden, Switzerland, and France, during the summer of 1950.[2]

EUROPE'S SOCIAL BACKGROUND

A few simple, basic facts about Europe have tremendous impact on health service organization. Some of these are so obvious to the American visitor that their great importance may be overlooked.

First, relative to the United States, Europe is old. The organization of society toward the solution of individual problems has proceeded for centuries; collective efforts have grown more extensively than here in every field. Leaving aside the full-blown communism of Eastern Europe, the economies of Western Europe have become increasingly planned. In Great Britain there is the vast domestic program of the Labour party, involving national ownership and operation of transportation, public utilities, coal mining, and now the basic steel industry. In Sweden, cooperatives have been a basic feature of the economy—in both the production and consumption of goods—for over a century. In Switzerland, cooperatives have also figured prominently and the all-important transportation system is nationalized. In both these countries, cooperative nonprofit exterprises are fostered and subsidized by government. In France, the individualistic tradition runs deeper, but there is still a system of social security far more sweeping than ours.

Second, relative to the economy of the United States, Europe is poor. Its natural resources in land, metals, timber, chemicals, coal, oil, and (except for Soviet Russia) manpower are much smaller than ours. For centuries most of its nations have depended on the exploitation of "underdeveloped" areas of the earth, and colonial empires have been fading away. National rivalries have long stifled the development of free trade, and currently the East-West political conflict has added new barriers to the exchange of raw materials and manufactured products. European cities, industries, homes, and people have been devastated by two World Wars in a generation, not to mention the centuries of lesser wars before these. By comparison the wastage and destruction of American resources caused by wars have been trivial.

Third, relative to the United States, Europe is small. Millions live in areas which on this side of the Atlantic contain only thousands. While there are sharp differences in nationalities and national traits, people are thrown together. A few hours' travel brings one into another nation and another culture. As a result, there is an extremely active exchange of ideas. People love to talk; the "strong, silent type" is not so popular. Arguments are not regarded as impolite, but as stimulating; yet there is great courtesy and it seems genuine. In this setting, although the force of tradition is great, new ideas grow rapidly— ideas in art, science, philosophy, and politics.

Fourth, relative to the United States, Europe has suffered. In recent years, virtually every family has been struck by tragedy. The suffering has been so deep and has affected so many millions of people that there is a demand for security far greater than in the United States. Europeans look for compensations to their sufferings and their discomforts through art, music, literature, travel, wine, good conversation. But they also seek various forms of assurance of economic security, through collective action. It is this search that leads Europeans now to various social programs, including measures for medical care. The suffering of Europeans has made them politically mature; the percentage of the population voting in elections is far higher than anywhere in the United States. The average citizen is sensitive to political issues, reflecting as they do social problems and collective ways of meeting them.

It is against this social background of Europe's relative age, its small size, its poverty, and its suffering that one must view and evaluate the structure and trends of health service organization. Observers who evaluate European medicine on the basis of bland comparisons with American medicine give conclusions no more scientifically accurate than an evaluation of the attributes of two plants without regard to the climate and soil in which they grew.

ECONOMIC SUPPORT FOR MEDICAL SERVICES

Throughout Great Britain, Sweden, Switzerland, and France, the economic support for medical and related services has become predominantly (though not entirely) socialized. The term "socialized" is used in its broad sense to mean: organized by group action, whether governmental or voluntary. It encompasses governmentally controlled financing whether by the device of social insurance or general taxation. Historically considered, these various forms of group financing—that is: voluntary insurance, compulsory insurance, and general revenue support—vary only in degree, each representing collective rather than individual economic arrangements, and one form leading frequently into the other. Only a minority fraction of total medical care costs remain to be borne through personal, individual responsibility in Western Europe.

Yet, there are great differences in the approach to the social support of medical care costs. Great Britain, after a limited program of social insurance from 1911 to 1948 (financing general practitioner services for employed workers), has now gone farthest in socialized financing—almost as far as Soviet Russia and the countries of Eastern Europe. Virtually all medical services for the entire population are financed collectively; about ninety percent through general revenues and ten percent through social insurance. In Sweden and in Switzerland, there are combinations of widespread voluntary insurance financing through local plans and general revenue support, somewhat along the lines of recent legislative proposals in the United States. In France there is a combination of national compulsory insurance and general revenue support.

Important distinctions must be made in the description of the financial support for hospital services, as against ambulatory medical care. The proportion of general revenue support for the former tends to be much greater than for the latter. As will be seen, the entire sphere of hospital services, including both the financing and the pattern of organization of professional services, has been subjected to much more social control than have the services of physicians in the home or office. Ambulatory care is associated more with the individual entrepreneur and contributory insurance financing.

The line between governmental and voluntary group action is much less sharp in Europe than in the United States. In Sweden and Switzerland, for example, the insurance plans for physician's care are voluntary.[3] The plans are organized on an area basis, rather than by occupation or industry, and administration is in local nongovernmental hands. But these plans are heavily subsidized by government, in Sweden by the national government and in Switzerland by the canton or state governments. In Sweden, the premiums for membership in voluntary "sickness funds" are fixed (not varying with the subscriber's income), but about fifty percent of the total costs of benefits is supported by government grants; this allows premiums to be quite low, offering little impediment to the enrollment of low income persons. As a condition for receiving these grants, the plans are closely supervised by the government with respect to their rules of eligibility, extent of benefits, administrative procedures, and so on.

The voluntary insurance plans give substantial but not complete protection against the cost of medical care. In Sweden they encompass only about seventy percent of the population and in Switzerland about the same. There are various restrictions to membership, similar to those of voluntary plans in this country; the Stockholm plan, for instance, excludes initial enrollment of persons over fifty years of age and denies benefits for the care of preexisting conditions. The full cost of physician's care, moreover, is not provided. In Sweden and Switzerland, the plans indemnify the beneficiary for two-thirds or three-quarters of the doctor's fees (for home and office service) according to government-approved fee schedules. Even in France, where the insurance is compulsory and nationwide for all employed workers, the social security fund reimburses the worker for about eighty percent of medical and hospital fees; in practice, it often amounts to less than this since doctors are permitted to charge fees in excess of the established schedules. Requirement of these partial payments by the patient is designed to discourage abuses, but it may discourage the procurement of needed services by low income families. Only in Great Britain is there complete freedom from financial impediments to medical care.

It is especially interesting to American observers to discover that voluntary insurance plan directors in Sweden have no objection to a system of compulsory enrollment. They would actually prefer it, believing that only in this way could protection be given to the entire population. Many healthy young people—good insurance risks—now fail to join plans, thereby compelling restrictions on "bad risk" persons for actuarial reasons. Compulsory enrollment requirements would not drive the voluntary plans out of business, but would give them a larger job to do, as was the case in the earliest compulsory health insurance program in Germany (since 1883) and in England from 1911 to 1948.

The present coverage of the social security program in France is a great extension over the prewar program, covering the entire employed population in the cities and their dependents. A separate comprehensive health insurance program covers agricultural workers, but all self-employed persons must depend on voluntary insurance. Since the war, Sweden too has passed a law which would encompass not only employed workers but the entire population under a compulsory health insurance scheme. The law was to have been effective in July 1950, was postponed to July 1951, but now has been further postponed indefinitely.[4] The law would levy a small fixed insurance tax on all persons, regardless of income, but most of the cost would be borne by general revenues. It is now felt that the cost would be excessive and the nation cannot "afford it." Is this attitude related to the fact that Sweden did not take part in the Second World War and that its people did not suffer? Great Britain also knew that its National Health Service would be expensive—and it proved even costlier than anticipated; yet the money has been appropriated without any significant opposition. The British people had suffered greatly and the demand for health security was enormous—enough to justify, in British opinion, the extremely high taxes involved.

HOSPITALIZATION AND AMBULATORY CARE

The social organization of hospital services in Europe has proceeded along very different lines from that in America. In the United States, the general hospital has been in the main an extension of the private practice of medicine. It has been regarded largely as the "doctor's workshop" where the physician takes his private patients who are seriously sick. In the average American community, the great majority of doctors have "hospital privileges." This has been undergoing gradual change here, with the crystallization of the specialties and tightening of hospital staff organization, the extension of governmental institutions, the development of great teaching centers and regional hospital plans, and so on. In most towns, however, the general hospital is still a part of the world of private medical practice.

In Europe, from the beginning hospitals have been predominantly public institutions. In Sweden and in Switzerland, nearly all hospital beds are in institutions owned, operated, and largely financed by units of government, usually local authorities. In France, while there are many voluntary institutions, most of the general hospital beds are in public facilities. Moreover, the voluntary hospitals have operated very much the way public hospitals do here, the great majority of their patients getting "ward care" paid for by combinations of insurance, general revenue, and charity. In England, long before the National Health Service Act, the proportion of general beds in governmental hospitals exceeded that in voluntary institutions and was continuing to rise; the pattern of care in voluntary hospitals was like that in France. Since July 1948, virtually all British hospitals have come under complete governmental control. Being costly, general hospital services in Europe have been largely assumed as a public responsibility, like grade school education or, indeed, hospital care for tuberculosis and mental disorder in the United States.

With the overwhelmingly public character of European hospitals, medical staff organization is naturally quite different from that in America. In Great Britain and Sweden, nearly all medical and surgical services in the hospitals are rendered by organized staffs of salaried specialists. This is hard for many American physicians to believe, so closely is the hospital tied to private fee-for-service medicine in our country. In France and Switzerland this is not the general rule, although a growing proportion of inpatient care in the governmental general hospitals is performed by salaried men. When professional services in the hospital are rendered by specialists in France or Switzerland, the average patient seldom pays a private surgical or medical fee. A general payment is made to the hospital—usually from the insurance system—and the physician is paid a relatively small honorarium (part-time salary).

Only a small percentage of physicians have any direct access to the hospitals, either governmental or voluntary. The patient is cared for by the physician who is "on service" at the time, as in the average ward service in the United States.

The sharp separation of general practitioners, constituting the majority of physicians, from the hospitals is a source of dismay to many American observers. The "closed staff" is far more tightly closed than here. From the viewpoint of maintaining a high level of medical performance in the general practitioner, his isolation from the stimulating influence of the hospital is surely unfortunate. But there is a good side to it: the level of professional work in the hospitals is high. As a rule only well qualified specialists render service and there is assurance that the patient is getting expert care. Patients do not seem to object to the loss of free choice of doctor that hospitalization and care by a specialist usually mean. A small proportion of people, perhaps less than five percent, insist on free choice of specialist and can pay the private fees for care rendered, usually in a "nursing home," outside the public medical system or the insurance system. Most important, the European patient seldom if ever has to avoid needed hospitalization because of the institutional and professional costs involved.

In Sweden, the public hospital system is particularly well developed. Less tied to tradition than England or the continent, Sweden has erected some of the most magnificently functional hospital structures in the world. About ninety percent of the cost of service is borne by the tax funds of the Swedish cities or counties, and only ten percent by the patient. This ten percent charge, moreover, is usually paid for the patient by his voluntary insurance society, or if he is indigent, by a welfare agency. Yet, in the new Swedish hospitals one does not see huge wards with impersonal management of cases. In the great South Hospital, Stockholm's newest, the largest wards contain four beds and there are many rooms with only one and two beds. The choice of a room is not made by the patient, in proportion to his affluence, but by the doctor, on the basis of the medical needs of the case. All services are rendered by salaried specialists and an active research program is conducted. These policies symbolize the general trend of hospital services in Europe.

Despite this high degree of organization of hospital services, physician's home and office care in Europe is rendered predominantly along individualistic lines. While the insurance systems have organized economic support collectively, the pattern of care for ambulatory patients is based on private office practice. Polyclinics attached to hospitals are busy because patients can get specialist services in them without paying the charges left uncovered by insurance benefits (since indemnification is eighty percent or less in France, Switzerland, and Sweden). The great bulk of care for ambulatory illness, however, is rendered by family doctors who receive private fees for each unit of service. In Great Britain, general practitioners are paid on a capitation basis and practice in private offices, even though financial support is almost entirely from general revenues.

PUBLIC HEALTH ADMINISTRATION

Administratively, the organized programs of medical care—both hospital and ambulatory—are quite separate and distinct from public health activities. The governmental or voluntary agencies responsible for supervision of the medical care or social insurance programs are different from those providing preventive health services. Theoretically, this seems unfortunate, but it follows from the separate historical origins of the two movements. Medical care insurance programs grew from the experience and demands of the labor movement; social security was a response to the insecurity of the industrial worker dependent on wages and faced always with the hazard of unemployment. Hospitals sprang from the public welfare movement, an outgrowth of monasteries and almshouses for the care of the sick poor; they were part of the charitable tradition of Christianity to help the unfortunate. Public health, on the other hand, had foundations in general community development, as urbanization created problems of crowding and spread of communicable disease. It was not tied so closely to the labor movement or to charitable efforts for the poor. While the early public health thinking, prior to about 1870, was motivated by efforts to improve the lot of the lower economic classes (Frank in Italy, Chadwick in England, Pettenkofer in Germany)—including improvement of housing and working conditions—after the rise of bacteriology, it acquired more technical foundations in engineering, immunology, statistics, and legal restraints.

As a result, it is not surprising that public health services, hospital services, and health insurance should have generally distinct administrative frameworks. This is unfortunate because certain opportunities are lost for preventive medicine. The insurance programs have become largely fiscal operations, with few active measures to prevent disease, and the hospitals likewise do little by way of case finding (tuberculosis, venereal disease), health education, or other preventive services. Yet, despite the administrative dichotomy, the basically preventive

value of any medical care program should not be overlooked. The elimination of economic barriers to early medical attention has great preventive value, especially in the control of chronic illness. Considering the overwhelming importance of the chronic, degenerative diseases, compared with the acute infections, programs providing easy access to medical and hospital care in Europe, as well as in America, have perhaps greater preventive value than anything else within present knowledge.

A partial exception to the dichotomy of public health and medical care administration is found in Great Britain, where at the national level all health services are centralized in the Ministry of Health. The unity virtually stops here, however, for at the local level throughout Britain, the administration of medical care and public health under the National Health Service is divided among four separate agencies. Public health services are administered by the local medical officers of health, as prior to the National Health Service Act; general medical and dental practitioner services are administered by newly organized local executive councils; hospitals and specialist services are under regional hospital boards; and the large teaching hospitals (associated with medical schools) have a separate administrative framework. While the local medical officer of health makes some effort to coordinate services, it is obviously difficult under such separations of authority. Critics of the unwieldy caaracter of the National Health Service organization sometimes overlook the fact that this divided system was not the wish of the government and especially not that of the Ministry of Health. It was set up in this way to satisfy the demands of special professional groups: the general practitioners of medicine and dentistry, the specialists, and the medical educators. Compromise yielded complexity in administration and correction of the problems would require a more radical, rather than a more conservative approach.[5]

In Sweden, while public health and health insurance programs are administered by separate agencies, there is some integration of preventive and treatment services at the point of delivery of clinical care in rural areas. The great problem of attracting doctors to the rural stretches of Sweden has been tackled through a system of rural medical officers. These physicians are paid a governmental salary for providing public health services—such as immunizations, school health examinations, operation of well-baby clinics, attendance of communicable disease cases, etc.—and for treating the poor. They may also engage in private and insurance practice. One of these rural medical officers is available for about every 3,000 to 5,000 people. While this seems like a poor ratio in terms of American standards, the effectiveness of the Swedish physician is extended greatly by three circumstances: (1) an excellent system of public health nurses (about one per 2,500 people—far more than we have in the United States nationally) for home visiting and auxiliary medical services; (2) a much greater supply of hospital beds, both rural and urban, than in America, saving the doctor considerable travel time; and (3) coverage of larger population units of about 75,000 with full-time "county" public health officers for sanitary, administrative, organizational, and educational duties.

To risk a large generalization, public health activities in Europe seem to be deeper than in the United States, though not so broad. The public health agencies do fewer things, but they do them more completely. English and French well-baby clinics, for example, are said to reach eighty percent of the infants born in their areas. In the United States, an excellent program may reach twenty percent of the babies, the rest being seen by private physicians or getting no systematic attention at all. The same sort of general comparison applies to tuberculosis and venereal disease control activities. On the other hand, the variety of programs promoted in the United States, at least in the better developed public health jurisdictions, is not found in Europe. In the four countries visited, the public health agencies do little in health education, mental hygiene, industrial hygiene, and chronic disease control (cancer, heart disease, or diabetes detection); mass case-finding surveys of all kinds are not so common as here. The reason may be that these personal health services are regarded as within the scope of clinical medicine, already more or less available through health insurance. In the United States, there is much evidence that the broad interests of public health agencies in new fields—especially the chronic diseases—are partly a result of pressures for organized medical care programs not being adequately met in other ways.

The thoroughness of much public health activity in Europe is due in part to a stronger "police power" tradition than characterizes American health work. Nontreatment of venereal disease for example, is usually a crime, punishable by imprisonment. In England, school health services are provided for every schoolchild in the land, since every school authority is compelled by national law to provide such services. Mandatory legislation of this type, even on a state-wide basis, is unknown in the United States. Because of the same legal tradition, the whole field of housing sanitation is far better developed as a public health function in Europe. Health departments in Great Britain, Sweden, and France inspect rented dwellings and can prosecute violations. On the other hand, public sanitation functions, like supervision of the water supply or the pasteurization of milk, are not so well developed on the Continent as in America. In France, one cannot be sure whether the water and milk supplies get inadequate protection because of the engineering costs involved or because of the terrific importance of a third beverage; even Coca-Cola was sacrificed for the welfare of the wine industry.

The administration of public health in France is strangely divided between two official agencies in each community: the public office of social hygiene and the office of public health. The former agency conducts personal health service programs like venereal disease control, tuberculosis control, and maternal and child health work. The latter handles environmental sanitation, statistics, laboratory services, quarantine, and medico-legal work. At the ministry level these are united, but in the local communities they are separate because of their historic origins. While this may seem peculiar to Americans, it is perhaps no more bizarre than the dispersion of administrative responsibility for health services among scores of governmental and voluntary agencies in this country. In one West Virginia county the writer found 155 separate agencies, governmental and voluntary, to be involved in organized health services for either the prevention or treatment of disease. In Europe, the frequent practice of governmental subsidy and partial supervision of voluntary agencies—for example in tuberculosis and child health work—assures teamwork between private and public action.

PROFESSIONAL EDUCATION

Medical education is quite different in Europe from that in the United States. To understand the differences, one should trace the doctor's training from its childhood beginnings in the primary grades, for the content of primary and secondary schooling in Europe differs appreciably from that in America. While it varies in different countries, it is generally believed that by the completion of high school (twelfth school year), the European student has had training equivalent to the first two years of college in this country. Then, following secondary school, medicine usually requires one continuous program for six or seven years, rather than four years of college followed by four years of medical school. One of the striking differences within this system is that clinical work usually starts earlier; almost from the beginning the student sees patients. This may have the effect of integrating theory and practice more successfully than is often the case here. The European student may see his patient more "as a whole" than does the American student who meets his patient only after years of pure theory in the lecture hall and laboratory, and then quite naturally views him merely as an example of some pathological process.

With this approach in medical education, it is not surprising that the role of the teaching hospitals is relatively even greater than here. Most of the teaching throughout the six years is done at the hospitals and one university, like the University of London or the University of Paris, may contain several medical schools, each associated with a separate hospital. As a result of his training, the English, French, Swedish, or Swiss physician may be more empirical in his practice, less well grounded in solid scientific theory. In France, this is complicated further by the fact that a majority of graduates do not have a period of postgraduate hospital training, equivalent to our internships and residencies.

Despite the great development of social services in Europe, the teaching of public health and preventive medicine seems to be less well developed than even in American medical schools. Little formal instruction is given in public health, which is regarded chiefly as a postgraduate subject to be studied in one of the schools of hygiene. It may be that the physician is expected to learn public health medicine from experience, as soon as he is in practice. Likewise little or no instruction is given to the undergraduate in the theory or operation of health insurance programs, perhaps because this represents elementary "civics" taught in secondary schools and experienced in everyday life. The teaching of "social medicine" consists mainly of instruction on the effects of poverty, poor housing, heredity, malnutrition, etc. in the epidemiology of specific diseases, rather than discussion of organized programs of medical care. In the graduate schools of hygiene or public health, American observers are surprised to find almost exclusively physicians, and virtually none of the nurses, engineers, health educators, statisticians, and others who constitute a major portion of the enrollment in American schools of public health.

Throughout Europe, and especially in Great Britain, the midwife has a respectable and integral place in medical service. A large portion of deliveries in the home have long been performed by women trained in midwifery and doing a good quality of work. Physicians are called for difficult cases, but the availability of the midwife for the normal obstetrical case has helped to compensate for Europe's relative shortage of physicians. With increasing hospitalization of maternity cases, the role of the midwife has changed, but even in hospitals most normal deliveries are done by nurse-midwives (except in primiparae). The arm of the physician is extended also by nurses, who perform a wider range of medical tasks in the hospital and in the patient's home than is conventionally permitted in the United States. In Sweden, it is commonplace for nurses to discuss the management of cases with physicians, and Swedish nurses visiting American hospitals are surprised at the subordinate role of their American counterparts. In France, the emphasis on psychological and sociological viewpoints in the training of the nurse is heartening. Nurses going into public health work receive training equivalent to one year of social work and all French social workers receive the equivalent of one year's training in nursing.

THE QUALITY OF MEDICAL SERVICE IN EUROPE

The previous discussion, while far from an adequate account of health service organization in Great Britain, Sweden, Switzerland, and France, may help to provide a background for evaluation of European medical care compared with American. It is very often said that the quality of medicine deteriorates under governmental medical care programs—whether insurance- or tax-supported—and the evidence often offered is that "medicine in Europe has gone downhill." This is a serious and damaging charge, but it is difficult to find corroboration of it among responsible bodies of European physicians. Individual European practitioners have broadcast unfavorable descriptions of perfunctory work done in the office of a doctor working under compulsory insurance legislation, but the professional societies, the academies, and the teaching centers do not confirm these accounts as a fair picture of general conditions.

While European medicine, on the average, has probably not deteriorated, it cannot be denied that it has failed to advance as rapidly as has American medicine. Europe, once the world center of medical science, has given way to the United States; American medicine, once weak, has in many respects come to surpass European medicine in technical excellence. The meaning of such comparisons, however, is deceptive. How much are these evaluations influenced by the quality of work done in the great teaching centers of the two continents and how much by a sober evaluation of the level and scope of service available to the average citizen, rich, poor, and in-between?

Much of America's technical superiority is due to our research programs. We are doing more research in almost all fields of medicine and public health than is any European country. Research costs money and we have more to spend. Great fortunes have been accumulated in the United States, yielding large philanthropic research endowments; industrial profits have made possible huge research programs under commercial auspices; government has increasingly subsidized research with tax funds. We have not been impoverished by the ravages of two World Wars. Yet we must be humble when we realize that even in recent years—let alone in past decades—some of the most important discoveries in medicine and public health have come from Europe: sulfanilamide from Germany, penicillin from England, and DDT from Switzerland.

If we attempt to focus, nevertheless, on the quality of medical service available to the average European, what can be said? There are undoubtedly many real problems; most of them relate to the conditions of general office practice, rather than hospital service. The insurance programs have enabled large numbers of people to have access to a doctor's office, but what happens to them when they enter the door? Keeping always in mind that a smaller proportion of Americans enter the doctor's office at all, those that do are likely to receive a better medical examination than does the average European. X-ray and laboratory work is less likely to be done for the European. Most, though not all, doctors are pressed for time. A quick prescription may be handed out in order to make room for the next patient. The doctor may lack interest in keeping informed on the latest scientific developments and may send his patient off to the hospital if a problem of the slightest complexity arises.

These criticisms of European medicine are frequently made by American observers. The same applies, however, to much general medical practice in the United States, especially for the 60,000,000 people living in rural areas and for the millions more living in the crowded slums of our big cities. These problems are substantially the result of a high demand for service relative to the medical manpower available. Whenever the effective demand for service exceeds the supply of medical time, perfunctory care may result. The situation is complicated further by the sharp separation between the office and hospital practice of medicine. But are these problems a result of the insurance and public medical care programs in Europe?

SHORTAGE OF MEDICAL PERSONNEL

To gain an understanding of the qualitative problems of European medicine, it is necessary to view it against its total economic and historical setting. Why is there a relatively insufficient supply of doctors in Europe? The supply of doctors in a nation basically is economically determined. A nation can support only a certain number of physicians with the money it has to spend on physician's care, relative to other needs of daily living. If the number of doctors is increased beyond the economic capacity to support them, doctors will not survive and men and women will not undertake the study of medicine. China and India can only support one doctor to 50,000 people or more; France about one to 2,000; England about one to 1,200; the United States about one to 750. Other important factors enter, like the adequacy of professional schools and limitations that may be placed on acceptance of candidates for training, but the most fundamental determinant of the supply of medical personnel in a nation is its national income and the share of it available for medical service.

The systems of health insurance, rather than decreasing the supply of doctors relative to population, have stimulated a steady increase in the relative supply since the 1880s, when the first governmental programs were enacted. In the United States, the relative supply of physicians has actually declined in the same period. Health insurance and public medical care programs have reserved larger shares of the national income for health services and made possible great expansion of the supply of both doctors and hospital beds. At the same time, the reduction of economic barriers for the consumer has obviously increased the effective demand for medical service. The question then becomes: has the increase in the supply of personnel kept pace with the increased demand for service? Idealistically considered, the answer is probably "no." The difficulty is that the insurance systems have not spent enough money, for there are still not enough doctors. Expenditures within the insurance- and tax-supported medical services have risen steadily—with the expanding demands for medical service and the increasing complexities of medical technology. But there is a limit to the expenditures a nation can support for medical care, just as there are limits to the reasonable expenditures of a nation for houses, bathrooms, or four-lane highways.

These rising costs of governmental medical care programs have, indeed, been attacked by American critics as evidence of the "extravagance" of compulsory health insurance. It is difficult to reconcile this viewpoint with the fact that greater expenditures make possible an expansion of personnel and facilities. The problems have been created not by the abundant expenditures of the programs, but by their frugality. Despite the rising expenditures, European economies still seem to put less money proportionately into medical care than does America. The total cost of the British National Health Service—even after the large increase in costs beyond the initial estimates—amounts to less than four percent of Britain's national income, while expenditures in the United States are estimated at over four percent of our income.[6]

Fundamentally, the insurance and related programs have helped to ameliorate the difficulties in European medical service caused by economic facts, rather than having produced these difficulties. Striking evidence of this is the fact that the British, French, Swedish, and Swiss medical associations have not advocated the abolition of the insurance programs, but rather their expansion to cover larger proportions of the population and wider scopes of service. The British medical profession remembers the "two-penny doctor" in the large cities before the first National Health Insurance Act of 1911 who, to make a scant living among his poverty-stricken clientele, had to charge ridiculously low fees. The insurance programs brought a better assured income for him, just as they did for doctors throughout Europe and just as Blue Cross plans in the United States, for example, have helped the hospitals financially. Not that physicians have been satisfied with the fees they receive under insurance programs. In France, today, there are bitter complaints about the government fee schedules and the British Medical Association has been battling hard for higher capitation payments to general practitioners. But these complaints are within a framework of acceptance of the total medical care program and they mean that more insurance is wanted, rather than less. To satisfy them would require adjustments in the remuneration of other classes of personnel or facilities (such as dentists who have been earning disproportionately high incomes under the British program) or the reduction of other expenditures in the total economy to reserve more funds for medical care.

If elevation of fee payments led to a greater aggregate national expenditure for medical care, it is obvious that increases in the overall supply of physicians would do likewise, or else average physician's earnings would decline. The persistent question remains how large a sum a nation can reserve from its national income for medical expenses, in relation to housing, food, clothing, and other essentials? One may then ask: "Why institute programs of compulsory health insurance or public medical service if a nation cannot afford to support adequate numbers of personnel and facilities to meet the demands for services?"

The answer must be found in the general social facts about Europe epitomized in its age, smallness, poverty, and suffering. These conditions have given rise to a strong demand for social improvement. The attitude of the governments elected to power has become: *we may not have enough resources, but what we have will be more or less evenly divided among us.* This has undoubtedly resulted in a situation—seen most sharply in England—in which a small percentage of persons of relatively high income cannot obtain as much medical service as they could when they paid for it privately, simply because the doctor has more demands on his time. But there can be no doubt that, under the governmental programs, the far larger number of persons who are of low or moderate income receive more medical care than they could possibly have afforded privately.

PATTERNS OF MEDICAL PRACTICE

Aside from the inadequacy of personnel, the relationship—or lack of it—between general medical practice and hospital services creates serious problems for the quality of European medicine. Is the isolation of the general practitioner, however, a consequence of the governmental insurance programs? The fact is that the independent development of hospitals, and specialist services within them, long antedates the insurance programs. It relates to the historic origin of hospitals as places for the sick poor. Sweden has operated public hospitals since about 1790 and Paris' Hotel Dieu or London's Guy's Hospital were established long before this. As both public and voluntary hospitals came to serve the great majority of the population at the expense of taxes or charity, the system of full-time salaried specialists attached to the institutions developed in the interests of both economy and efficiency. Even when the hospital specialists were not full-time, as in France, their services were seldom remunerated on a private fee basis. The opportunity for the average physician to use the hospital as an extension of private office practice, with private fees, was rare. (A separate system of "nursing homes," of small aggregate capacity, developed to serve this purpose for the small class of high income patients.) This economic foundation of the American doctor's "hospital connection" lacking, it is natural that general office practice should have become increasingly isolated from hospital medicine.

If anything, the European insurance programs have probably strengthened office practice by making private physicians accessible to patients who might formerly have gone to the free outpatient hospital clinics. Moreover, the ready access of the general practitioner's patients to hospital service is, after all, a tremendous help to both doctor and patient. It is conventional for the hospital to send the general practitioner a full report on his patient, helping to provide some continuity of care. Nevertheless, the stimulating professional influences of hospital affiliation are not available to most European physicians. This is an organizational challenge yet to be faced; the same problem, in reverse, is being faced in the United States, with general practitioners increasingly losing hospital connections which they once enjoyed.

Even within the limited supply of doctors in Europe, a better quality of service might be possible if certain organizational changes were made. Such changes, however, would make European medicine more socialized rather than less. Thus, while many physicians are overworked and give perfunctory care, others are not working to capacity, exactly as under private practice in the United States. This is not necessarily a reflection of competence but may be related, as in America, to length of time in practice, location, social connections, "bedside manner," or professional competition. As long as free choice, private office practice is the rule, as it is throughout Western Europe, these disparities will probably continue. Only a completely salaried medical service could make full utilization of all available medical manpower, on a rational basis. Despite the acceptance of this pattern for most hospital service, it is generally opposed by the physicians for office practice.

It is proposed in England that the quality of general medical practice will be elevated by the eventual construction of health centers, in which groups of general practitioners will work together, aided by auxiliary personnel and diagnostic equipment. This is, of course, different from the American conception of group practice, involving a team of general physicians and numerous specialists. With specialism tied to the hospitals, it is natural that the American type of private medical group for ambulatory patients should be very rare in Europe. The British plan, nevertheless, would correct much of the unhealthy isolation and individualism of solo office practice; it would also promote closer organizational connection between general practitioners and hospitals, since health centers would be professionally related to hospitals in a regional scheme. For the present, the construction of health centers is delayed by the requirements of general public housing and military mobilization.[7]

The quality of office medical practice might also be improved by fuller utilization of auxiliary personnel to conserve the doctor's time for essential duties. This could be most economically done in group med-

ical clinics; in solo practice it would be feasible on a large scale only if larger aggregate payments were made to doctors to enable them to support auxiliary workers. In Great Britain, almost fifty percent of patients coming to doctors' offices are not seeking direct medical service, but rather disability certifications, permits for certain rationed products, etc. These professional services are essential for other important programs, but their performance could be greatly expedited through a screening of cases by auxiliary health personnel. The same applies to the general record keeping and reports necessary to systematic medical service. It should be added that the volume of "paperwork" in the British National Health Service, itself, is small. No reports to the government are required on diagnosis, treatment, fees, volume of service, or other details of medical care; only referrals for specialist service, prescriptions of drugs, disability certifications, and the like call for written forms, exactly as are required in the usual American practice. In Sweden, Switzerland, and France, where payments to physicians are on a fee-for-service basis, vouchers must be filled out for reimbursement—equivalent to private physicians' bills here—but even these tasks could be simplified by clerical assistance.

Systematic postgraduate education of physicians would be another entree to an elevation of the quality of service which warrants further development in Europe. The use of standard drug formularies would be an additional device, consistent with practices in the finest medical centers. These and other measures, which might elevate the quality of service, would be steps toward greater rather than lesser organization of the European medical professions. Western Europe has more and more oganized the financing of medical care by the population, without a commensurate organization of the pattern of providing services. In the hospitals, where the latter has been carried much farther, the quality of service is high and, except for the shortage of beds, the problems are few. Yet, it is significant that the organized medical professions in various nations have few complaints about the place of physicians in the hospitals. Salaried positions on hospital staffs are eagerly sought and there are far more candidates than openings. The complaints of European physicians relate almost entirely to the rates of remuneration for office practice and the heavy demand on the time of successful general practitioners, problems already discussed.

SOCIAL TRENDS

Today in Europe we are seeing great social movements. Consider the significance of the British income tax of ninety-nine percent on earnings over 5,000 pounds ($14,000) per year; castles and estates everywhere are being converted to rest homes and parks. Consider the French social security levies of thirty-five percent on wages and salaries (twenty-nine percent paid by the employer and six percent by the worker), used mainly for an elaborate system of family allowances which yield, in effect, higher wages to persons with more dependents. Increasing classes of industry are being nationalized, prices are controlled, scarce goods are rationed equitably, social services of all types are being extended. Whether or not these changes will lead gradually to complete socialism, as the British Labour party envisages, remains to be seen. Difficulties in international relations still complicate internal social policies. Nevertheless, democratizing social change is the order of the day; there is little talk of war and much talk of constructive planning, such as that which characterized the American scene at the height of the New Deal in the 1930s.

The organization of health services is only one part of this movement, but it is a very important part because medical care is so intimate a need of everyone. In health services, the social movement takes the form of spreading the available services to all people in such a way that, while the supply of personnel and facilities is limited, the criterion for priority becomes not the extent of purchasing power but the extent of medical need. The transition is obviously difficult for the doctor, compelling him often to work much harder for only a slight increase in financial reward. But the people everywhere have demanded it. It will be recalled that one of the few things in the Labour party program in Great Britain not attacked by the Conservative party was the National Health Service. The same multipartisan unity toward health service organization has characterized the other nations of Europe.

Ultimate evaluation of the impact of the European medical care programs on the quality of service depends on how "quality" is defined. What happens to the quality of service for 1,000 persons when all of them are provided some essential care, compared with a situation in which 100 receive a "luxury" volume of care, 400 receive a moderate volume of care and 500 receive hardly any at all? Considering all 1,000 persons, does the quality of service go down or up; can quality be separated from quantity? This is perhaps a somewhat oversimplified formulation, but it symbolizes the nature of the developments in European medicine and the difference between European and American conditions.

There can be no doubt that Great Britain, Sweden, Switzerland, and France are proceeding toward a time when medical services will be a right rather than a privilege for everyone. There remain serious problems complicating the attainment of this goal, but at rock bottom these problems are mainly economic and historical. It is the economic difficulties, expressed principally in shortages of personnel, and the historical development of European hospitals that have caused the medical problems, and not the systems of insurance or public support of medical services. The latter have been corrective measures designed to adjust to the underlying social situation, and without them the professional problems would be more serious. The ultimate attainment of Europe's health service goals will depend on the achievement of world peace and the improvement of general economic conditions.

NOTES

[1] This chapter is based principally on observations during a survey in August-September 1950, sponsored by World Study Tours (Columbia University Travel Service).

[2] The party consisted of four physicians (a general practitioner, a specialist, a full-time public health administrator, and a teacher of public health), two private dentists, a nursing supervisor in a mental hospital, a podiatrist, two general social workers, a medical social worker, a research worker from an insurance company, and two medical economists from the federal government (the Social Security Administration and the Bureau of the Budget).

[3] In 1956, Sweden made membership in a local sickness fund mandatory for everyone, thus achieving universal coverage.

[4] See note 3.

[5] See chapter 11 for an account of the major integrative changes made in the British National Health Service in 1974.

[6] Since 1950, the percentage of national income devoted to health services has risen in both countries, but is still appreciably higher in the United States.

[7] As discussed in chapter 11, governmental health centers, staffed by general practitioners and other health personnel, began to expand rapidly in the 1960s.

Chapter XI
The British National Health Service and Its Recent Changes

Chapter 10 included references to the National Health Service of Great Britain, soon after its establishment in 1948, along with the health service systems of several other Western European countries. The structure of the British system, however, and its recent (1974) reorganization have such great importance in the world scene, that a closer examination of this experience should be made. Because of the great dissemination of British culture not only to America, but to Asia, Africa, and other places where the Empire had once extended, the policies of the United Kingdom in health and many other sectors exert influence on every continent. Even in Chile, part of a continent with relatively little British colonial involvement, the Servicio Nacional de Salud of 1952 was substantially influenced by the British model.

This chapter traces the origins of the National Health Service from the previous National Health Insurance Act of 1911, the experience of World War II, and other influences. It analyzes its triparite administrative structure, the several vested interests responsible for this design, and some of the achievements and problems. Then it describes the reorganized system formulated in the 1970s to bring about greater integration. This text has not previously been published.

The British National Health Service has in many ways set a model for the entire world. Although developed in a capitalist democracy, indeed a parliamentary kingdom, it embodies concepts of equity, of establishment of health service as a social right of everyone, which have influenced health planners in every nation. Its very structure has helped to clarify the anatomy of the health service industry in any country and the dynamic interplay among the ambulatory, the institutional, and the community preventive services.

In the United States, born out of a revolution against the British crown, the lingering influence of the former mother country is visible in countless ways—in public health policy, welfare systems, higher education, the common law, and many other sectors. It is no accident, therefore, that American medicine has long had special interest in the British National Health Service (NHS)—its successes and difficulties, its costs, medical profession attitudes, its

service trends—although reportage of the experience in American medical journals has seldom been unbiased.

NATIONAL HEALTH INSURANCE, 1911-1948

To understand the NHS and its recent sweeping changes, one must appreciate, of course, that it did not arise de novo in 1948. As in all of Europe, trade unions, fraternal associations, and "friendly societies" had been providing disability and sickness care insurance since the early nineteenth century. Germany and several other Central European countries had made enrollment in such protective bodies compulsory since the 1880s, and the influence was bound to be felt in the more western European countries and the British Isles. Back in the 1840s, upper class employers had encouraged and assisted the mutual aid societies, as a way to get lowly paid workers to look after themselves during sickness, instead of becoming a burden on the Poor Law authorities, supported by general revenues.

When the first National Health Insurance Act was passed by the British Parliament in 1911, it was not under the leadership of the Labour party. As in the German regime of conservative Chancellor Bismarck, it was under the moderate political leadership of the Liberal party's Lloyd George that the law was enacted. Only the British doctors opposed the idea, favoring—as in America today—continuation of the purely voluntary health insurance system for the self-supporting, coupled with a strengthened public medical service for the very poor.[1]

The 1911 Act required insurance protection to meet the costs of medical care and wage loss during sickness for all manual workers earning less than a certain amount (160 pounds or about U.S. $780) per year. While membership in an "approved society" was not specifically mandated, all but a small percentage of workers met the legal requirements through such membership. The worker's dependents did not have to be insured, but could purchase protection voluntarily through the same mutual aid societies. Payment of insurance contributions was required from both workers and employers, and government provided funds for the support of administration and the coverage of very low income or indigent persons. The benefits were limited to the services of general practitioners and prescribed drugs. Specialization was, in any event, not highly developed at the time. If the G.P. thought his patient required a specialist, the case could be referred to a hospital outpatient department where such services were free. Hospitalization was not insured, since open ward service in many public hospitals or some large voluntary ones was provided anyway through local government support or charity. If specialist care in a private office was desired, it had to be obtained privately. Dental or other special services were not covered at all.

The general practitioners, under the original law, were not paid for their services directly by the approved societies, but rather by insurance committees set up by statute in each county or county borough; these committees had to contain a majority of elected representatives of insured workers, with the balance representing the local doctors, local government, and the Ministry of Health. The approved societies were responsible for the enrollment of workers and for the payment of cash disability benefits but not for the basic medical and pharmaceutical benefits; if they had accumulated surplus funds they could finance supplemental benefits, such as part of hospitalization costs.

Under the law, the doctors in each insurance committee area could decide how they wished to be paid—whether on the basis of "attendances" (fee-for-service), by capitation according to the number of persons who chose to be on each doctor's list, or by a combination of these two methods. It is not always understood that it was the British doctors themselves who increasingly chose the straight capitation method, so that by 1927 this pattern had become universal.[2] This method was preferred because it involved less bureaucratic "red tape" and was least subject to competitive abuse among the insurance doctors in each area. It was only later, with the National Health Service, that capitation remuneration of general practitioners became mandatory.

In addition to the statutory G.P. and drug benefits, as well as cash disability payments, approved societies could sell insurance for other benefits, such as dental care, or for voluntary medical coverage of persons not coming under the social insurance law, such as dependents or higher income employees. Many approved societies had been set up by commercial insurance companies as nonprofit subsidiaries, and they enrolled several millions of persons on a voluntary basis, including coverage of specialist attendance in hospitals. G.P. services in small private hospitals (the British "nursing homes") were also sometimes insured for, especially to handle maternity cases and relatively simple surgery.

A study in 1923 showed that the average insured person in Great Britain received 3.5 attendances per year. It is noteworthy that at about the same time (actually 1928-1931), the Committee on the Costs of Medical Care showed that persons of equivalent income in the United States, without insurance, were receiving 2.2 physician services per year. Thus, the British doctor was giving fifty percent more service under capitation insurance arrangements than was the American doctor, having fee-for-service incentives but without insurance.

PRELUDE TO THE NATIONAL HEALTH SERVICE

Over the years, the income threshold for mandatory insurance coverage in Great Britain was elevated, so that more workers were covered. Additional persons and benefits were also insured on a voluntary basis. On the eve of World War II, however, the health insurance protection of the British population was obviously far from complete, both as to persons covered and benefits provided. It was not surprising, therefore, that during the war—among the goals of which was "freedom from want"—an Inter-departmental Committee on Social Insurance and Allied Services was set up, under the chairmanship of Sir William Beveridge to "survey the existing national schemes of social insurance and allied services . . . and to make recommendations." In late 1942, under Winston Churchill's Conservative government, the famous Beveridge Report was issued.[3]

This classic document explored the deficiencies and need for expansion of all the branches of social insurance, including old-age pensions, unemployment benefits, disability benefits, and so on, as well as health services. Regarding the latter, in summary the Plan for Social Security recommended:

> Medical treatment covering all requirements will be provided for all citizens by a national health service organized under the health departments (of England and Wales, Scotland, and Northern Ireland) and post-medical rehabilitation treatment will be provided for all persons capable of profiting by it.

In further elaboration of this goal, the Beveridge Report stated that:

> A comprehensive national health service will ensure that for every citizen there is available whatever medical treatment he requires, in whatever form he requires it, domiciliary or institutional, general, specialist, or consultant, and will ensure also the provision of dental, ophthalmic and surgical appliances, nursing and midwifery and rehabilitation after accidents.

The Report explicitly avoided discussion of "the problems of organisation of such a service" as falling outside its scope.

These were the objectives recommended under a wartime Conservative party government in 1942. It remained for a Labour party government, elected after the War, to implement them with the passage of the National Health Service Act in 1946. Allowing a tooling-up period of about eighteen months, the Act took effect in July 1948.

As in any sweeping social legislation, there was intense debate in the period between the introduction of draft legislation and enactment of the final law. The Minister of Health was Aneurin Bevan, a rugged former Welsh coal miner, who soon found himself at loggerheads with the British Medical Association. The B.M.A., anticipating the postwar mood, had set up its own Medical Planning Commission which had recommended achievement of the Beveridge goals through extension of the existing National Health Insurance to cover higher income persons, government grants to voluntary hospitals in order to enable them better to serve the poor, but retention of the private medical market for higher income persons. Mr. Bevan's bill, on the other hand, would not only cover all residents of the nation for comprehensive services, but would provide a basic salary for all general practitioners (to be

supplemented by capitation payments) and a network of health centers from which both preventive services of local health authorities and primary services of GPs would be furnished—as proposed back in 1920 by the Dawson Report. All beds in public hospitals, moreover, would be solely for NHS patients; while specialists could continue private practice on a part-time or full-time basis, they would have to hospitalize their patients solely in private institutions.

In the ensuing debate, which involved a threat to strike by the doctors, many compromises were naturally made by both sides. Universal population coverage was retained, but basic salaries—which general practitioners opposed for fear that they would gradually be extended to lead to full government employment—were abandoned. Public hospitals were authorized to maintain about five percent of their beds for the private patients of consultants. The network of health centers was not to be established, except for a few experimental facilities. On the other hand, financing was to be derived mainly from general revenues, and only a small fraction from social insurance contributions. Top authority was vested in the national Ministry of Health. And nearly 100 percent of hospital beds were put under the control of the national government.

The most important compromises—or perhaps adjustments to the forces at play would be more accurate—in defining the administrative lines of the National Health Service were in the design of its tripartite structure. Past developments in Britain up to 1948 had given rise in the health services to several principal sets of vested interests: the general practitioners, the community hospitals with their staffs of specialists, the medical school-affiliated teaching hospitals, and the local public health authorities. To achieve an operational program, that would be adapted peaceably to these clusters of power, required an administrative structure in which substantial sovereignties were retained by each of these groupings. Coordination among the interests, for the sake of good patient care and efficiency, was a secondary consideration to be tackled deliberately only later.[4]

AMBULATORY SERVICES AND THE EXECUTIVE COUNCILS

The first interest group, general practitioners, were already represented, and their remuneration handled, by the insurance committees operating since 1911 under the old National Health Insurance law. These committees already had subcommittees for doctor services and for prescribed drugs. It was a relatively smooth transition, under the NHS, to establish a network of executive councils—138 of them in England and Wales—which would assume the functions of the former insurance committees; in the new program, these functions would be broadened to administer services for the total population and also to widen their duties to handle dental care and optical services.

The average executive council administered these ambulatory services for about 350,000 people, although the range was highly variable; one council for part of London covered 3,000,000 population. Most important were the council's responsibilities for capitation payments to and monitoring of the general practitioners. Each month the G.P. was paid a fixed amount for every person on his list, irrespective of a patient's use or nonuse of services. At any time a person could change to another G.P., whereupon his name would be transferred to the other doctor's list. In order to protect quality, the maximum number of persons permitted on a G.P. list was 3,500, although in recent years the average was about 2,200. Moreover, the rate of capitation payment went according to a slightly descending scale, so as to discourage excessively long lists. In many ways, the general practitioner or family doctor, as the primary point of entry into the Service, underwent many changes in his mode of work, but more will be said of this below.

Also under the responsibility of the executive councils were the dental services. Unlike the GPs, dentists were paid on a fee-for-service basis, but not all procedures were covered by the NHS. For partial dentures, bridgework, crowns, and certain other prostheses the patient had to pay extra fees personally, although complete dentures were fully covered. The supply of dentists in Great Britain, as in all of Europe (and, indeed, most countries) is relatively low in relation to the needs, the demands for care were high, and dentists' incomes in the early years of the NHS were greater than those of the general practitioners. (Later, adjustments in G.P. remuneration changed the relationship.) Priority was accorded to children through a free, public dental service furnished by salaried dentists under the local health authorities.

Prescribed drugs obtained at local chemist shops or pharmacies were another benefit administered by the executive councils. At first, these were entirely covered through NHS fees, calculated by a formula (accounting for the wholesale cost, overhead, dispensing service, etc.), paid to the pharmacist. When the Conservatives were returned to power in 1952 they imposed a copayment charge of one shilling (fourteen U.S. cents) on each prescription, and later this was raised to two shillings. With the generally rising consumption of drugs, and higher costs per item, certain constraints were introduced around 1960; a "recommended list" was issued by the Ministry of Health, and doctors could order products not on it only if they were specifically justified; otherwise the patient would have to pay the full cost. The deterring effect of copayments was transitory, and when the Labour party was reelected to power later, these charges were dropped. All the while, nonprescribed or "over-the-counter" products remained available to the British people, at their personal expense, and great quantities were indeed purchased. With advertising and old wive's tales, self-medication does not disappear even under a publically financed health service system.

Finally, under the executive councils, were the responsibilities for optical services. These included vision examinations by prescribing opticians (optometrists in America) and eyeglasses furnished by dispensing opticians. Fees for standard model spectacles were paid by the councils, but the patient was charged extra for unusual or fancy models. Hearing aids, prosthetic limbs, wigs (when medically ordered), or other special medical devices were further benefits.

REGIONAL HOSPITAL BOARDS AND SPECIALIST SERVICES

The second major pillar of the NHS structure was a network of regional hospital boards (RHBs)—fifteen of them to cover England and Wales. Just as the executive councils had evolved from the former insurance committees, the RHBs had antecedents, though more recent, in the system of emergency services set up during World War II while Britain was being bombed. The wartime experience obviously educated British hospitals about the feasibility of communications and teamwork among institutions in a region.

British general hospitals, for some years before the War, had been confronted with financial difficulties. The public hospitals, depending mainly on local revenue support, were chronically underfinanced. The voluntary hospitals, despite the long and distinguished traditions of many of them, were likewise hard-pressed from the dwindling of charitable contributions and the difficulty of private patients in meeting the ever-rising charges. When, therefore, on the "appointed day" in 1948, the Minister of Health took over control of all but a handful (mainly religious) of British hospitals, there were no significant objections. With the nationalization, the government acquired all the property of the hospitals and assumed all their debts and obligations. Overnight Britain's 2,700 hospitals with about 480,000 beds (about eighty percent municipal) attained financial stability. The nationalization included all mental, tuberculosis, and other chronic disease facilities, as well as the general hospitals, but not old people's homes or convalescent units.

The hospital regions were mapped out to contain about 2,000,000 to 3,000,000 people and roughly 30,000 hospital beds of all types. The regional hospital boards were appointed by the Minister to represent the general population, the medical profession, and the former hospital owners or sponsors. To actually administer the hospitals, the RHB appointed hospital management committees, which were typically responsible for institutions containing a total of between 1,000 and 2,000 beds; this might mean two or three large units or as many as fifteen or twenty small ones. The funds for both operation and capital costs of all hospitals in a region were allotted by the central government to the RHB, which in turn distributed them to the management committees. Because of Britain's postwar financial difficulties and competing obligations for housing construction, schools, roads, military purposes, and so on, new hospital construction until quite recent years was not undertaken, and capital expenditures went almost entirely for renovating the old structures. As a result, many American observers have been struck with the antiquated physical features of most British hospitals; the dedication of their staffs and the efficiency of their operations, however, have been equally noteworthy.

British specialists in medicine and surgery, unlike their American counterparts, are attached mainly to the hospitals. Leaving aside the younger doctors in training (registrars, junior registrars, etc.) about sixty percent are on full-time salaries and forty percent spend part of their time (typically twenty to thirty percent) in outside private practice. General practitioners, however, who constitute about half of Britain's doctors seldom have hospital appointments under the NHS, nor did they have such appointments before. In other words, the patient requiring hospitalization (except in emergencies) is referred by his G.P. to a hospital outpatient department, where the examining specialist decides if he should be admitted. Likewise, he may be referred to the hospital OPD simply for a diagnostic work-up. In either case—whether admitted to a bed or not—a report is sent back to the referring practitioner on the hospital specialist's findings.

This separation of general practice from the hospital has been the subject of much criticism in North America, where nearly all doctors, generalist and specialist, have hospital ties. This "closed staff" pattern is by no means unique to Britain, but prevails in most of Europe and, indeed, most countries of the world. While it means that the community family doctor is deprived of the stimulation of hospital experience and is temporarily separated from his patient, it assures technically high quality service within the hospital walls. Moreover, under the NHS, the general practitioner was brought closer to the hospital by giving him access directly to the hospital's laboratory and x-ray services for diagnostic tests (without necessarily sending his patient through the OPD), by inviting him to participate in the hospital's educational programs, and by sometimes appointing him to work in the outpatient department or other sections of the institutions.

Until quite recently, specialist salaries in hospitals were typically higher than the earnings of community doctors in general practice. All specialists and consultants (the highest rank) are appointed by the RHBs, and there is great competition for these positions. When an opening occurs, it is widely advertised in the medical journals, and the specialist appointed usually acquires permanent tenure. Those not appointed may be frustrated and must face the decision of going into general practice or emigrating. (Quite a few of the ex-British doctors in North America who broadcast the defects of the NHS are those who failed to win a specialist appointment.) Periodically, specialist salaries are raised, with increased tenure or responsibility, and merit awards are granted for outstanding performance. In the light of the conventionally negative attitudes towards salaries in American medicine, it is noteworthy that the most prestigious and coveted positions in Britain's NHS, and indeed in all of Europe, are those offering salaried hospital employment.

THE TEACHING HOSPITALS

In tracing the origins of the NHS, the special interests of hospitals linked to medical schools were noted. Usually associated with a long tradition, and exceptionally qualified medical staffs, these hospitals in England and Wales objected to coming under the control of regional hospital boards. The thirty-six of them (twenty-six in London), therefore, each with its board of governors, were made directly responsible to the Minister of Health.

From the outset, this perhaps elitist posture did not apply to the teaching hospitals in Scotland, and these were integrated into their respective RHBs. In the reorganization of 1974, as we shall see, such integration has been finally achieved on a nationwide basis.

Medical student education which is invariably associated with a teaching hospital is simultaneously under the wing of a university. Unlike the American pattern, British medical students take a continuous six-year course, rather than a four-year university baccalaureate, followed by another four-year medical curriculum. Contrary to some forebodings, after initiation of the NHS the volume of applicants to British medical schools did not decline, but rose. The majority of medical and other health science students are supported by government scholarships.

LOCAL HEALTH AUTHORITIES

The final major branch of the British NHS was the network of local health authorities—146 of them in England and Wales. These were responsible for traditional preventive public health services, but also for several other activities. While the NHS withdrew from local authorities their responsibilities for public hospitals (which, in a sense, weakened their role), they were assigned new functions for ambulance transport, for visiting nurse services (bedside care at home, which had been traditionally offered by voluntary agencies), for homemaker care to the chronically ill, and for the operation of long-term facilities for the aged or chronic sick not needing hospitalization.

The preventive services long included a major emphasis on maternal and child health. The vast majority of pregnant women and infants in Great Britain have been periodically checked by health department clinics. This applies to all social classes, not only to lower income families, as in America. One must recall that the general practitioner, being paid on a capitation basis, is happy to have his patients so attended; he loses no fee, it saves him time, and the mother and child are seen by experts in this preventive work. At the child welfare stations, as they are called, infants and small children receive all necessary immunizations, and the mothers are advised on childrearing practices. Sick children are referred back to their family G.P. To lighten the heavy load on these health department clinics and to promote integrated care, in recent years general practitioners have been offered supplementary fees, beyond the capitation payments, for immunizations and certain other preventive services.

Local health authorities also conducted other special clinics for tuberculosis and venereal diseases. Health services for schoolchildren were still financed by the educational authorities, but the local medical officer of health (MOH) in most jurisdictions was appointed likewise as school health officer. (Under the recently reorganized NHS, these school health services have become administratively brought into the general program.) Environmental sanitation has been another major responsibility of the local health authorities. In the water supply and sewage disposal systems of Britain, less modernized than in America, close surveillance is necessary. Inspections of housing, for enforcement of minimum standards, were another responsibility of the MOH and his sanitation staff, and occupied a good deal of time.

OTHER SPECIAL SERVICES

Separate large hospitals for the mentally ill and retarded had evolved in Great Britain, as in most of the world, but with the NHS they were brought under the integrated supervision of the regional hospital boards. Psychiatric commitment was changed from a judicial to a medical procedure; the vast majority of admissions became voluntary, as to a general hospital, or in the minority that were mandatory, certification was by two doctors (one had to be a psychiatrist), rather than a court of law. After admission, the patient was still entitled to a judicial review, but most mandatory admissions were later converted to "informal" ones. Increasing emphasis was placed on community service for mental illness: mental health clinics of many types under the local authorities, mental sections in general hospitals, day care centers, and a variety of other special arrangements. The average length of stay in mental hospitals, as well as the total census, greatly declined—as was, indeed, also happening in America.

Workmen's compensation for on-the-job injuries was greatly modified under the NHS. The payment of cash benefits for wage loss, financed solely by employers, was continued as before under the social security system. All medical services, however, were simply integrated with and provided by the NHS system. Since medical care for all illness was fully covered, there was no reason—as so often criticized in the United States—to falsely attribute a worker's symptoms to an employment cause in order to gain financial protection. Great emphasis was put on rehabilitation, and a special center was developed for the psychosomatic treatment of those few workers, often called "malingerers," whose persistence of disability was mainly on a neurotic basis.

Medical inspection of factories for safety and occupational disease hazards was one of the few health-related activities not integrated into the NHS, but retained as a function of the Department of Labour. First aid in the factories, preplacement examination of workers, safety standards, and the like were enforced through periodic visits, and imposed a responsibility on management. Medical treatment of sick or injured workers, of course, was through the NHS.

Public assistance for the poor, in its financial aspects, was administered by welfare authorities. But the medical care of the indigent was through all the normal procedures of the NHS, as for anyone else. No special enrollment or identification of the recipients of public aid, as in America, was necessary. Likewise any temporary visitor to Great Britain, who happened to be struck with illness or injury, would be treated by the resources of the NHS, exactly as the police force would be expected to protect a visitor against crime.

FINANCIAL SUPPORT AND VOLUME OF SERVICE

These were, then, the main features of the British National Health Service as it was set up in 1948, and they were attainable only through the substantial assumption of financial responsibility by the Exchequer or general treasury of the nation. Because employer and worker contributions to the old National Health Insurance had become customary, however, and because they were set up to cover many other cash benefits (old-age pensions, unemployment compensation, maternity and disability allowances, etc.), a share of these funds was still assigned to help support the NHS, along with monies from some other sources.

The exact proportions of funds derived from different sources were not identical over the years. In 1970-1971, they were as shown in table XI.1.[5]

Table XI.1	
Sources of funds for British National Health Service: 1970-1971	
Source	*Percentage*
Central government	80.0
Insurance contributions	9.0
Local government	6.5
Payments by patients	4.5
Total	100.0

The central government funds included allotments to local governments to help them carry some of their responsibilites. The payments by patients included charges for prescribed drugs, for prosthetic dental services, for private beds in NHS hospitals, for special spectacles, and for other miscellaneous purposes. Altogether the NHS cost 2,384,000,000 pounds in 1970-1971. Expenditures outside the NHS were estimated at about 100,000,000 pounds for self-medication and about 25,000,000 pounds for privately purchased medical care. For the

55,400,000 population in the United Kingdom (48,500,000 being in England and Wales), this amounted to an annual per capita outlay for health services of about 45 pounds or, at an exchange rate of $2.80 per pound at the time, of about $125 per person per year. This compares with an expenditure in the United States for all health service in 1970 of about $325 per person per year. Even if one were to allow an exchange rate of $3.00 per pound, in recognition of actual purchasing power differentials in the two countries, the British per capita expenditure for health services was less than half the American.

Yet, for this lesser expenditure, British health manpower and facilities provide a volume of personal health services very similar to the levels in the United States. With 4.2 general medical, surgical, and maternity beds per 1,000 population in Britain, the figure is about the same as for the United States. Counting all types of hospital beds—including mental and long-term chronic—in 1970, the British supply of 9.5 per 1,000 compares with America's of about 8.0. In general hospitals, British admission rates are somewhat lower than American, but the average stay per case is longer and the occupancy percentages greater, so that the aggregate days per 1,000 population per year in Britain are slightly more than in the United States.

Patient-physician contacts are somewhat higher in Britain for primary or general practitioner care than in America, and lower for specialist care. Dental services are less frequently received in Britain, especially for adults, than in the United States, because of a lower supply of dentists. Preventive services, on the other hand, especially for children, are undoubtedly more frequent in Britain than in America.

A propos of services, it is significant to note that the rate of elective surgery in Great Britain is much lower than in the United States. It has been pointed out that the ratio of surgeons to population in England and Wales is about half the level of that in the United States, and the rate of elective surgery is correspondingly about half.[6] There can be little doubt that this finding relates to the methods of paying surgeons in the two countries: high fees for each operation in the United States and fixed salaries based on merit in Great Britain. The abundance of unnecessary surgery in the United States has been frequently demonstrated, but whether there is, in fact, too little surgery in Britain might be argued. In any case, the life expectancy for both males and females is longer in Great Britain than in America, in spite of their average per capita incomes (and presumably levels of living) being lower.

SOME SPECIAL FEATURES AND DEVELOPMENTS

Over the years, the rate of services and volume of expenditures in the British National Health Service have risen, as they have in the health care systems of most other countries, especially the industrialized ones. Yet, the striking fact is how slowly the rise has occurred in Great Britain. Ten years after the NHS started operation, concern for the rise in costs generated a commission of enquiry—yielding the Guillebaud Report in 1960. The surprise was that, while absolute expenditures had risen, as a percentage of gross national product (GNP) the outlay had actually declined from 3.9 percent in 1947-1950 to 3.6 percent in 1958-1959. By 1968, this proportion had risen to 4.6 percent of GNP, but at the time, Americans were spending about 6.5 percent of their larger GNP for health services.[7] In 1974, the American health expenditure had risen to about 8.0 percent of GNP.

Some point to this relatively constrained expenditure for health purposes in the United Kingdom as a defect, in comparison with the freewheeling escalation of outlays in the United States. The former is attributed to the largely unitary public source of funding in Britain, not easily expanded, compared to the pluralistic sources in America. But it is not difficult to show that most of the American increase in expenditures is accountable not to a rise in the volume of services, but rather to a climb in the prices of hospitalization, physician and dental care, drugs (prescribed and over-the-counter), and other services—not to mention the large overhead costs of hundreds of private insurance agencies. One must conclude, therefore, that in balance the Briton is getting more for his money under the NHS than the American under his predominantly laissez-faire system.

Trends over the years in the British NHS involve many developments beyond money. As in all industrialized nations, the relative importance of hospitals has increased, in tandem with the expansion of medical and surgical specialization. As a reflection of this, the expenditures for hospital care in the NHS rose from 55.7 percent of the total in 1951-1952 to 62.6 percent in 1970-1971. Still, compared with the American scene, this rise in the proportion of resources allotted to the hospital sector was not very great.

More significant are probably the major changes that have been occurring in British community general practice. At the time of NHS enactment, the vast majority of general practitioners held forth in their private one-man "surgeries." The Ministry of Health, however, gave financial inducements to medical grouping. The quality of isolated general practice had been criticized in several studies, and group practice, it was believed, could upgrade it; the engagement of office assistants—to relieve the doctor of many simple tasks—would be more feasible, and a team of doctors would mean convenient opportunities for consultation and general professional stimulation. Government policy was successful and the grouping of GPs increased steadily. By 1970, over sixty-five percent were in offices of two or more, most being in groups of three or more. In such settings, each practitioner would usually develop skills in some special aspect of general practice, such as child care, minor surgery, gynecological problems, emotional difficulties, or the like.

Another government objective was to improve the geographic distribution of doctors. This was done principally through a ban against settlement of new graduates in areas designated as "overdoctored" (for purposes of payment under the NHS); the result, of course, was to channel physicians to areas where they were needed. As a result, the British population in "underdoctored" areas was reduced from about fifty percent in 1948 to twenty percent in 1963. Moreover, the "sale" of medical practices—a traditional custom in Britain, through which a retiring doctor acquired money to live on—was prohibited and replaced with a social insurance pension program for doctors. Accordingly, the high price of "buying a practice" would no longer inhibit the young doctor from spending money on modern medical office equipment.

Improvement in the quality of general practice was also encouraged by supplemental government grants for engagement of allied health personnel, by higher capitation payments for aged patients on a list, by supplemental fees for various office procedures and for home calls, and by other methods. There was a serious pay dispute between GPs and the government in 1965, resulting in a substantial boost in their earnings and making the whole field of general practice more attractive. By 1970, about half of G.P. income came from the various special fees and grants, rather than capitation. A Royal College of General Practitioners made "specialist" status possible in general practice, and this was associated with an intensified program of continuing education, along with establishment of professorial chairs for general practice in the medical schools.

Perhaps the most significant trend affecting general practice, or indeed all ambulatory health care, in the British NHS has been the movement, starting about 1965, for establishment of health centers. As noted earlier, such centers figured prominently in the early planning of the system, but they were not implemented except in a few experimental projects.

Then in the mid-1960s, first in connection with development of "new towns" and later in most large cities, buildings were constructed or redesigned for housing groups of general practitioners, complemented by public health nurses, social workers, office or practice nurses, sometimes laboratory technicians, psychologists, dieticians, clerks, or other allied health personnel. Usually built by local health authorities, the quarters were rented by GPs who had their regular lists of patients, but most of the ancillary personnel were furnished at local government expense.

By 1971 there were 475 such health centers in operation or under construction, housing about 1,500 general practitioners, with space available for about 1,000 more. In the centers in full operation, there were an average of five or six GPs, and these doctors tended naturally to cooperate with each other, cover the practice of a colleague who was away, consult among themselves, and make much greater use of the allied health workers than would occur when these personnel were stationed in the traditional health department. While some centers used the office or practice nurse as a screening agent more than others, and there was great variation in other features, it appeared in the early 1970s that the health center was in time likely to change the entire image of ambulatory care in the NHS.

ATTITUDES AND OTHER CONSEQUENCES

Almost from its onset, the NHS encountered problems in the sphere of remuneration of doctors, both specialists and general practitioners. A series of enquiries led to continual readjustments, but on the whole the British medical profession became gradually supportive of the essential principles of the Service. Among the population as a whole, the NHS was probably the most popular program that had been launched by any political party. A British Gallup opinion poll in 1964 found eighty-nine percent of the population generally satisfied with the NHS, and in 1967 a survey by another organization found ninety-five percent of the people to express general approval, and of these sixty percent rated the Service as "very good" or "excellent."

Large bureaucratic structures, like the NHS, are often charged as discouraging local initiative and any incentive for volunteer work to strengthen the program. Yet British voluntary agencies have not declined. Hospital administrators point out that their committees of volunteer workers are as busy as ever. Instead of spending so much time on fundraising as in the past, however, they devote their energies to rendering services in the hospital, to help the patients or lighten the task of the staff.

The charge of "deadly uniformity," so often leveled against large governmental systems, does not stand up to scrutiny in the British setting. As one visits different hospitals and health departments in Britain, the striking observation is the diversity found. While each hospital, for example, is administered by a sort of "troika"—the hospital secretary (or administrator), the matron (or director of nurses), and the medical chief—whose members obviously must work closely together, the variations in style and emphasis among the different clinical services and departments of an institution are countless. There is plenty of room for innovation, as long as basic minimum standards are met.

In terms of resources generated by the NHS, the effect has clearly been to yield an increased supply of physicians—from about one to 950 people in 1948 to about one to 830 twenty years later; the availability of about 25,000 midwives for obstetrical services (both inside and outside hospitals) must be noted if one is to compare this with America's 1:730 ratio around 1968. Over this same span of years, in fact, the ratio of doctors to population in the U.S. had remained almost constant (increasing only after about 1967), while the British ratio improved. Medical incomes meanwhile, for both general practitioners and specialists, have risen substantially, and doctors now fall in the uppermost two or three percent of the British income ladder.

The general hospital bed ratio to population has not significantly increased in Britain, but lengths of stay have steadily shortened so that rates of admission have risen. They rose from about sixty-seven per 1,000 annually in 1949 to ninety-two in 1960 and to about 110 per 1,000 in 1970. As noted earlier, this lower rate than in America (about 140 per 1,000 in 1970) is associated with greater use of hospital outpatient departments, admission of more serious cases (clearly in need of hospital care), and a much lower rate of elective surgery. Waiting lists for hospital treatment of elective conditions are still a difficulty, but their length has declined, and there is no problem about admission of emergency cases.

Perhaps one of the best reflections of the general adequacy of the NHS is the relatively small percentage of the population seeking care through private arrangements outside the official structure. Voluntary health insurance schemes to finance private care have been free to operate, and though intensely promoted by private carriers, their enrollment had grown to only 883,000 or less than two percent of the population by 1969. In fact, between 1965 and 1967 the rate of disenrollments exceeded that of new enrollments. Although less than one percent of NHS beds are reserved for private patients, in the last few years this arrangement for "breaking the queue" with affluence has been intensely debated in Labour party circles and the loophole may soon be closed. In any event, whether it is left open as a safety valve for placating the consultants and wealthy patients or not, it would appear that not many patients are displeased with the waiting times or other limitations of the NHS to the point of deciding to pay for private medical care.

PROBLEMS OF COORDINATION

Despite this generally favorable picture of achievements, the British NHS has not been without problems. Controversies about medical remuneration have been mentioned, constraints on the construction of new hospital beds (because of competing demands for government funds) have caused waiting lists for elective conditions, complaints of some patients about the brevity of their visits to the general practitioner, and the general rise in costs (despite its being slower than in America and most other countries) have all been causes for concern. The basic concept of the NHS, nevertheless—with a strong primary doctor, who provides convenient entry to the system and serves to oversee his patient's use of the back-up specialist and hospital services, the preventive program, and the several other parts—is nevertheless a basis for pride by the architects of the whole structure.[8]

If any feature of the NHS was continually vexing to the responsible authorities, it was the maintenance of the segmented administrative structure, described earlier. A pregnant mother, for example, would get prenatal care from a local health authority clinic, treatment of illness from her family G.P., and delivery of the baby by a hospital doctor or midwife. Similar fragmentation of patient care applied to the care of children, many chronic disease cases among all age groups, the management of mental disorders, etc. Moreover, economic trends in the NHS showed a gradual escalation of the resources allotted to the hospital sector, while the general practice and other components remained static or declined.

Since the 1948 beginnings, there were various coordinating committees, to attempt to achieve integration among the executive councils, regional hospital boards, and local health authorities, as well as the teaching hospital boards of governors; some overlapping of board or committee memberships was designed deliberately for the same purpose. As early as 1962, the Porritt Committee under the British Medical Association had advocated unification of all the three or four vertical components at the local community level.[9] Politically, however, in terms of the power centers responsible for the original divided structure, the time did not seem ripe. Not until 1968 did the national government, then under the Labour party, issue a first "green paper" advocating, for discussion purposes, a merging of the three main sectors of the Service at the local level through forty to fifty area health authorities.

Responses were quick to come, and the proposal was criticized as vesting responsibility still too remotely from the local areas, while not making adequate provision for larger regional planning. In 1970, a Conservative government was elected, and a second green paper was issued in 1971, responding to the criticisms of the first. Then a government "white paper," laying out the ruling party's final official plans, was issued.

THE REORGANIZATION OF 1974

In recognition of demands for greater local controls, ninety local area health authorities were contemplated, with a second tier—largely for planning purposes—of fourteen regional health (not hospital) authorities. Area health authorities (AHAs) would range in size from 250,000 to 1,500,000 population, and would be congruent with (but independent from) simultaneously reorganized general local government authorities. The regional health authorities (RHAs) would range from 1,000,000 to 5,000,000 population; thus each RHA would contain from one to eleven AHAs, and usually more than three. The larger AHAs would be further subdivided into districts of about 250,000 population—or the catchment area of a district general hospital. The law putting this general plan into effect was passed in 1973, to take effect April 1, 1974

True to British tradition, the new reorganization still takes account of past realities. While the AHA is responsible for all types of service—ambulatory, hospital, and preventive—within its borders, advisory to it will be a family practitioner committee, successor to the former executive councils. The AHAs take over the functions of the former hospital management committees—to administer the hospitals—and the RHAs retain the former responsibilities of the regional hospital boards for planning the construction of facilities. The teaching hospitals will finally be absorbed into the system, but in the areas where they are located they will have especially strong representation on the AHA board. The school health services, formerly controlled by educational officials, will also be made a responsibility of the AHAs. Only the industrial health services remain separate.

Nonmedical representation on governing bodies,

although the meaning of this point is debated, would be somewhat greater than formerly. A majority of members of AHA boards will not be health professionals, but—in the interests of improving efficiency—they will be required to be persons with managerial experience. Perhaps of greater importance is provision for, not a traditional MOH, but a new type of medical leader: a "community medicine specialist" as advisor to each AHA.[10] His duties will be not only administration of the preventive services (communicable disease control and environmental hygiene—as done by the former MOH), but also consultation and evaluation for the AHA on the efficacy and efficiency of all health services in the local hospitals and doctors' offices. He will be expected to provide health education to the people and also epidemiological information to the doctors. He will offer planning guidance to other local government authorities, particularly in education and social services, as well as to voluntary bodies.

Consumer representation will also be assured through community health councils at the health district level within the AHAs. These councils will be advisory, as well as a channel for patient complaints, to the district management team, composed of the community medicine specialist, a district nurse, a chief administrator, and two clinicians (one a G.P. and another a specialist) elected by their peers. Specifically to cope with patient complaints will be an ombudsman, called the health services commissioner.

It is expected that local health centers will continue to be built and, along with extension of group practices, will provide a setting for linkage of the district public health nursing, social work, and other local government personnel with the general practitioners. Indeed, to some the overriding objective of the NHS reorganization is to enhance the importance of the ambulatory and primary care services as a reaction to the enlarging role that was being assumed by hospitals. The elevated status and strengthened educational support for general practice, with the same objective, have been noted earlier.

To others, the major purpose of the NHS reorganization is to achieve greater managerial efficiency.[11] A single hierarchy of authorities from health districts, to area health authorities, to regional health authorities, up to the central Ministry of Health is deemed more efficient and administratively economical than three or four separate vertical bureaucracies. Strengthened administrative responsibilities at the local level through AHAs and community medicine specialists, backed up by various advisory committees of both providers (family prac-

titioner committees) and consumers (community health councils), will presumably mean more effective decentralization of the execution of policies that are formulated at the national level.

Obviously only time will tell to what extent these various objectives of the NHS reorganization are actually achieved. Some have viewed the whole metamorphosis skeptically as a set of new labels for the same old mechanisms. Certain of the role definitions of different entities in the new structure are not crystal clear, and their final implementation will probably depend on the strengths and weaknesses of diverse groups in each local area. Nevertheless, in my opinion, the latest action for the redesigning of the British National Health Service is further confirmation of a point made in other chapters of this book: the worldwide trend toward unified and comprehensive health service planning and delivery. Whether through social revolution or incremental changes, the movement seems to be in the same direction.

NOTES

[1] G. G. McCleary, *National Health Insurance*. London: H. K. Lewis and Co., 1939.

[2] I. S. Falk, *Security Against Sickness: A Study of Health Insurance*. New York: Doubleday Doran & Co., 1936, pp. 155-156.

[3] William Beveridge, *Social Insurance and Allied Services* (American Edition). New York: Macmillan Co., 1942.

[4] Almont Lindsey, *Socialized Medicine in England and Wales: The National Health Service 1948-61*. Chapel Hill: University of North Carolina, 1962.

[5] Gordon Forsyth, "United Kingdom," in I. Douglas-Winston and Gordon MacLachlan (eds.), *Health Service Prospects: An International Survey*. London: The Lancet and The Nuffield Provincial Hospitals Trust, 1973, pp. 1-35.

[6] John Bunker, "Surgical Manpower: A Comparison of Operations and Surgeons in the United States and in England and Wales." *New England Journal of Medicine*, Vol. 282, January 15, 1970, pp. 135-144.

[7] T. E. Chester, "How Healthy is the National Health Service? *District Bank Review*, September 1968. Also U.S. Social Security Administration, *National Health Expenditures, Fiscal Years 1929-70 and Calendar Years 1929-69* (Research & Statistics Note No. 25). Washington, D.C.: December 14, 1970.

[8] George E. Godber, "The Future Place of the General Physician" (The 1969 Michael M. Davis Lecture). Chicago: University of Chicago, Center for Health Administration Studies, 1969.

[9] Roger M. Battistella and Theodore E. Chester, "Reorganization of the National Health Service: Background and Issues in England's Quest for a Comprehensive-Integrated Planning and Delivery System." *Health and Society*, Vol. 51, Fall 1973, pp. 489-530.

[10] George A. Silver, "The Community-Medicine

Specialist—Britain Mandates Health Service Reorganization." *New England Journal of Medicine,* Vol. 287, December 21, 1972, pp. 1,299-1,301.

[11] Keith Barnard and Kenneth Lee (eds.), *NHS Reorganization: Issues and Prospects:* University of Leeds (England): Nuffield Centre for Health Services Studies, 1974.

Chapter XII
Health Care in a Province of Canada

Despite its closeness to the United States and the similarities of its historic origins, Canada has organized its economic resources for providing medical care much more completely than its southern neighbor. In 1958, Canada legislated a nationwide program of universal hospital insurance, and in 1966 this was extended to provide social insurance for all physician's services. The impetus for both of these important social programs came from the prairie province of Saskatchewan, which enacted hospital insurance for all its residents in 1947.

This chapter traces the general development of the remarkably innovative Saskatchewan program of health services up to 1958, including its early municipal doctor plans, its health regions, its cancer treatment service, its air ambulance, and other "firsts" in North America. Four years later, in 1962, Saskatchewan ushered in a social insurance program for physician's care, after coping with a "doctor strike" of twenty-three days that made front-page news around the world. The account is based on the author's three years of administrative service in the provincial Department of Health; it was published as " 'Socialized' Health Services in Saskatchewan" in Social Research (Vol. 25, Spring 1958, pp. 89-101) and is reprinted here by permission. In the 1970s, most of Canada's ten provinces were no longer satisfied with simple insurance for hospital and doctor's care, and were exploring more fundamental approaches toward reorganizing medical care delivery through community health centers and regionalized networks for maximizing the quality of all services.

When Prince Edward Island agreed, in April 1957, to adopt a scheme of universal hospital care insurance, the requirement was met for a Canada-wide program that is of enormous importance to the United States. Now that assent has been given by a majority of Canada's ten provinces (Ontario, British Columbia, Alberta, Newfoundland, P.E.I., and Saskatchewan), with a majority of the national population, legislation will take effect by which the federal government will finance about half the cost of any provincial plan providing general hospital care to the whole population. While this would be regarded as "socialized medicine" by many in the United States, the new program, which will probably take effect in 1958, is being greeted enthusiastically by all political parties in Canada. In fact, the law was passed under the Liberals and is to be carried out under the present government of Conservatives.

The movement that has culminated in this sweeping measure for social financing of the high costs of hospital care had its beginnings not in the legislative halls at Ottawa but in the drab village meeting rooms in one of Canada's lesser known provinces. It was the prairie farmer of Saskatchewan who launched the movement that may eventually have an influence on how everyone in North America obtains hospital care. Unbeknown to most Americans, he and some 900,000 of his fellowmen in this province just beyond the North Dakota border have been living with a system of compulsory health insurance in various forms for over thirty years—and thanking their lucky stars for it.

The Canadian prairies were settled hardly seventy-five years ago, and Saskatchewan graduated from its wild and woolly status in the Northwest Territories to a self-governing province only in 1905. In the Golden Jubilee celebration, held in 1955, pioneers recalled the sod huts, the Red River wagons, the horse-drawn plows that helped them open up this forbidding, cold, flat land.

Once a settlement developed—made up of a few houses and a grain elevator to store the wheat, which grows well in the dry soil—and once children came along, people began to feel the need for a doctor. A handful of medical men came to the main cities of Regina or Saskatoon, but how could they be attracted to the grim, isolated little villages, with no pavements, no piped water or sewage, hardly a house to live in? The prairie farmers, with their European background and faced with the rigors of the environment, were bound to turn to cooperatives for marketing wheat and buying consumer goods. Why not apply the same principle to medical care? Better yet, why not expect everyone in the village and in the rural municipality around it to pay toward the salary of the doctor, so he could be assured a living and would therefore remain in the area? As they say in this semiarid country, the idea seemed as right as rain.

In 1918 the local government unit of Sarnia (population about 1,700) imposed a tax to pay for a general medical practitioner who would then treat everyone in the area without charge. The plan was an immediate success, and other municipalities soon followed suit. By 1930 there were thirty-two such plans operating. Through the bleak depression years these local compulsory insurance plans kept up a minimum level of medical care for rural Saskatchewan families, when drought and misery were driving people away by the thousands.

With provincial aid the plans multiplied, and today there are over 100 in operation, protecting some 170,000 people with general medical and surgical care. They don't meet all the needs for specialist care and they don't cover all the rural people in the province, but these "municipal doctor plans" have helped thousands of rural families. Moreover, they have enjoyed staunch cooperation over the years from several hundred country doctors.

After the Second World War and the "dirty thirties"—compared with which the dust-bowl period in the United States was no more than a mild setback—Saskatchewan voters were ready for a change of government. The two old political parties had lost their appeal, and the vacuum was filled by a new party, the CCF—Cooperative Commonwealth Federation. This movement was a sort of agrarian socialism, something like the old Farmer-Labor party of Wisconsin, but ideologically akin to the British Labour party. In its campaign for election the CCF called, in so many words, for "a system of

socialized medical services." It stood also for a moratorium on farm mortgage debts, provincial aid to cooperatives, government operation of all public utilities, expansion of welfare services and education, and development of industry and natural resources. On this program the CCF was swept into power in 1944, capturing forty-five out of the fifty seats in the provincial Legislative Assembly.

With such a mandate, the Premier of the province (a former Baptist preacher) took for himself the Health Ministry and set about carrying out the campaign pledge. Professor Henry Sigerist, a distinguished medical historian of Johns Hopkins Medical School, was called in for advice. After a summer of on-the-spot study and village meetings at all hours of the day and night, a sweeping program of "socialized medical services" was outlined.

One of the first acts of the new government was to strengthen the old municipal doctor plans. On the basis of the bit of "socialized medicine" that already existed, provincial standards were set up to protect patients and doctors, and grants of money were given. Next was the launching of a province-wide system of medical care for the poor. This had formerly been a local government responsibility, and the level of medical care received by most indigent persons (mainly the elderly) was meager. A scheme was set up that permitted a recipient of public assistance to see any doctor of his choice, and to receive drugs, hospitalization, dental care, even physiotherapy or private nursing—with all fees paid.

Every state in the United States has, of course, a program of public medical care for the poor. These schemes, however, are usually characterized by limitations on the services received: there may be no access to private dentists; drugs may be limited; it may be necessary to use public medical clinics; or prior approval may be required from an administrative officer before calling a doctor to the home. Moreover, in the average state only about two percent of the population qualifies for such public medical care. In Saskatchewan the figure is about four percent, and it rises to some fifty percent of persons seventy years of age and over.

Since 1906 there had been a health department in the provincial capital of Saskatchewan, concerned with environmental sanitation and control of communicable diseases. The record on tuberculosis was outstanding, but there were few other notable achievements. In 1945, "health regions" were organized, to bring preventive services closer to the people. In regions of about 50,000 population, councils of citizens were elected to supervise all health activities. To the traditional services were added activities in nutrition, child health, dental hygiene, health education, and accident prevention. Mainly because of personnel shortages, not every section of the province is covered with these health regions as yet, but nine are now in operation and there will be fourteen of them when the job is done.[1]

In the first health region organized, around the city of Swift Current, people were interested in more than the old-line public health activities. They wanted day-to-day medical care, beyond what some residents had from the local municipal doctor plans. Therefore, when the region was established by popular vote, the regional council promptly enacted a universal insurance plan for general medical care. A contract was made with all the doctors in this southwestern district of the province to provide all needed medical services, with specified fees to be paid by the insurance fund. On July 1, 1945, the 50,000 people in the Swift Current health region became entitled to physician's care in the office, home, and hospital, supported by a compulsory tax.

After well over a decade this unique medical care program continues to operate successfully. There have been quarrels with the doctors about the fee schedule, but they have always been resolved in the interest of keeping the program going. Proof of the pudding is that the number of doctors in the region has doubled since the plan began, an increase greater than that in any other rural section of the province. Doctors have been attracted from all over Canada *because* of the insurance plan and the fact that their incomes in the region are higher than the provincial average, especially for young medical graduates. The support of the people has been reaffirmed each year with virtually unanimous votes by the elected regional health council, which must impose the annual tax.

The volume of medical and surgical services received by these rural families seems to be the highest in Canada (judging by the national Canadian Sickness Survey of 1951). As for the quality of services, the plan has been studied and favorably appraised by the Canadian Medical Association. The little town of Swift Current, and its health region office in small quarters above the government liquor store, have been visited by medical officials from all over the world. But this remains the only program in North America which encompasses all residents of a large geographic region (about 10,000 square miles) under governmentally controlled insurance for medical care.

Hospitalization is even more costly, and nearly always more critical, than care by the physician in his office or the patient's home. Happily, the Blue Cross movement and commercial insurance have protected millions of Americans against the bulk of these hospitalization costs. Nowhere in the United States, however, is the whole population of a city, county, or state fully protected. Being voluntary, these hospital insurance programs leave uncovered many families of low income, most persons past sixty-five years of age (when employment has ceased), and the great majority of residents of rural areas.[2] Moreover, there are often limitations to the period of time for which hospital services are financed (usually thirty days at the full rate), waiting periods for certain services, like deliveries or tonsillectomies, and less than complete payment of the cost of each hospital day.

In 1947 Saskatchewan inaugurated a program of hospitalization insurance covering its entire population. Every self-supporting person must pay a tax to finance it, except those who, like Indians or disabled veterans, receive hospital service through some other organized program. The indigent are covered automatically, without payment of a tax. There are no limitations on the length of stay in the hospital, except the decision of the attending doctor. There are no exclusions of care for preexistent conditions, no "waiting periods," and no limits on x-ray or laboratory tests. The only extra charges are for certain nonessential drugs and for the use of a private room, for which one pays $1.00 or $2.00 a day extra.

The hospitals are paid their full costs of operation by the government, but they remain independent institutions, operated by local boards of directors or Catholic sisterhoods. Hospital deficits, necessitating campaigns for community funds, are practically unheard of; in 1956 the aggregate deficit of all 160 general hospitals in the province was less than one-quarter of one percent of total hospital budgets.

To say that the Saskatchewan Hospital Services Plan has been a success would be the height of British (Commonwealth) understatement. Anyone will tell you it has been the most popular thing done by the government in any sphere. The volume of hospital service received by Saskatchewan residents (2,100 days per 1,000 persons per year) is today the highest in North America. This is over and above the services provided in tuberculosis sanatoria, mental hospitals, or nursing homes, and it is about double the United States average, although the Saskatchewan per capita income is considerably below that found in the richest country in the world. There is no evidence that Saskatchewan people are any sicker than others; it is simply that their needs are being met. Some believe that much hospitalization is medically "unnecessary," but there is no question that a hospital must often meet social as well as medical needs, especially in aged persons.

Easy access to hospitals has greatly eased the burden on the busy, hard-working country doctor, and improved the quality of his diagnosis and therapy. By protecting the patient's pocketbook, the Hospital Plan has also helped to assure prompt payment of the doctor's bill. Saskatchewan doctors, though they were skeptical at first, with the familiar fear of "entering wedges to socialized medicine," are now as enthusiastic about the Hospital Services Plan as patients and hospital boards. In fact, their chief complaint is that there are still not enough hospital beds.

When the CCF government came to power in Saskatchewan in 1944, there were about 4.2 beds in general hospitals for each 1,000 people in the province. This is about the ratio now prevailing throughout the United States, after several years of the Hill-Burton hospital construction program. It was known, of course, that hospitalization insurance would greatly expand the demand for beds, and therefore a program of constructing new hospitals and expanding old ones was launched, even before the hospital insurance plan was started.

A "master plan" was drawn up, with the cooperation of town and village leaders throughout the province. Where distances for a scattered population were great, small "community" hospitals of eight or ten beds were built. In the towns of 2,000 or 3,000 people, "district" hospitals of thirty or forty beds were established. In the cities of 5,000 or more, the hospitals were expanded to serve as "regional" centers, with seventy-five or 100 beds. And in the province's two main urban centers—Regina (70,000) and Saskatoon (60,000)—the existing institutions were greatly enlarged and improved to serve as "base centers" of 300 to 800 beds each.

Most of the costs of this construction were borne by local land taxes, but the province facilitated the organization of "union hospital districts" (representing unions of several municipalities), with special taxing powers. In addition, provincial grants were given, later matched by federal construction grants. Under all this steam the supply of general hospital beds rapidly increased, and stands today at 7.4 per 1,000 of population.

But quantity of beds is not enough, and a government providing some ninety percent of all hospital income must be concerned also about the quality of hospital service. Farmers and merchants on the board of directors of a community hospital may be the salt of the earth, but without adequate numbers of technically trained staff their institution might not give good service. Therefore consultants were engaged by the provincial Department of Public Health in every aspect of hospital management: nursing service, dietetics, pharmacy, x-ray, laboratory service, medical social work, construction, ac-

counting, and general hospital administration. These consultants are continually on the road, visiting the hospitals, answering requests for help, rolling up their sleeves and demonstrating new techniques. They help to elevate standards of patient care and, at the same time, to see that the people who are paying for the Hospital Plan are getting their money's worth.

It's all very well to have good hospitals, but what happens when sickness strikes the home of the isolated farmer who lives plunk in the middle of the prairie, the roads blocked by snow in the dead of winter or by mud in the spring thaw? How can he get to the hospital? Or suppose he can get to the nearby community hospital in a snowmobile, but really needs the technical services of a regional hospital 200 miles away. In the prairies rapid transportation is essential.

To cope with this the Saskatchewan Air Ambulance Service was organized, in 1946. A Royal Canadian Air Force pilot and a flight nurse were provided with a single-engine plane, to fly anywhere in the province on mercy calls. Demands were immediate and expansion was rapid, with the result that today the corps consists of four pilots, four flight nurses, and the maintenance crew—equipped with four single-engine and two double-engine planes, converted to accommodate stretchers. Flight missions are made at the rate of two a day, year round, dark or light, rain or shine. Emergency cases of every medical classification have been carried—fractures, hemorrhages, appendicitis. Blood may be given en route, as well as oxygen or drugs. Polio victims have been transported in iron lungs, and babies have been born in midair.

The average flight costs the government about $180.00, but the patient is charged only $25.00, or nothing if he is indigent. No flight is denied on account of money. In over ten years there has not been a single accidental fatality, or even serious injury. Saskatchewan farm families swear by the Air Ambulance Service for the sense of security it gives them.

Air Ambulance may also be used to take a disturbed psychotic patient to a mental hospital. There are two large mental institutions in Saskatchewan, and, like those everywhere else in North America, they are seriously overcrowded. The situation was eased by the recent completion of a 1,200 bed training school (in the city of Moose Jaw) for feebleminded persons—the newest and, according to expert observers, the most ingeniously designed such institution in Canada. In addition, there are two short-stay mental hospital units attached to general hospitals. In five cities there are government-operated mental health clinics, with full-time psychiatrists, for diagnosing and treating less serious mental and emotional disorders, especially in children. When the American authority, Dr. Karl Menninger, visited Saskatchewan a few years ago, he said the psychiatric program there was the "outstanding" governmental service on the continent. He was particularly impressed with the fact that scientific research was being conducted into possible organic causes of schizophrenia—and this within an active mental hospital set-up.

In psychiatric services one of the most serious problems faced everywhere is the shortage of trained staff. Mental hospital attendants have often represented the bottom of the manpower barrel, so far as education and human sensitiveness are concerned. Only a handful of registered nurses are found in the average mental hospital, because the salaries and working conditions in general hospitals are usually more attractive. Moreover, nurses are seldom trained adequately in psychiatric patient care. In Saskatchewan the problem was solved by instituting a new course of training for "psychiatric nurses"—a full three-year course, based in a mental hospital and granting the graduates legal status equivalent to that of registered nurse. With such increased staffing the level of mental patient care has been enormously improved.

In other fields, too, ingenious methods of training personnel have been developed to meet serious needs. For example, laboratory technicians and x-ray technicians to staff the scores of new and expanded hospitals were in very short supply. Students graduated from the training schools in eastern Canada are seldom attracted to cold prairie villages, even for above-average pay. Therefore the provincial Department of Public Health took the bull by the horns and organized its own seven-month training course for "combined technicians"—young men and women who can give a modest level of both x-ray and laboratory service in the small rural hospitals. For other disciplines, like physiotherapy, hospital administration, or dietetics, in which needs are great and local training resources lacking, the government provides fellowships for training elsewhere, on condition that the graduate will return to work in the province for a stated period.

Some health gains are made not by improving general medical and hospital services, but by concentrating efforts on certain diseases. Saskatchewan's achievements in tuberculosis have already been mentioned. In 1954 the TB death rate had been reduced to the phenomenally low level of four per 100,000 of population. This was the lowest rate of any province in Canada, and compared with a United States average for that year of about twelve per

100,000. Moreover, this rate includes the large number of deaths among the depressed Indian population, who are the medical responsibility of the federal government of Canada. Much original research in BCG vaccination against tuberculosis has been conducted in Saskatchewan.

Another disease summoning important social action in Saskatchewan has been cancer. In line with what is being done today in many states of this country, there were organized in 1931 two cancer clinics, to which patients could be referred for diagnostic work-ups and, if necessary, radiation therapy. The service was free only to the indigent, and surgical operations were entirely at personal cost. But in 1945, building on these clinics, the complete diagnosis and therapy of cancer were made a public service for everyone, rich or poor.

Any patient with a suspicion of cancer is sent to one of the two well staffed and equipped cancer clinics. The complete diagnostic work-up is done without charge—unless the patient proves not to have cancer, when a charge of $10.00 is made. When surgery is required (as is nearly always the case) the patient goes to the surgeon of his choice, whose fee is paid by the government. Hospitalization, of course, is covered by the Hospital Services Plan. If radiation therapy is required it is given directly at one of the cancer clinics, free of charge. Extra services, in the way of special drugs, nursing, and even ambulance transportation, are also provided free as needed.

In the opinion of cancer specialists throughout America, the standard of radiation therapy in Saskatchewan is second to none. Radioactive cobalt therapy is now applied as the newest technique in the great medical centers of America, but it is not widely known that the first cobalt bomb was developed by the cancer clinic staff in Saskatoon, Saskatchewan. American radiologists who visit these government clinics are amazed at the technical level achieved.

Poliomyelitis is still another disease for which special measures are taken. As in the States, there is a Polio Foundation in Canada, with its March of Dimes. Long before this voluntary effort got going, however, the government of Saskatchewan had established public responsibility for the costs of treating infantile paralysis. With the advance of the whole rehabilitation movement after World War II, this responsibility was expressed through direct operation, by the Department of Public Health, of two rehabilitation centers for the treatment of polio and other crippling conditions. Free services are also provided for any child with cerebral palsy. In cooperation with the voluntary Council for Crippled Children and Adults, mobile clinics are held at rural points around the province, to diagnose all types of crippling condition and, when appropriate, refer the patient to one of the rehabilitation centers.

The striking thing about all these disease-centered programs in Saskatchewan is that they are open to everyone, not just to the lower income groups. This is true, for example, of the chest clinics for tuberculosis and the well-baby conferences. The Provincial Laboratory makes free tests not only for communicable diseases, as in the United States, but also for blood chemistry determinations and other clinical purposes that typically command private payments in this country. When the Salk vaccine against polio was reported as a success, the Saskatchewan government promptly announced that free immunizations would be given, once the vaccine became available in sufficient quantities—not simply to children but to all persons up to thirty-five years of age. No American state has gone this far.

Not that government does everything in Saskatchewan. Doctors and dentists are still in private practice, and hospitals are locally owned and controlled. Voluntary effort has by no means been squelched. In fact, it has expanded. Despite the sweeping governmental treatment service for cancer, there is still a strong Saskatchewan branch of the Canadian Cancer Society, which devotes its attention to raising funds for cancer research, public education on early cancer detection, and personal assistance to the families of cancer patients. Even insurance plans for medical care under voluntary auspices have flourished. Prepayment plans sponsored by the physicians now cover some 150,000 persons, not only for surgical care in hospitalized illness—as in the Blue Shield plans in the United States—but also for ordinary medical care by general practitioners or specialists, in the office and in the home.

Altogether, counting the coverage of persons in government-sponsored prepayment plans, public assistance categories, and voluntary plans, *comprehensive* medical care insurance is enjoyed by about fifty percent of the Saskatchewan population. This compares with about three or four percent in the United States. The trend is toward still greater enrollments, and there can be no doubt that eventually the whole population of Saskatchewan will have prepaid medical care, to match the prepaid hospital service.[3]

When Dr. Sigerist made his survey in 1944, he recommended the organization of a full-term medical school (a preclinical science school already existed) and a university hospital. These centers were proposed not only to help train more doctors for

Saskatchewan, but also to inspire a higher quality of medical practice throughout the province. It is no easy matter to organize a new medical school, and the cost is high. In rural Saskatchewan the sources of private philanthropy are few. Nevertheless, a magnificent 500 bed university hospital opened its doors in 1955, and thirty-five physicians, fully trained in Saskatchewan, were graduated in 1957.

Thus the arrangements for the maximum availability of health services to the greatest number of people have not obscured concern for the highest possible quality of services. The overall effect of the Saskatchewan health program has been to improve the quality of medical care received by the average person as well as to greatly extend its quantity.

Let it not be thought that all these organized health programs were started as easily as rolling off a Canadian log. It may be true that in a pioneer setting the role of government is more readily accepted, since private resources have not yet had a chance to develop. But despite this, there was opposition from certain professional and political groups at every step of the way. It took imagination and fortitude to work out the organizational problems, and much remains to be done. An idealistic and hard-working American physician, Dr. Fred Mott, who served Saskatchewan from 1946 to 1951, deserves the main credit for providing this leadership. Credit must also go to a medical couple, Drs. Mindel and Cecil Sheps of Manitoba, for early work in the program, and to Dr. Burns Roth of Ontario for current leadership. The government ministers at the helm were native sons of Saskatchewan, Premier Tommy Douglas and Health Ministers Tom Bentley and Walter Erb.

The general reader may be less interested than the professional public health worker in the fact that almost the entire Saskatchewan health program is administered by one department of the provincial government. Dispersion of authorities for various preventive and curative segments of a health program is the bane of most health officials' existence. It leads to waste, inefficiency, and often ineffective efforts, although there may be serious social and psychological obstacles to coordination of services. The unification of Saskatchewan's health program in a single provincial Department of Public Health has, among other things, inculcated a preventive viewpoint into the administration of all the curative services. It has also made possible a dynamic program of operational research into health problems. Public health and hospital experts throughout the world have profound respect for the statistical data that flow from Saskatchewan and are frequently reported at scientific conferences.

The data from the Saskatchewan Hospital Services

Plan, the Swift Current Regional Medical Care Program, and the public assistance medical service are of such value to the national government of Canada that special federal grants are made to Saskatchewan each year to facilitate their compilation. It is no secret that these reports have been used for the calculation of future costs of a national plan for all of Canada, covering hospital and medical care insurance.

More important, of course, is the practical influence that the Saskatchewan experience in health service organization has exerted on the rest of the country. Two years after the Hospital Services Plan started in 1947, the province of British Columbia followed suit. A year later Alberta adopted a hospital insurance scheme, with modifications. Finally, in 1955, the federal government proposed a nationwide system of universal hospital insurance, to be administered by the provinces.

Under this plan the government of Canada offered to assume approximately fifty percent (higher proportions for the poorer provinces) of the costs of any provincial plan of hospitalization insurance covering the entire resident population. The plan was to take effect when a majority of the provinces with a majority of the national population complied. Saskatchewan and British Columbia, with schemes already in operation, declared their participation immediately, followed by Alberta, Newfoundland, and Ontario. Now that the little Atlantic island named after Prince Edward has come into the fold, the legislation will take effect. (As mentioned, the Conservative party,

now in control nationally, favors the legislation as much as the Liberals, under whom it was passed.) There can be little doubt that the remaining four provinces will soon pass qualifying laws, so that all 15,000,000 Canadians will have the protection of hospitalization insurance.

These and other Canadian developments in health service can be credited to or blamed on (depending on your viewpoint) the Saskatchewan farmers and their CCF party.[4] A national hospital insurance scheme across the border is bound to have an influence on American thinking. But in any case the unique program of health services in Saskatchewan may make this prairie province of interest to more Americans than those who fly north each summer for a week of angling in wonderful Lac la Ronge. It may be sobering to observe that on this continent a jurisdiction of nearly a million persons seems to be moving toward a system of "socialized medical services," and liking it.

NOTES

[1] By about 1965, all health regions were organized and staffed.

[2] This was corrected in large part, of course, by the U.S. Medicare Law of 1965.

[3] This was legislated in Saskatchewan in 1962, and nationally in Canada in 1966.

[4] Renamed about 1965 as the NDP or New Democratic party. By 1972, the NDP had gained control in three provinces.

Chapter XIII
New Zealand's Health Scheme:
Problems and Trends

One of the first industrialized and capitalist countries to launch a national health service covering the entire population for virtually complete health services was New Zealand–an island nation of hardly 3,000,000 people in the Southwest Pacific. Ten years before the British, New Zealand started such a program, initially under social insurance financing, and later shifted to general revenues.

As a visiting Professor of Social Medicine at the University of Otago, an opportunity was offered to me to study this program, and report on its current problems. These were summarized in "New Zealand: GPs Ask Time and Help, Not Money," an article published in the Medical Tribune *(September 28, 1970), which is reprinted here by permission. Since then, the interest expressed by general practitioners in working in health center teams has been encouraged by construction of such centers by a number of regional hospital boards.*

The chief problem of the New Zealand National Health Service, after thirty years of operation, is the work situation of the general practitioner. Unlike his American counterpart, he does not covet hospital connections, which he lacks, nor does he seek a higher income, which is often greater than that of the hospital-based specialist. What he wants is help in doing a good job of family medicine—more ancillary personnel, more time, better office equipment, further continuing education—and greater respect from his high-status specialty colleagues in the hospitals.

New Zealand's 2,750,000 people are served by a doctor-population ratio of 1:830—slightly poorer than that of the United States, but better than that of most European countries. Of the approximately 3,300 doctors in New Zealand, roughly thirty-five percent are specialists, attached mainly to hospitals on full-time or nearly full-time salary, forty percent are in general practice—for a ratio of about one G.P. to 2,100 persons—and the remainder are in public health, teaching, research, administration, or inac-tive. This 1:2,100 ratio is actually better than that of Great Britain, to which New Zealand's medical profession looks for most of its standards, but the southern hemisphere G.P. claims to be doing better quality work and his expectations are evidently higher.

The New Zealand general practitioner is not paid by capitation, like his British counterpart, but by fee-for-service. The Social Security Act of 1938, which launched the health program the following year, originally contemplated capitation remuneration, but objections led to a change in 1941 to the fee system, permitting either straight payment of a statutory amount by the government (Department of Health) or reimbursement of the patient who has paid directly. The latter method eventually dwindled out, but the G.P. gained the right to charge his patient an extra amount beyond the governmental fee, so that today his earnings are roughly half from the statutory "general medical benefit" fees and half from patient payments.

On several occasions, the government has pro-posed that the "general medical benefit" be raised to reflect contemporary costs, with elimination of extra billing, but the doctors have refused the offer. They cherish the independence that they feel is associated with private charges, even though these are not permitted to specialists in public hospitals. In those hospitals, where eighty-five percent of the specialty work is done (the remainder being in small private hospitals or part-time private offices), the specialists enjoy great prestige along with their salaried employment. There is also general consensus that the technical quality of service in public hospitals is much higher than that in private units, which are largely devoted to simple elective surgery (hernial repairs, tonsillectomies, etc.) and normal deliveries.

In spite of his cherished independence, the New Zealand general practitioner has increasingly been turning away from solo practice toward partnerships of two to five doctors. Surveys indicate that only about forty percent of GPs are now practicing alone, these being mainly in small towns and rural areas. Unlike the American conception of "group practice," however, specialists are never involved (their "groups," so to speak, being in the hospital outpatient department), and there are various formulas for income sharing. The grouping is designed, of course, to give the family doctor periodic relief on weekends and evenings, to permit continuing education, and to render economically feasible the engagement of more ancillary personnel.

The most frequent ancillary health workers sought by the G.P. are not, interestingly enough, laboratory or x-ray technicians, but visiting nurses, social workers, and physiotherapists. The traditional G.P. role of family health advisor, with plenty of home calls and tender psychosomatic attention, is obviously still alive in New Zealand medicine.

In the same spirit, one of the general practitioner's commonest complaints is that he doesn't have enough time to give his patients all the sympathetic care they may need. Critics point out that some of the time pressures are of the doctor's own making; studies have shown that in areas with fewer patients per doctor, the number of services per patient is higher, due apparently to an effort to maintain professional incomes.

In spite of this, there is general agreement in the Medical Association of New Zealand that the nation needs more doctors. The lone medical school at the University of Otago in Dunedin (on the more sparsely populated South Island) was recently supplemented by a new school at the University of Auckland in the nation's largest city. There is current debate about starting even a third school at Wellington, the capital city, but this is being countered by the Dunedin and Auckland faculties through increases in their student enrollments.

It is remarkable to observe the full agreement among all parties about the need for more doctors, in contrast to the usual controversies on this issue in America and Western Europe between government and the medical profession. This may reflect the striking egalitarian nature of New Zealand society, in which a reasonably comfortable life seems to be favored over high incomes with a seventy-hour medical work week. In the face of a sixty-seven percent income tax on earnings over $8,000 a year, doctors would rather not drive themselves to exhaustion.

Still, physicians are in the topmost income group in this land which has few very rich and few very poor. The relatively large tax revenues are used mainly for a social security program of exceptionally wide scope and coverage. In addition to the medical care and old-age pensions, there are children's allowances, disability benefits, and even special grants for housing. Virtually everyone is covered, without benefits being related to insurance contributions but rather to needs. The health care program, in fact, is not supported by social insurance any more, but by general revenues.

Costs, of course, have been rising in New Zealand, like everywhere in the world. As in the United States, the rise is referable mainly to hospital services, which account for two-thirds of the total governmental health expenditures. Except in some small isolated rural facilities, the quality of hospital care appears to be very good, with the rigorously appointed and highly structured medical staffs, the excellent nursing service, and modern equipment.

With the rising costs in the hospital sector, it is not surprising that the national Health Department, which administers the whole program, agrees with the general practitioners that the ambulatory services should be strengthened. At a conference held in Dunedin July 22-24, it was advocated that the growing number of G.P. group practices be developed gradually into fully staffed community health centers, that the government build and equip these facilities and subsidize the payment of paramedical personnel, and that continuing education of general practitioners be promoted through the public hospitals. These proposals came not from a public health official, but from Dr. S. J. Carson, a leading spokesman of the general practitioners.

To construct and develop local health centers for ambulatory health care—both curative and preventive—it has long been advocated that the hospital boards, elected bodies which control all public hospitals, provide leadership. A law authorizing these boards to establish and operate such centers has, indeed, recently been passed. In addition to upgrading general practice, this widening of hospital board authority should help to achieve closer integration of the ambulatory and the hospital services. The district medical officers of health (MOHs), with their preventive focus, are also expected to be tied more closely to the curative services. Eventually the hospital boards would hopefully evolve into regional health boards, with the MOH as their agent, for integrated supervision of all health services in an area.

In spite of its problems, the health record of the New Zealand National Health Service is outstanding. Compared with the far wealthier United States, New Zealand has a lower infant mortality, lower maternal mortality, and higher life expectancy (especially for males). Nor can this be attributed—as is often done to explain the superior health record of the Scandinavian countries—to a "homogeneous all-white population." Ten percent of new Zealand's population is made up of nonwhite races, mostly the Maoris, whose health records are indeed poorer than those of the whites.

Health is due, of course, to many factors beyond medical care. It may be that the slower pace of New Zealand life has something to do with its surpassing the American record. On the other hand, with its rich lamb and dairy industry, the population's consumption of saturated fats is exceptionally high. International comparisons are always risky, but the available evidence would seem to favor the New Zealand system over the pluralistic American health services.

In one health care sector, the child dental services, New Zealand's record is indisputably superior. While the incidence of caries is nearly as high in New Zealand as in the U.S., the rate of teeth extracted or unfilled is far lower. This is clearly attributable to the School Dental Nurse Service, under which some 1,300 young ladies, with two years of training after high school, are authorized to give virtually complete dental care (except orthodontia or root canal work) to all children up to age thirteen.

Some twenty other nations have now emulated the New Zealand dental nurse concept, since it was launched in 1921, and one wonders when our country, with its miserable dental care record in children, will do likewise.

A propos of sensible use of paramedical personnel, it may be noted that the great majority of childbirths are attended by trained midwives, working in hospitals. Only primiparae and complicated cases are handled by doctors. Yet in 1963-1965, the maternal mortality rate was 3.13 per 10,000 births in New Zealand, compared to 3.36 in the United States.

All in all, the National Health Service of New Zealand has proved its value in an island nation, with high mountains and difficult land transportation. Its rural-urban health care disparities are not so serious as in most other countries because its farmers are among the most prosperous occupational groups. Yet even in the cities, where the minority racial groups of lower socioeconomic level concentrate, there are no visible slums. Except for cost sharing on general practitioner services, medical care is essentially available free to all, and this includes prescribed drugs.

If public opinion about medical care is a reflection of merit, surveys have shown an extremely high level of satisfaction. While introduced by the Labour party in 1938, the program has been under the control of the conservative Liberal party for most of the years since then, but there has been no reduction of benefits. The problems of general practice, which are prominent today, concern the one sector of health service (among hospitalization, ambulatory treatment, and public health) which has remained essentially private in its delivery. The solution, advocated by both the government and the profession, is in the direction of organization of general practitioners with teams of paramedical personnel. As G.P. leader Dr. Carson put it, "Health centres are the order of the day."

Chapter XIV
Australian Health Services in Transition

Australia, for many years, demonstrated a concept of health insurance advocated by certain interest groups in the United States–namely, voluntary agency programs, with substantial governmental subsidies to encourage people to enroll. The subsidies came from both state and federal government levels, and were greater for persons of low income.

For this and other reasons, Australia–along with Canada, Norway, and Belgium–was the subject of a study undertaken 1973-1976 for the Bureau of Health Manpower of the Health Resources Administration, U.S. Department of Health, Education, and Welfare. The objective was to learn lessons for America about health manpower policies and practices–in education, functions, and regulation–associated with various types of national health insurance legislation.

The full report of the Australian sector of the study was written jointly with Ruth Roemer, J.D. and published by the U.S. Department of Health, Education, and Welfare in 1975 as Health Manpower in the Changing Australian Health Services Scene. *This chapter is a brief synopsis of the observations on overall Australian health service patterns made during this research. It was written in October 1975–about a year after the field investigation, that had been made at the height of the ferment in the health care system under the new Labour party government (elected in late 1972). This text has not been previously published.*

After twenty-two years of Liberal party control, in December 1972 the Labour party of Australia won the national election in this large but thinly settled nation of the South Pacific. With this electoral victory, a health service system, which had long been unique in the world, began undergoing sweeping changes. Just three years later, in December 1975—following an unprecedented intervention of the Governor-General (appointed by the British crown)—an election was called which returned the Liberal party to power. Whether this shift will lead to reversal of the recent health system changes remains to be seen, but the account below analyzes the Australian health scene as of October 1975.

THE HEALTH INSURANCE PROGRAM

American physicians had come to look to Aus-

tralia's health insurance program as illustrating many principles they had long advocated here. It was based on voluntary enrollment, but with numerous subsidies to encourage people, especially those of low income, to join. Copayments by the patient, varying from twenty to higher percentages of charges, were required, with the intention of discouraging "unnecessary utilization." Day-to-day administration was by scores of local voluntary health benefit funds, very much like our Blue Cross and Blue Shield plans. Virtually all hospitals were heavily subsidized by federal and state governments, so that—with or without insurance subsidy—the voluntary health fund premiums were relatively low. For the aged of low income there was a separate "Pensioner Medical Service" providing general practitioner care out-of-hospital and public ward service in hospitals, through direct federal financing and control.

Despite these arrangements, so generous to the population and so supportive of private enterprise, there were many difficulties. In 1968, therefore, while the Liberal party was still in power, a Committee of Enquiry into Health Insurance, chaired by Mr. Justice Nimmo, was appointed by the federal government to investigate the program that had evolved since 1950. The Nimmo Report, issued in 1969, was a long and detailed analysis, but its principal conclusions may be summarized as follows below.

CRITICISMS AND RESPONSES

(1) The health insurance scheme is unnecessarily complex and beyond the comprehension of many. (2) There is often a wide gap between financial benefits received by patients and the costs of hospital and medical care that they must pay. (3) Premiums have become so high that a significant proportion of people cannot afford to enroll in the voluntary funds, and for others they are a hardship to pay. (4) The rules of many funds permit disallowance or reduction of claims in too many cases. (5) Administrative expenses of some funds are unduly high. (6) The financial reserves held by numerous funds are unnecessarily large. (7) Allied health services, like podiatry, optometry, or dentistry, while important, are not included among any of the fund benefits.

In all there were forty-two recommendations in the Nimmo Report, and in the next two years many of them were acted upon, such as eliminating exclusion of care for "preexisting conditions" after six months' membership in a fund, setting a ceiling on doctor's fees, simplifying hospital benefit procedures, placing top limits on health fund administrative expenses and reserves, increasing the subsidies for low income families, and so on. Nevertheless, some ninety voluntary funds continued their quite autonomous operation, with indemnification remaining the pattern for covering doctor's fees. So long as a doctor notified the patient in advance that he did not observe the "common fee" (we might say, the official fee schedule), the patient could frequently end up paying much over the statutory twenty percent copayment.

By mid-1972, about fifteen to twenty percent of the Australian population (depending on whose estimates one accepts) remained uninsured. Many of the balance were covered by the Pensioner Medical Service, but with restricted benefits (such as no ambulatory specialist service nor hospitalization outside of large public wards). Also there was the Australian Pharmaceutical Benefits Scheme, financed from federal general revenues and covering everyone since 1950 for almost all necessary prescribed drugs (with a $1.00 copayment, which is waived for pensioners, veterans, or indigent). Following the Nimmo Report, despite improvements in the health insurance system, and also in the associated federal benefit programs, by the time of the 1972 election the Labour party could point to the complete nonprotection for health of "over one million" out of Australia's 13,000,000 population. Dental and optometric services, appliances, and other health needs were quite lacking in insurance protection. Copayments were still considerable, with studies demonstrating their inhibiting effect being greater in low income families, where illness rates were higher. Costly and cumbersome administration of the ninety insurance funds and the complex funding of hospitals from federal, state, insurance, and private sources were still contentious issues. Surveillance of quality of or charges for medical service by the insurance funds was meager.

LABOUR PARTY CHANGES

Therefore, soon after its December 1972 victory, the Labour party set to work planning a national health insurance program that would cover everyone under a unified fund, with equal benefits for all (i.e., no restrictions for the aged or indigent). Free choice of doctor would still be assured, along with some copayment, but this was limited to fifteen percent of the official fee or a maximum of $5.00 (regardless of the charge—even for a complex surgical operation). There is no cost sharing in hospitals, if the patient uses "standard ward" service. The existing voluntary funds would still be free to sell supplemental benefits. In August 1974, the new National Health Act was passed, but by a very slim majority—and even this was achieved only by invoking a special constitutional provision under which both houses of Parliament were assembled to vote together. In fact, a further vote required for financing the program, through an intended annual 1.35 percent levy on all individual taxpayers' incomes (up to a $150 ceiling), failed narrowly to pass; as a result, the whole program is being financed from general or "consolidated" revenues.

AUSTRALIAN MEDICAL PRACTICE

Of probably greater long-term importance were the deliberate actions taken by the Labour government in 1973 to modify the traditional Australian health care delivery system. As in the United States, private medical practice has long predominated, but general practice is proportionately stronger. About forty percent of the nation's 16,000 doctors (1:813 population—a poorer ratio than in the U.S.) are general practitioners, compared with hardly twenty percent in America.

Yet, there is much concern about the declining proportions of general practice, and several movements have arisen to strengthen it. One has been a mounting rate of group practice—now encompassing about thirty-five percent of GPs in teams of three or more. Another has been a specialty College of General Practice (similar to the American specialty Board of Family Practice), and a dynamic Family Medicine Program subsidized by the government to provide a rich schedule of continuing education courses. Thirdly has been the important movement to develop as a locale for primary care community health centers, staffed by GPs and several allied health personnel (see below).

Another long-recognized problem in Australian medical service has been the sparsity of doctors in the thinly settled rural areas—especially the vast interior or the "outback." One solution has been the world-famous Flying Doctor service, with physicians at airplane terminals connected by radio to hundreds of posts in the interior. Another has been to send young residents to isolated stations, visited periodically by their teaching hospital chiefs. Bursaries (fellowships) have also been given to Australian medical students, who would agree to serve for a corresponding number of years in rural locations. In Tasmania, rural district doctors on relatively high salaries have long been employed by the health department. Probably most important is the "bush nurse" who is trained to handle minor ailments, give preventive services, and call for medical help when she considers it necessary.

HOSPITALS

General hospitals in Australia are much more under the sponsorship of government than in the United States. As of 1971, over eighty-two percent of beds were in "public hospitals," and ninety percent of these were in state-government operated facilities. The remaining ten percent of public hospital beds are in what we would call "voluntary non-profit" institutions, but they are regarded as "public" because the great majority of their beds are reserved for "public ward" (recently renamed "standard ward") patients and the great bulk of their support comes from government sources. Thus, the average public hospital—regardless of its original founders—derives fifty-three percent of its support from state government, fourteen percent from federal government, twenty-three percent from volun-

tary insurance, and ten percent from private payments or other special sources.

In this setting, very much like the traditional European hospital, the majority of patients, who are on the ward service, have been treated by physicians without charge. Traditionally, the doctor received only an honorarium from the hospital, but his principal rewards were the prestige of the hospital appointment and the right to admit his patients to the minority of private beds. Recently, this "charity pattern" had been changing toward hospital payment of "sessional fees" to the doctor for his service to the ward patients. Under the new health insurance legislation, such sessional payments will become general, and it is expected that hospitals may find it more economical and efficient to engage many full-time salaried physicians.

HEALTH CENTERS

The community health centers, noted above, have been a source of controversy and have taken many forms. Generally, they have been developed by local public authorities in low income areas, like the U.S. "neighborhood health centers," but occasionally—as in Canberra, the national capital itself—they have been established in any newly settled area and are open to anyone, without a means test. Doctors work in them by either fee-for-service or salary remuneration, whichever they prefer. Some centers stress preventive services to mothers and children, some concentrate on geriatric care, and some are truly comprehensive. It is expected that with the new health insurance legislation, patterns will be developed (perhaps like those of the U.S. "health maintenance organization") to encourage multiplication of health centers as a commoner model for delivering ambulatory care.

THE HOSPITALS AND HEALTH SERVICES COMMISSION

The major administrative mechanism for promoting these and numerous other changes in health care delivery patterns is the recently established Hospitals and Health Services Commission. Although under the Minister for Health, the Commission is independent of the traditional public health structure and has a free hand to develop new ideas. It must work, of course, through the state health authorities in this federated republic, and the configurations for management of hospitals, public health services, mental hygiene, and other fields differ in each of the six states. The Commission, chaired by a dynamic former private practitioner who came to Australia from South Africa, has a sizable annual budget to distribute in grants for innovative programs.

HIGHER EDUCATION

Another channel for influencing the Australian health care system has been through the assumption by the federal government of 100 percent (it had formerly been fifty percent) of the costs of tertiary education. This includes not only the universities and their medical schools, but also a second echelon of "colleges of advanced education" and a third one of "schools for technical and further education." In all three of these types of postsecondary school institution, health personnel are trained. While faculty appointments, student admissions, course content, etc. remain autonomously under the control of each institution, the offering of stronger federal support in selected fields naturally exerts an influence. Thus there has been increased support for all medical schools (to enable them to enlarge enrollments) and also for departments of family practice within them. As in the United States, the training of nurses is being shifted from the hospitals to academic settings, and this is being fostered by substantial grants for the purpose to the colleges of advanced education. Increased training of technicians, rehabilitation therapists, and other allied personnel is being promoted in the same way.

With the high importance attached to family medicine, the "nurse practitioner" concept of America has little enthusiastic support in Australia. The need is felt for more "community nurses" to help in the care of families at home, especially the chronically ill, and stronger training programs for such personnel are being supported. But these are more like our public health or visiting nurse than like the clinical nurse who actually substitutes for the American doctor in management of patients with simple ailments. The male "physician's assistant" is not being promoted at all in Australia.

SCHOOL DENTAL THERAPISTS

On the other hand, in the dental field, Australia has begun to emulate New Zealand by training young women in a two-year course to become "school dental therapists." The shortage of dentists in Australia has been so great and the demands on those available have been so heavy that several of the states have been able to launch these programs with virtually no opposition from the dental societies. These young women, working in the schools under only the limited supervision of a dentist, are now serving to elevate the dental health of Australia's children to a level well above that of the past—and at a relatively low cost.

REGIONALIZATION

Another new development being promoted by the Hospitals and Health Services Commission is the regionalized organization of all health services. In the large land areas of each of Australia's states, plus its Northern Territory, some form of decentralized administration of various branches of government has long been necessary. The emphasis now, however, is on integrated planning and operation of all aspects of the health services, including hospitals and community health centers, as well as the preventive public health services, mental health programs, health manpower education—both basic and continuing, and eventually health insurance administration.

REGULATION AND MALPRACTICE

Licensure in Australian medicine is perhaps simpler than in American, because of the basically public character of higher education. Graduates of all Australian medical schools (nine currently and two more in the planning stage) are automatically registered for practice in any state, as are graduates of British or New Zealand schools; no "second examination" by a state board is required. The same applies to most other health professions. It is only for other foreign graduates that a special examination (like our ECFMG exam) is required. As for quality controls over medical performance, the voluntary health insurance funds have done little, and under the new insurance law Australia is looking to America's professional standards review organization program with interest. In-hospital medical services, on the other hand, tend to be more highly structured than in America.

The more disciplined medical staff organization in most hospitals may help to explain the very low rate of malpractice suits and low malpractice insurance premiums (averaging about $100 per year) in Australia, compared with America. Another factor is probably that, with the population's high rate of health insurance protection, few patients get angry with their doctors over fees. Also doubtless contributory is the legal system, which does not provide for jury trial in noncriminal tort cases, nor does it allow contingency fees to lawyers.

THE NATIONAL HEALTH ACT

The new National Health Act took effect in Australia on 1 July 1975. As of that date, all Australians were entitled to financial protection for comprehensive physician's care, although with various degrees of cost sharing. It is still too early to know how well the program is operating, but by 1 October 1975, all six Australian states had concluded agreements with the federal Ministry of Social Security on the sharing of hospitalization costs; whether the return to power of the Liberal party ten weeks later will mean any reversion of these actions remains to be seen. The Australian Medical Association had been strongly opposed to the whole new law—more perhaps for what it feared might evolve from it than for the provisions of the Act itself.

Basically, the conversion of Australia's previous subsidized voluntary health insurance scheme into one with universal coverage has simply followed worldwide trends. The inadequacies of voluntary enrollment and highly fragmented administration had led finally to the kind of unified social security system that virtually every industrialized nation has now adopted. The United States remains now alone, among the world's affluent nations, to lack such a health care system, and we know that some form of national insurance is not far off. As in Australia, it is altogether likely that the area of major contention will shift from the principle of collectivized money raising to issues surrounding the patterns by which doctors and allied health personnel provide their services. Also as in Australia, a great deal depends on the outcome of the next national elections in the United States.

Chapter XV
Highlights of Health Services
in the Soviet Union

While all of the industrialized, as well as the developing, countries have organized the financial support and the delivery of health services to a substantial degree, none has gone further than Russia, following its 1917 Revolution converting this large nation into the Union of Soviet Socialist Republics. The Soviet health services have been analyzed in several books, which describe in detail the fully governmental and centrally planned character of the system. In many respects the health planning now being actively undertaken in most developing countries is modeled implicitly, if not explicitly, on the Soviet pattern.

This chapter does not recapitulate the entire structure and function of the Soviet health system, but rather analyzes its main features according to twelve pervasive concepts. Based largely on a field study made in 1961 by a party of ten American and British physicians and social scientists, it was published as "Highlights of Soviet Health Services" in the Milbank Memorial Fund Quarterly *(Vol. 15, October 1962, pp. 373-406) and is reprinted here by permission. While the fundamental socialist model, with its emphasis on comprehensive public services, universal coverage, and integration of prevention and treatment continues, the intervening years have seen a substantial increase in health manpower (or more accurately womanpower) and facilities.*

The formal structure and function of Soviet health services have been described abundantly over the last twenty-five years. As the first fully socialist nation, its approach to problems of health and the organization of medical care has interested hundreds of Western observers, and we have available as a result of this interest many excellent and thorough accounts, from the Sigerist volumes of the 1930s to the recent study tour reports of the World Health Organization and the United States Public Health Service.[1]

The excuse for another exposition would not be to add further details to the picture of Soviet medicine. A two-week observation could hardly do that anyway. It is, rather, to attempt to analyze the Soviet health service system in terms of certain key concepts that are of interest in the United States and perhaps in all countries. Under each concept, one may explore the Soviet approach in several of the formal subdivisions of the health services.

One need hardly be reminded that the Soviet Union is a huge country—the largest land area of any nation in the world, with a population of 220,000,000. Because it is built from fifteen republics and an enormous diversity of local national and ethnic groups, one should hardly expect a simple, clear picture of uniformity, in the health services or any other aspect of life. This would be true even had the past forty years since the 1917 Revolution been times of quiet social development. But since the overthrow of czarism, almost half the time has been spent in periods of war and reconstruction. After the First World War the country experienced a period of hostility from the rest of the world, with armies of a dozen nations at her borders for several years. Then came the Second World War, from 1939 to 1945, and with it the loss of 20,000,000 men and women—far more than the losses of any other country—with untold destruction of villages, towns, and cities, from Leningrad to Stalingrad. Then came the postwar reconstruction period, ushering in the era of the cold war with its enormous military expenditures which the Soviet economy could ill afford to make.

The hospitals, clinics, and sanitary facilities of the czarist period, and the personnel to staff them, were meager—the poorest in Europe; in Asiatic Russia conditions were comparable to those of India or China. In the fifteen years from 1924 to 1939, improvements were enormous. Resources in health personnel and hospitals increased five- and tenfold. But the Second World War destroyed a great part of these. Much of what we see in 1961 has been rebuilt in the last decade. The vast need for rebuilding also of homes and schools and railroad stations has naturally influenced the rate at which medical facilities and equipment could be provided.

Observations of Soviet health services must be made against this background, which a visitor from North America—physically untouched by either world war—may find it hard to appreciate. Any particular observation can be interpreted in different ways, depending on one's sensitivity to factors of this sort. In a hospital ward, it will affect whether one notices most the frugality of the low flat beds or the cleanliness of the linens and the energetic attitudes of the nurses. Almost any experience is felt differently by the sympathetic and the critical visitor. The twenty minutes' wait between courses in a Moscow restaurant may be relaxing to one tourist and exasperating to another. The observations recorded here will try to strike an objective balance between the extremes.

Here then, are twelve key concepts which it is hoped will contribute to an understanding of health service organization in the Union of Soviet Socialist Republics.

PUBLIC SUPPORT

The first, the most obvious, and probably the most important feature of Soviet health services is that, with a few exceptions, they are free to all. Health service is regarded substantially as a public responsibility, an obligation of the government to the entire population.

The exception is drugs taken at home and certain appliances (dentures, eyeglasses, etc.), which patients must purchase from governmental stores at very low prices. (More of this later.) But all services

of physicians and hospitals, dentists and technicians, all forms of diagnosis and therapy and rehabilitation are provided without personal charge. There are no limitations with regard to the duration or frequency of medical attention. There are no exclusions of maternity care, tonsillectomy, or preexistent conditions. There are no qualifications for eligibility like a specified time of employment, payment of a membership fee, or residence for a given number of years in an area. There are no prior authorizations required and no deterrent fees, even for house calls of a doctor by day or night. The utter simplicity and inclusiveness of this financial support can perhaps be appreciated only by those of us who have been brought up in a free enterprise medical economy. When the international organizations list the coverage of social security and health insurance systems in the nations of the world, the space required to describe the Soviet eligibility is shortest of all; it says simply: "all residents." And under the benefits it says merely "complete medical service."

Nothing in this world, of course, is "free," and the real question is how are the services financed. The answer is by government revenues derived from the income of all enterprises which are, of course, government-owned-and-operated. Soon after the Revolution, the Soviets made medical services freely available to all, but they adopted first the Western European pattern of financing them through health insurance for employed workers and through general revenue funds for the rural population (based on the old system of "zemstvo" doctors in the villages). This system, however, permitted great inequalities between urban and rural resources, and in the 1930s it was changed to one of complete and general governmental support. On the whole, this means funds come from the central government and are allocated outward to the republics and *oblasts* (provinces). Initial budgets are prepared locally and sent into a central office. The decisions made at this higher level determine the resources in personnel, equipment, and facilities that will be available in the local community—and these will be examined below. Whatever resources are provided locally, however, are available to everyone without charge.

But is there any private practice, everyone asks, for which individuals actually pay? The answer is extremely little, although it is not legally prohibited. A physician may not use public facilities to see private fee-paying patients, as he does for example in the Philippines or in Egypt. But he may see them at his home in the evening. Recent Soviet reports give hint of a slight rise of private practice in the cities, particularly for calls to the patient's home. From all that one can learn, however, very little of this goes on. In

Latin America and elsewhere, physicians employed "full-time" in a public system usually engage in private practice to supplement their low salaries, and the weaknesses of the system yield a clientele for them. These forces do not seem to operate in the USSR.

SCOPE OF SERVICES

The medical services offered to the Soviet people are comprehensive, but they differ greatly in their pattern from the American custom. The basic scheme is that all persons are expected to get care from a team of doctors at the health center near where they live. In this sense, there is little "free choice of doctor," just as we have no choice of public schools for our children—since they go to the school in the neighborhood. The physicians at the local health center or polyclinic, however, serve as true family doctors; each is responsible for the families in a district. The general practitioner is backed up by a team of specialists in pediatrics, surgery, ophthalmology, and so on. He sees these families in the clinic or, when urgent, in their homes. As in the United States, the ratio of home calls to clinic visits is relatively low, about one to ten or one to twelve. The local polyclinic also provides dental services, given either by a dentist or by a stomatologist. The latter is a physician specializing in diseases of the mouth and is trained more thoroughly than the dentist. Soviet taste runs to dental prostheses of gold, which must be paid for, although the services of personnel are without charge.

Drugs given in a polyclinic or hospital are free, but others prescribed must be purchased in a local drugstore, somewhat as in other countries. The difference is that in these stores only drugs are sold. Life-saving preparations required for ambulatory patients, like insulin, are provided free from special endocrinology clinics. In any event, prices are low for all prescribed items. Other drugs may be purchased "over the counter" without a prescription, and their prices are higher. The "Bayer aspirin" that we saw in one drugstore, imported from abroad, was apparently for this use. The vast bulk of Soviet drugs, however, are manufactured in the country in government factories supervised by the Ministry of Health. There tends to be only one preparation of each chemical composition. Appliances—from eyeglasses to artificial limbs—also must be purchased privately, unless the need grows out of military service or industrial accident.

Admission to a hospital is without limitation, except that a hospital physician must participate in the decision as well as the doctor who sees the ambulatory patient. This is, of course, the prevailing system in Western Europe where general hospitals have closed and salaried medical staffs, distinct from community doctors. Once hospitalized, the patient gets a range of services much like that in other countries. There is perhaps more emphasis on physical therapy, exercise, and diet, somewhat less on diagnostic laboratory and x-ray examinations, than in the United States.

Hospital services are offered predominantly in general hospitals, but there are also some mental hospitals—large institutions in the main cities. The definition of need for mental hospital care, however, is very different from that in the United States; while we have roughly one mental hospital bed for every bed in a general hospital, the Soviet Union has only about one-tenth of a mental bed for each general bed. How much of this large difference reflects a lower relative prevalence of mental disorder and how much represents a different approach to the problem, demands study.

For other long-term care there are sanatoria of various types. Some of these are for old people, but very little stress seems to be put on this group—unlike the situation in America. The focus is more on the types of disease: cardiovascular, cancer, neurological disorders, children's care, and so on. In addition, there is a wide network of rest homes for short stays of persons in need of some release from their work, and of spas and similar resorts for stays of about a month.

Finally, the scope of services includes those of a purely environmental and preventive nature, which will be discussed later. It should also be mentioned that cults like Christian Science are not known in the spectrum of Soviet health services. There are some drugstores, however, that claim to specialize in homeopathic medications, and there is a marginal fringe of chiropractors who make home calls—a subject on which *Izvestia* published a recent attack. Cultist medicine, nevertheless, is of much smaller proportions than in the West where it is a part of the legal medical establishment.

QUANTITY COVERAGE

A third feature of Soviet health services is their great emphasis on mass impact. The central philosophy is to attempt to provide a reasonably satisfactory level of service for everyone, instead of high-level service for a few. The attitude is that qualitative improvements "will come later." This passion for quantity is evidenced in many ways.

Most prominently it is seen in the enormous production of medical and allied personnel. By the standards of other countries, the output of physicians has been fantastic. There are now over 402,000 doctors in the USSR, or a ratio of one to every 540 persons—the highest relative supply of any country in the world (the United States ratio is about one to 750). This was achieved by great expansion of the medical school enrollments; there are eighty-four schools—about the same as in the United States—but each class has several hundred students. The educational process is doubtless less individualized than in America. The length of training also was shortened, having been fixed at five years beyond high school for some time, although now it is six years. (While this is shorter than the usual American eight-year course, it is similar to the practice in most European countries.)

As in Western Europe, only a small percentage of physicians have internships. Instead they go right to work in a polyclinic, hospital, or health station—some organized setting where their work is subject to review by other doctors. The Soviet Union is very proud of achieving a short work week for all employed persons, and this applies to doctors as well. A six- or seven-hour day, which with a six-day week usually amounts to about forty hours per week, is the norm. This may be contrasted with the American medical practice in which doctors tend to be proud of their fifty- to sixty-hour week. Some Soviet physicians, however, may hold second part-time jobs. Moreover, they do not lose time going between an office and one, two, or three different hospitals or other facilities each day; each Soviet doctor is located at one center.

Everyone has been struck by the very high proportion of women doctors in the USSR. Undoubtedly this has been one of the consequences of the emphasis on quantity output; thousands of men were needed for other fields like engineering, the sciences, and education. It has also been due to the emphasis on child health service (see below) for which women are believed particularly well suited. Then after the Second World War, the proportion of women medical students went up from about fifty to seventy-five percent, because so many men had been killed. Still another factor has been the policy of encouraging advancement in the ranks of health workers, so that many medical students are former nurses. The Russians explain that, contrary to Western conceptions, this female predominance does not imply a lower status for physicians.

It has been said that the vast numbers of Soviet physicians are partially wasted by assignments to tasks which in Western countries are performed by auxiliary personnel. This is certainly true in the field of public health, since there are relatively few sanitary engineers or sanitarians, and much of the surveillance of environmental sanitation is done by medically trained "hygienists." (See below.) (There were actually some 28,000 sanitary and epidemiological assistants in 1960.) In the clinical fields, however, I could see no evidence of squandering medical skills. On the contrary, there are large numbers of auxiliary personnel in the hospitals, polyclinics, and various health stations—adding up to about 1,350,000.

In 1960, there were 623,000 nurses—more than in the United States, and a higher ratio to population. In addition, the Soviet health services have a special type of auxiliary health worker not found in other countries—the feldsher. Unlike the nurse, the feldsher is not simply an aide to the doctor, but works with greater independence on the basis of "standing orders." He or she (about one-third are men) is often stationed at an isolated rural point (the pattern started in the nineteenth century under the old zemstvo medical system), and is authorized to give drugs for common ailments like diarrheas or respiratory infections, to give first aid to injuries, to vaccinate, to make sanitary inspections, and to offer health education. In 1960, there were 334,000 feldshers. In addition there were 76,000 feldsher-midwives and 139,000 regular midwives. Technicians of all types number about 84,000 which is fewer than exist in the United States. Other personnel include about 80,000 pharmacists and almost 31,000 dentists (not counting about 16,000 stomatologists who are numbered with physicians).

The mass impact applies also to hospital facilities. In 1960, there were about 1,740,000 civilian hospital beds of all types of which only 162,000 were for mental patients. (The number of military beds is not reported.) Thus, the overall ratio was about 8.0 beds per 1,000 people. Beds are classified in different ways than in the United States—for example, there are many separate maternity homes—but it is quite evident that the supply of *general* hospital beds is well in excess of the American ratio of under 4.0 per 1,000 population. (This is not counting the beds in sanatoria or rest homes.) Attached to practically every hospital is an outpatient department or polyclinic, serving everyone in the area. In addition there are several thousand separate health stations at collective farms or industrial enterprises.

The quantity coverage, however, is associated with many deficiencies in quality, at least by American standards. The diagnostic work-up of cases appears to be less thorough than prevails here. Routine screening laboratory tests (urinalyses, hemoglobins, etc.), which we have come to consider essential in the United States, are not done on all hospital admissions. Even the mass periodic health examinations (see below) are weak on laboratory procedures like chest x-rays or serological tests. The training of medical and surgical specialists is done in special postgraduate institutes, but it tends to be less elaborate than that required by the twenty-odd American specialty boards. Physical facilities in the hospitals and polyclinics are certainly modest by United States standards. The beds are simple, flat cots, usually without the mechanical features—bedside lamps, call-buttons, and other gadgets—that add to patient comfort in the United States. On the other hand, there is the sputnik complex, with artificial kidneys, operating room television, and electronmicroscopes to be seen in hospitals that have only rudimentary diagnostic x-ray equipment.

Still, it may not be fair to compare Soviet resources with those of the wealthy United States. The technical level of hospitals is certainly as good as much that one sees in Western Europe, not only in France and Italy, but also in Great Britain. Moreover, the Soviet doctors never tire of telling you that the quality will be improved later on.

GEOGRAPHIC SPREAD

Tied to the rapid expansion of health personnel and facilities is a policy of equitable distribution of these resources through the vast stretches of the Soviet Union. Not that full success has yet been achieved, but there is no question about the deliberate policy of getting physicians, middle-medical personnel, and facilities into the remotest villages, wherever people live, and regardless of the local affluence of the region.

Physicians are attracted to the rural districts in several ways. Every new medical graduate is, first of all, theoretically required to spend a period of three years in one of a list of localities posted by the ministry of health of his republic. His medical education has been completely subsidized (including living expenses), and this is a way of paying back his obligation to the state. The new graduate is given a list of places needing physicians, from which he makes a selection, but the higher-ranking students get the first choices. Such periods of rural service, incidentally, are required also in Turkey, Greece, and several Latin American countries.

A certain proportion of these young doctors remain in rural health service, but there is no question that in the USSR, as in other countries, the cities have greater attractions. To counterbalance these, rural medical positions pay higher salaries than urban posts of comparable responsibility.

The basic key to geographic coverage of the vast Soviet lands is simply the "table of organization" of the health services. Even if the great majority of

medical and allied personnel preferred to settle in the cities, they could only go where there are job openings. It is not a question, in other words, of physicians and dentists settling where they wish and opening offices—a policy which in most countries has resulted in great overcrowding of the main cities and critical shortages in the hinterland. While there is free competition for all medical posts, the virtual absence of private practice means that personnel go where there is an established need, whether in city or village.

Another instrument of wide geographic coverage is the extensive use of auxiliary personnel. The feldsher is specifically suited to meeting rural needs, especially in thinly settled areas where it would be very costly to provide physicians. Thus, a village of a few hundred persons or less will be served by a locally stationed feldsher, who can refer cases to a physician when necessary.

A built-in regionalization of hospitals and polyclinics is the ultimate basis for providing a reasonable quality of services throughout the Soviet system. Thus, the hospitals are conceived as a network of small rural units of ten to fifty beds, (*uchastock* hospitals), which feed into *rayon* hospitals of about 100 to 200 beds; and these, in turn, orient toward the large *oblast* (provincial) or municipal hospitals in the main citites. There is no hestitation to refer a patient from a peripheral to a central unit, since all the physicians are on salary and no loss of a fee is involved. A specialist from a central hospital occasionally goes out to a smaller hospital to see a case, but much more often it is the patient who is moved. In this way, the better equipment and technical staff of the whole central facility are available to him. At one small rural hospital which we visited, however, there was striking pride that difficult cases—even gastric surgery—could be handled locally, without having to send the patient to a city institution. To provide transportation for patients, there is an ambulance attached to every urban and rural hospital. For transportation from very remote places, there is an airplane ambulance system with special nurses. This service is all free.

PREVENTIVE EMPHASIS

Another striking and pervasive feature of the Soviet health services is the great emphasis on prevention of illness and promotion of health. This is not simply a responsibility of the "public health"-type agencies, although these exist, but is built into the whole system.

It starts with medical education which includes much more attention to instruction in environmental sanitation, health education, and preventive concepts than is found in the West. The status of these subjects and their teachers is obviously higher than in Western medical schools. Moreover, the basic scheme of Soviet medical education calls for a decision after the second year among three major specialties: "therapeutics" (i.e., medicine and surgery), pediatrics, and hygiene. The next four years are then spent with a concentration in one of these fields. The hygiene concentration gives attention not only to sanitation but to all social aspects of medicine, including occupational health, epidemiology, biostatistics, medical administration, etc. A physician may also take postgraduate work in this field, although there are no special "schools of public health" such as we have in the United States.

The physicians trained in hygiene staff the "sanitary-epidemiological stations" of the Soviet health system. These are the equivalent of our public health agencies. Until very recent years, Russia was a very backward country, especially outside the main cities, and environmental conditions were primitive. The main emphasis of these stations, therefore, is on environmental sanitation. The medical hygienists, as well as their assistants (feldshers, nurses, sanitary assistants, etc.), are engaged in sanitary work involving food, water, waste disposal, vermin control, and especially housing. They also supervise control of the communicable diseases with isolation, quarantine, disinfection, and immunizations. They give much attention to general health education of the public. Not much is done, however, in the field of chronic disease control, mental hygiene, or administration of medical care, for reasons we shall note below.

The entire territory of the Soviet Union is said to be covered with these sanitary-epidemiological stations, manned with full-time staffs. There are no "noncovered" counties or districts. In the main cities, like Moscow or Kiev, there is a central sanitary-epidemiological station that supervises smaller ones around the city and operates various laboratories for chemical or bacteriological analyses. Generally, however, the station—as we shall discuss later—is part of a hospital center.

This aspect of the Soviet health services is not very different from Western public health, especially as seen in Europe, but it is in the day-to-day program of medical care that an extraordinary emphasis on prevention is seen. The heart of this is the national policy of "dispensarization," which entails provision of periodic general medical examinations to well persons, and the follow-up of those found to have any significant symptoms. The national goal is to examine every person every year, with children being done more frequently. The goal is far from reached, however. In 1960, there were 44,000,000 persons given prophylactic examinations, which is about twenty-two percent of the Soviet population. Of these, about 8,000,000 were called back for further care of some sort. Priority in these examinations is given to industrial workers, pregnant women, and children—groups which, of course, also get more preventive service in other countries.

The examinations are evidently not too exhaustive because we were told that they included x-ray and laboratory tests "only on indication." The goal, however, is to make them more complete. The point emphasized is that people are called in for these examinations, or they are done at the place of work, without waiting for patients to come with complaints. Much time is devoted also to health counseling. A record of the findings of all examinations is kept at the polyclinic attended by the person; if he should move, it is sent on to the clinic nearest to his new residence.

Health education is in evidence everywhere. The hospitals and polyclinics are lined with posters, and even outside on the hospital grounds there are billboards with health messages. Some of these are more matters of political propaganda about Soviet health achievements than hygienic education, like the bar chart indicating that the ratio of doctors to population in the USSR was better than in the USA or any other country. In the hospitals, however, the graphic presentations are devoted to child health, control of respiratory infection, insect control, nutrition, and so on. Much use is made also of simple leaflets. In one hospital we visited there was an elaborate system of audio-visual health education, requiring only the pressing of buttons on the wall. Most remarkable perhaps is the requirement that every Soviet physician in a polyclinic should spend a half-hour daily in specific health educational activities with a group or a family.

Health promotion is emphasized through a widespread program of physical culture. Everyone has seen the movies of vast masses of young Soviet men and women engaged in public spectacles of exercise and gymnastics. But these are not only for youth; in factories there are designated periods when the machines stop and everyone does some calisthenics—instead of a coffee break. Housewives are also encouraged to do this. There are various athletic leagues for different age groups. Even in hospitals, convalescent patients are encouraged to exercise at certain periods each day. Development of physical prowess is part of the national health policy.

INTEGRATION OF SERVICES

While it has been implied already, special recognition must be given to another pervasive feature of the Soviet health services. This is the principle of integrated organization.

Health is a goal of high priority, and it is conventional to quote the founding father V. I. Lenin, that "socialism will conquer the louse or the louse will conquer socialism"—the thought being extended beyond the problem of typhus fever. From the earliest postrevolutionary days, therefore, the USSR has had a separate Ministry of Health. One must emphasize the word "separate," for in much of Europe and elsewhere the health services do not command such a top cabinet post, but are included within a general welfare ministry of some type. (Witness the ministries of social affairs in Norway and Sweden or the Department of Health, Education, and Welfare in our country.) More important, all health activities are encompassed under this ministry, with the exception only of the military medical departments.

The full extent of this integration at the top level can only be appreciated by making comparisons with other nations. "All health activities," of course, include preventive and curative services, so that there is no separate administration of insurance for medical care under a labor or social insurance ministry, as one finds in most European countries. (The trade unions do supervise many aspects of the social insurance system, but in the health services their authority is limited to control of admissions to certain sanatoria and rest homes.) But the integration goes much farther. Medical education is not a function of universities and, as elsewhere, supervised by ministries of education, but is provided in special institutes supervised by the Ministry of Health. Research also is under the wing of the health ministry; there is a general Academy of Sciences that plans overall scientific research, but medical research comes under the national Academy of Medical Sciences which functions as part of the Ministry of Health. Even the production of drugs is supervised by the Ministry of Health, as well as their distribution through pharmacies.

Integration of health services is found not only at the top—as it is, for example, in the British National Health Service—but more particularly at the local, operating level as well. In most countries one can distinguish three fairly separate branches of the health services: that for ambulatory medical care, the hospital system, and the public health program. In Great Britain, as well as in most other countries, these three activities are quite distinct, with separate authorities and management, not to mention their physical separation. In the Soviet health system, national policy calls for unification of all three both professionally and physically at the local level. In practice this policy has not yet been achieved everywhere, but it is almost accomplished in the rural areas and is on the way to realization in the cities.

The facility around which all the local health services are built perhaps should not be described as the hospital, since it is much more than a building for the bed-care of the seriously sick. Attached to it usually is the polyclinic, in which are located all the physicians serving the population of the district. In order to avert narrow attitudes and to help each physician appreciate the problems of the other, there is a system of rotation between polyclinic and hospital duties. The schedule varies at different places, but usually involves a period of about three months a year when the polyclinic physician works in the hospital and vice versa. This system of rotating apparently does not operate universally—e.g., it was not found to be widely practiced in a large teaching hospital visited in Moscow—but it is the official goal of the system. It is significant that the Soviet literature defines these integrated facilities as "therapeutic-prophylactic institutions" rather than as hospitals. (We have already noted their attention to preventive medicine.)

More remarkable is the professional attachment to these medical centers of the preventive sanitary-epidemiological stations. Even when the personnel of these hygienic services are located at certain outposts, they come administratively under the center. The head of this tripartite service (i.e., hospital, polyclinic, and "san-epid" station) is typically a physician on the hospital staff, very often a surgeon. He is chosen for his general leadership abilities. At the *rayon* level, the deputy head is always the hygienist responsible for the sanitary-epidemiological activities; at higher levels, this is also usually the case.

In a city or a rural *rayon* (like a county), the head of the whole jurisdiction, which may contain several "therapeutic-prophylactic institutions," is said to be head of the "health department." But this must not be confused with the American or British use of the term, since it is meant to encompass all health services. Nevertheless, this executive is seldom full-time, but is ordinarily a highly respected clinician in the largest central hospital, aided by the hygienist in his district. Strictly administrative or bureaucratic duties are performed by a clerical assistant. The ultimate integration occurs within the work of the individual physician where, as noted earlier, preventive services play a major role, side-by-side with therapeutic activities.

CENTRALIZED POLICY AND DECENTRALIZED EXECUTION

While the whole Soviet health service is centrally planned and directed, the day-to-day or even the month-to-month orders do not all emanate from Moscow. There is great delegation of responsibility peripherally, and enormous diversity is found in local practices. The execution of policies is a responsibility of the health ministries in the fifteen republics, and is delegated further to hundreds of *oblasts*, municipalities, and *rayons*.

The fundamental requirement, for example, that the services of physicians and hospitals should be available to everyone without charge, but that drugs outside the hospital or polyclinic must be purchased, is national policy. The central ministry also issues recommended standards for proper ratios of physicians of different specialties, and hospital beds of different types to meet the needs of a population in cities and rural areas. The actual building of these hospitals and the staffing of them and of the polyclinics, however, is left up to local authorities. The great geographic variations in resources actually found are evidence of this decentralization. In 1959, there were 112 physicians per 100,000 population in the Tajik Socialist Soviet Republic, 242 per 100,000 in the Latvian Republic, and as many as 314 per 100,000 in the Georgian Republic. Georgia is an attractive place with a climate like California. Total hospital beds varied in 1959 from 6.2 per 1,000 population in the Tajik Republic to 10.5 per 1,000 in the Latvian. These are figures issued by the Soviet Ministry of Health, so it is perfectly obvious that there are great diversities across the nation.

The official curriculum for education of physicians, feldshers, and other personnel is spelled out in some detail, but again there are obvious diversities in the way a particular faculty handles the subjects. Originality in teaching methods, both didactic and practical, is encouraged. All new graduates are supposed to spend three years at a rural post, as noted earlier, but a vacancy in an urban polyclinic can draw a bright young man or woman from his country spot before the three years are up. Public health regulations on sanitation or communicable disease control are nationally uniform, but the degree of their enforcement will obviously vary with the energies and effectiveness of the local staff. Drug production is centrally planned; the distribution system, however, is not flawless and some drug stores are better stocked than others.

There is particular decentralization in the estab-

lishment of hospitals, polyclinics, industrial health stations, and other physical facilities. A substantial share of the capital costs of these is met from local, rather than central, revenue sources—particularly in rural areas. The collective farms are now expected to build hospitals and maternity homes from their own funds. Factories provide the space needed for health stations. Once established, however, the full costs of operation are met by funds allotted from the central government. The amount a particular local unit gets, however, depends directly on the budget proposal it submits. Thus, the first action on needs for personnel, equipment, and supplies is taken when financial estimates are sent up the line. These local budgets are reviewed at the *oblast* and republic levels before being submitted to Moscow, and there can be no doubt that there must be decreases or increases in funds requested along the way, just as in a federally supported program like the post office system in the United States. But it is equally clear that the persuasiveness of the account about local needs will influence the allotment that the local institution eventually receives.

Variations in local performance are seen in matters like the application of preventive measures. While every physician is expected to spend a half-hour daily in health education activities the diligence with which this is done obviously varies enormously. In one hospital we visited, particular stress was put on audio-visual education because, it was quite evident, one of the doctors on the staff was an amateur electronics fan and enjoyed rigging up various loudspeaker systems. There are also great variations in the rate of dispensarization of the population in different localities; at one rural center, the head physician insisted that all 6,000 people in the area (*uchastok*) had been examined twice in the last year, which would be much more than the national average achievement. The precise pattern of work of the feldshers and other personnel of the sanitary-epidemiological stations must vary greatly.

While the lines of authority from the *uchastok* to the *rayon*, *oblast*, republic, and central ministry are perfectly clear, a great deal of use is made of local committees. Much as one sees in the British civil service, these committees are made up principally of health service workers from the establishment; there may be a few nonmedical or public representatives as well. Such committees will be responsible for various phases of the operation of the health program and may influence greatly how general policies are carried out. Separate voluntary agencies, however, are not common, although the Red Cross and Red Crescent operate—primarily in conjunction with the military services.

This leeway in local operations—which has been especially prominent since the generalized Krushchev policy of 1957 on decentralization of industry—should not obscure the fact that Soviet health services are mainly characterized by their centralized planning. Indeed, the main function of the national Ministry of Health is probably best described as planning the health services. In this it is aided particularly by the Semashko Institute for the Organization of Public Health and the History of Medicine, a research unit named after the first Commissar of Public Health who worked at the elbow of Lenin. It is this institute that studies the supply of hospital beds needed for a region, that explores the value of closer relationships between polyclinics and hospitals, that analyzes the use of drugs, etc., and recommends changes which the ministry may promulgate.

Because of the basically centralized and uniform scheme of the Soviet health services, well understood by everyone, there is an impressive paradox to the American observer. This is the presence of much less in the way of full-time administration than we have come to expect in the United States. Almost all directors of local health jurisdictions are physicians who have active clinical responsibilities in a hospital or polyclinic. The full-time hospital administrator or local health officer is almost unknown. There are clerical personnel who keep the records and accounts, but top administration seems quite casual. It absorbs much less time and energy than in the United States, where health administrators are kept busy dealing with hundreds of agencies—public and voluntary, with boards of directors, scores of sources of money, and so on. The building in which the Ministry of Health of the USSR is housed in Moscow is a modest structure, such as might accommodate a health department in a small American state; the same applies to a republic ministry, such as the Ukrainian one in Kiev. Yet these agencies supervise not merely preventive health work, but all medical care as well. In other words, the very systematization and unification of the Soviet health system reduces rather than increases the administrative overhead and bureaucracy of the entire program.

POLITICAL OVERTONES

In the Soviet Union, one expects to see all sorts of political overtones in the health services, but the predominant impression is how very similar the services are technically to the modes of the West. Doctors diagnose and treat most illnesses about the same way they do in England or America. Substantially the same drugs are used and the same surgical opera-

tions are performed. The average duration of stay of hospitalized patients for a given diagnosis is much longer than it is in the United States, but this is true throughout Western Europe; British or Norwegian hospital practices are more like Russian than they are like American. The Soviet physician may use somewhat different forms of antibiotics or surgical sutures than the American, but the predominant principles of therapy and diagnosis are substantially the same.

Despite all this, there are certain political overtones to Soviet medicine which can be recognized while not exaggerated. In the professional education of all physicians and other personnel, for example, instruction in Marxism-Leninism is always included. This seems shocking to some Western observers, but one must keep in mind that the Russians would regard the ordinary instruction in "capitalist economics" or "bourgeois sociology" at our universities as essentially comparable indoctrination. The instruction in Marxism-Leninism is intended to inculcate in Soviet personnel a dedication to the collective goals of the health service. There is some evidence, however, that this instruction is not always taken seriously by the students, any more than are the compulsory courses in "military science" provided in many American universities.

The materialistic philosophy of Soviet society is seen also in certain aspects of medical theory and practice. Most striking is its influence in psychiatry. The predominant view seems to be that mental illness is associated with organic changes in the brain. Not that functional disorders are denied, but the major psychoses are believed due largely to chemical processes induced by metabolic disturbances, trauma, infection, or other physical causes. A virus etiology for schizophrenia has long been sought. The greatest emphasis is given, therefore, to physical forms of therapy—electric shock, drugs, hot baths, work regimes, and so on. Prefrontal lobotomies had been commonly done but have now been discontinued since they were found ineffective. There is virtually no acceptance of Freudian concepts or practice. Some interpersonal psychotherapy is used— both on a group basis and an individual basis—but it is largely directive, and aimed to encourage the individual to see his role in the larger society. To some extent the differences from American psychiatric concepts are due to different definitions of illness along the continuum from sanity to psychosis. The peculiar behavior of some old people, for example, which in America calls for hospitalization as senile dementia, is seldom regarded as mental illness in the USSR. Behavioral disorders in children, on the other hand, are treated through institutionalization, during which fairly rigid routines are designed to reorient the child in his group. One such institution that we visited was significantly called a "psychoneurological sanatorium." Despite the organic and the collectivistic philosophy, both children and adults in mental institutions seem to be served with great care and tenderness.

Another expression of Socialist materialism is perhaps the great emphasis on physical medicine in general. Not only does every hospital seem to have a well-developed department of physical therapy, but there is a great network of rest homes and spas where people may go for recuperation. Various regimes of exercise, baths, diet, and rest are followed in these places.

The Pavlovian theory of the conditioned reflex, developed actually before the 1917 Revolution, is given great emphasis in Soviet physiology and medicine, and it seems likely that this is partly because it was a native Russian scientific discovery and partly because it coincides so well with Marxist philosophy. Its basic implication, after all, is that modification of the physical environment can directly influence the behavior of human beings. In one hospital we visited, a central theme of the whole insitution was the principle of "Pavlovian therapy." This meant, for example, great attention to the colors of rooms and wall decorations, systematic physical exercise for almost all patients, a program of sleep therapy, a special department of climato-therapy, and much health education. It also seemed to include a department of acupuncture, which is worth special comment.

Acupuncture is a system of treating all disease by inserting needles of different lengths into the body at sets of points (usually three or four at a time) among some 250 designated spots on the human surface anatomy. Each disease calls for a special grouping of points, with a prescribed duration and schedule of insertions. Without examining the actual or supposed rationale of this therapy, its origin dates back to ancient China of at least 2,000 years ago. Since the victory of the Communist movement in China, acupuncture has been seriously reexamined on the ground that it is part of the national culture which may well have some value if it has survived two millenia. (The policy of India, which has set up institutes for the reexamination of Ayurvedic medicine with its ancient herb therapies, reflects a similar attitude.) In about 1955, an institute for acupuncture was established in Moscow with Chinese instructors, and there can be no doubt that this represents an extension of the hand of political friendship to China. Soviet medicine is obviously lending its resources to test out the theories of acupuncture, and

see if they have demonstrable merit. Three or four hospitals out of about 290 in the Kiev *oblast*, we were told, are now trying out acupuncture therapy.

There are other medical policies that seem to derive from a particular political philosophy. Just as religious influences in the West deeply condition our social attitudes, our practices, and even our laws on abortions, Soviet ideology has comparable though opposite influences. Abortions are quite openly sanctioned legally and medically; physicians may sometimes try to discourage a woman from having her pregnancy terminated, but if she still requests it, it is done as readily as other elective surgery. This policy has had its ups and downs; after initial legality following the Revolution, in 1936 abortions were prohibited on the ground that they were being done to excess and population growth was threatened. Now that the Soviet population and economy are robust again, abortions are again fully permitted. Of course, contraceptive information is also freely available everywhere.

The nonreligious attitude toward death may also be responsible, in part, for the achievements of Soviet medicine in blood collection and preservation. I do not know of any other country that removes blood from cadavers—except after fatal infections— and uses it for transfusions. It may be the nonsanctified attitude toward dead bodies that led also to the first transplantation of corneas by Filatov in the USSR.

Direct political influence on health policy in the Soviet Union is seen in such actions as the withdrawal from the World Health Organization, in the last days of Stalin and at the height of the cold war. Perhaps this is no more political than the nonrecognition of the People's Republic of China by the Western majority in WHO. The Soviet Union is now fully active again in this and many other specialized agencies of the United Nations. Within the country, the operations of the health services at all levels are subject to the surveillance of the Communist party, just as a kind of "watchdog," equivalent in some ways to legislative committees or voluntary accreditation agencies in America.

Another political overtone—priority for the proletariat—is so basic in Soviet health services that it requires a special discussion.

PRIORITY FOR THE PROLETARIAT

The Soviet Revolution was led by the Communist party on behalf of the working class of czarist Russia, and it is understandable that the top priority in health services should be accorded to the industrial proletariat. The vast impoverished peasantry was also involved, but as in all countries it was politically more conservative and sections of it were antagonistic. Moreover, the vast industrialization plans of the Soviet economy demanded a robust urban population, whose health would be constantly protected.

The priority accorded to industrial workers is evidenced in many ways. Most important is the network of health stations in the factories. Unlike the American pattern, these do not restrict their services to physical examinations and first aid, but may provide any medical care required. At the same time, they put much emphasis on occupational hygiene in the preventive sense. In the larger plants, there is a whole staff of physicians, nurses, and others; in smaller ones, it may be only a feldsher. In either case, this staff is under the wing of a hospital and polyclinic nearby, to which patients may be readily referred. The tendency lately, in fact, has been to get away from elaborate medical facilities in the plants in favor of better services at the general medical institutions in industrial districts. One purpose of the factory health unit is to make medical care convenient for the worker, so that follow-up therapy may be given at his place of work.

Within hospitals and polyclinics also, the worker is accorded priority. Polyclinic hours are scheduled to his convenience. He is put to the head of the line—ahead of housewives and oldsters. One does not see the attention to geriatrics in the USSR that marks the current American scene, and it may be that this reflects a lower priority for the aged. (It may also reflect a society closer to the rural model, in which old people stay with the extended family. The high proportion of married women who work is certainly facilitated by the custom of having grandma take care of the children.) In any event, the worker, both in cities and rural districts, gets the most energetic attention from medical centers.

The whole social security system in the USSR is geared to an attitude of high respect for and faith in the worker. All disability insurance systems in the West for example, pay to the disabled worker a cash benefit only after a waiting period—typically three to seven days. This is partly for economy, and partly is designed to discourage abuses. In the Soviet Union, the integrity of the worker, on principle, seems to be more fully respected. Cash disability benefits are paid from the first day of illness; there is no waiting period.

In the education of physicians, training in industrial hygiene and occupational diseases is given substantial attention. For those specializing in "hygiene," it is a major component of the training. The rest homes and spas mentioned earlier are largely controlled by the trade unions, and admission to them is first of all for industrial workers.

In medical establishments, the Soviet philosophy is also expressed in the unionization of the health workers, including everyone from janitor to chief physician. The union is intimately involved in the hiring and firing of workers, in settlement of grievances, welfare services, etc., although it does not negotiate for wages in the Western sense. There is great pride, as mentioned earlier, in the seven- or six-hour day for all health personnel, including doctors. Another key feature of personnel policy is the opportunity for health workers to rise from the ranks. About half the Soviet women medical students (or about one-quarter of the total) are former nurses or feldshers.

PRIORITY FOR CHILDREN

Another priority that permeates Soviet society is the enormous favor shown to children. Foreign visitors are always struck by the vigor and healthiness of the youngsters. The great Soviet attention to both elementary and higher education is well-known, and the same priority applies to the health services for children.

One of the three basic specializations after the second year of medical education is pediatrics. There are twenty-seven whole medical faculties devoted to the field. The great majority of doctors in pediatrics are women, and perhaps the very high proportion of women in medicine as a whole represents a favor for persons particularly sensitive to the needs of children.

The philosophy of Soviet childrearing is different from in the West. Babies are swaddled firmly—a practice seen also in some other European countries and found more generally in rural than urban parts of the Soviet Union. If lack of crying suggests a happy baby, the custom certainly has its advantages, and who knows if it perhaps contributes to a more secure child? (American pediatrics seems to have returned to pacifiers.) The question is surely worth careful comparative study. Greater use is made of crèches and nursery schools than in the West. In these the child learns cooperative behavior for the welfare of the group, from an early age. There are stations for free milk to families with small children.

Although the United States has moved away from specialized children's hospitals, the Soviet Union is still building them in the cities. There are also children's polyclinics, separate buildings associated with general hospitals as well as with children's institutions. The staff of such a polyclinic has within it all the specialties of surgery, dermatology, and so on that one would see in an adult medical center. A medical record of the child's whole development, as well as of any illness, is kept in the greatest detail. There are also special sanatoria for children with long-term illness or psychological problems.

The Soviet emphasis on children makes different impressions on different observers. To some it may be seen only as the breeding of "cannon fodder;" to others, it is pure humanitarianism. Doubtless it means many things, but above all it embodies the same concepts as those expressed by Bishop Berkeley for Catholicism when he said "give me the child before five...." It is the Soviet strategy in building a socialist society, by starting out with the shaping of a sound mind—socialist style—in a sound body.

SOCIAL MOTIVATION

Whatever one may think of the goals of Soviet society, there is no question about the energy and dedication with which the vast majority of people in the USSR seem to be working toward them. After forty years, a particular philosophy and way of life have become firmly established and the great mass of the population are identified with it. Almost all foreign observers get this impression today. In the health services it is quite apparent.

Physicians, nurses, and other health workers seem to be deeply devoted to their work. They are proud of everything and the morale seems high. Turnover of personnel in the hospitals is low, although people are free to leave for other jobs and, since unemployment is virtually unknown, there are plenty available. (Compared with the United States, the turnover of hospital personnel throughout Europe is low.) The attitude of doctors and nurses toward patients seems warm and sensitive. We saw a young woman who had just been treated with an artificial kidney machine for anuria, following a self-induced septic abortion. Since medical abortions are quite proper, her act was illegal, but the the gynecologist explained that she would only be scolded and not be reported to the police; she was just a foolish and unfortunate girl, he said. An Egyptian patient, with whom I was able to speak English, had been operated on a few days before for appendicitis. Although he was just a young tourist, not a high personage whom the Russians would be anxious to impress, he said he had never been treated so kindly. High Soviet officials or other important citizens, of course, get special attention from top-flight medical centers, as they do in any society, but it is within the framework of the regular medical care system.

One often hears the view that the high proportion of women in Soviet medicine implies a lower status for the profession than prevails in the West. Western observers seem frequently to get this impression, although the top Soviet medical leaders (most of whom are men) certainly do not admit to it. Reports on physicians' salaries are conflicting. Our group was informed officially that they are relatively high—approximately at the same level as engineers'. Other observers report them to be lower—more like those of schoolteachers or skilled workmen. Of course, there are great variations within the ranks of the system. The medical schools have two or three applicants for every place, about the same ratio as in the United States today, suggesting a high level of attraction of the field. Morale, as well as competence, in the medical profession is also maintained through continuous encouragement of postgraduate education and financial support for the physician while he is undertaking it.

There may be some of the attitude of condescension toward patients by Soviet doctors that one sees in many Western countries. In a speech made in December 1960, Dr. S. V. Kurashov, the Minister of Health of the USSR, called for many improvements in the health services. Among other things, he criticized the attitude of some hospital personnel toward patients as heartless and inattentive. This is mindful of recent attacks on American hospitals in popular magazines and probably means the same thing—that there is a rising consciousness of the importance of sensitivity in good patient care, and rising public expectations about it. In one hospital we toured, the visiting hours were on only one afternoon per week, on Sundays, except by special permission of the doctor. While this was justified as protecting the interests of the patient, it would seem to reflect a rather rigid institutional policy in which the convenience of the staff was put ahead of the feelings of patients and their families.

The social motivation of health workers is also reflected by their almost uniformly optimistic response to questions. Undoubtedly there is much exaggeration about the health services, and the story is told in glowing terms. As in other aspects of Soviet development, the achievements are usually presented in percentages of improvement over a previous level, which are usually quite impressive. Much detail is given on trends in the supply of health personnel and facilities, and very little on rates of death or illness for specific diagnoses or age groups, which would reflect the end results of the health service. (Data on the crude death rate and infant mortality are freely quoted and are impressive.) Nevertheless, there is an obvious enthusiasm about achievements which everyone seems to share. To elicit admission of shortcomings, one has to probe pretty deeply, and can seldom expect any negative comments except from high officials who are concerned with overall planning.

The relative simplicity of administrative machinery, discussed earlier, is another reflection of the basic motivation of the collectivity of Soviet health workers. In a well-knit team, everyone knows what to do and the role of the captain can be limited; in a team of individualists or prima donnas, it takes a lot of cajoling and directing to reach a goal. This is perhaps an oversimplification, but still may epitomize the Soviet health services and offer an interpretation of their paradoxical simplicity of administration. The men or women rising to key executive positions seem to be those with natural leadership qualities, regardless of medical specialty and whether or not the person has had any training in administrative matters (like the hygienists). The rules of the game are well understood, and the general social pressures toward collective behavior are so fundamental in Soviet society that they become internalized in the motivation of each individual in the health service.

THE VIEW TO THE FUTURE

A final characteristic permeating the whole Soviet health service is its persistent view to the future. Whatever may be deficient now, everyone will assure you, will be corrected in time. Soviet planning is a complex mechanism under the overall direction of a central agency of government known as "Gosplan." Health service goals, of course, are only a small part of the total, and must be fitted into the planning of resource allocation in industry, agriculture, housing, education, and all other fields. There is no question, for example, that the top priority given to the construction of new housing— thousands of new apartment houses in the cities— has slowed up the development of modern hospital facilities.

The goals for health service are still very ambitious by Western standards. While the Soviet supply of physicians, at one to 540 population, now exceeds that of all other countries, the goal for 1980 is to have one doctor to 333 persons. Whether this can be achieved, while at the same time improving the quality of the professional product (as many Soviet medical leaders advocate), remains to be seen. The goal for total hospital beds is 16.5 per 1,000 population, a level which—if achieved—will probably surpass that of all other countries. The important Third Program of the Communist Party, issued in 1961, specifies that all medical services will soon be free, which has been interpreted to mean inclusion of

drugs and appliances, as well as all the other elements of care, in the public service.

There is also continual discussion of improvement of the quality of service. Medical education, one hears, may eventually be extended to seven years. Postgraduate medical courses are to be expanded, so that more doctors may be included in them. The health examinations and dispensarization of the population are to be extended so that they reach everyone every year. By 1965, it is planned that there should be an increase in the supply of drugs, medical supplies, and equipment of 350 percent above the 1958 level.

An important sign of the high attention given to health services, as suggested earlier, is their independent place in the structure of both the national and republic governments. The Ministry of Health is a full-fledged cabinet department, on a par with agriculture or heavy industry or other major functions. The Soviet Union is very proud of its health achievements, and gives them top billing in its international propaganda on the benefits of socialism. I am not certain of the accuracy of its mortality statistics, but the crude death rate in the USSR (not age-adjusted) is now down to 7.6 per 1,000, or lower than that of the United States. The infant mortality in 1960, at thirty-six per 1,000 live births, was lower than that of any other vast and predominantly rural country, although still higher than that of Great Britain or the United States. In the International Fairs at Brussels and New York and elsewhere, the attainments of the health service enjoy prominent display, not as a byproduct but as a central purpose of Socialist society. And the emphasis is always on future improvements.

In interpreting Soviet health services, everything depends on one's points of comparison. Americans naturally are inclined to compare with conditions in the United States—even perhaps in the most advanced sections of our country. But the Soviet Union is European and, in fact, largely Asiatic. Many of the attributes of its medical system—which we may look upon either as weaknesses or as strengths—are indeed European rather than Communist. The central planning, for example, has much in common with the British National Health Service; prolonged hospital stays are found throughout Europe; emphasis on physical therapy and spas goes back to nineteenth century Germany; hospital organization with full-time salaried doctors has long prevailed in Scandinavia and elsewhere.

Many of the deficiencies are more Russian than socialist. The washrooms in restaurants tend to be grim and unsanitary—as they were before the Revolution and as they still are throughout France and

Italy. The American achievements in plumbing and cleanliness are simply not to be found in most of Europe. The design of hospitals and other public buildings seems terribly ornate, nonfunctional, and old-fashioned to American eyes—but the Soviet Union of 1945-1960 was in its Victorian age of great national pride and pretentiousness. It is mostly in the physical setting—the way walls are plastered or lawns are kept—that one detects a certain lack of workmanship, wherein one can contrast Russian standards with, say, Swiss or Swedish. This is a vast complex nation, only recently emerging from rurality and ignorance, and the style of life of an affluent industrialized society is not to be achieved overnight.

In so big a country, one must expect unevenness of local development. As everywhere in the world, much depends on the energy and initiative of leaders and health workers in each community. Perhaps the greatest achievement of all has been the provision of a reasonably good minimum level of health service everywhere, even in the most primitive sections of Asiatic Russia, where roads are yet to be built and the women still wear veils. In visiting some of these regions a few years ago, the Minister of Health of India, Rajkumari Amrit Kaur, said that she would be pleased if the great cities of her country could achieve the level of health service found in the humblest Soviet village. Perhaps it is most accurate to evaluate Soviet health service—or other aspects of this society—in terms not of the United States, nor of Western Europe, but of itself, as a nation that has emerged in a brief span of years from an underdeveloped to an industrialized society, and still has some rough edges.

The Soviet health workers are obviously anxious to smooth off those edges and are eager to learn from other countries how to do it. In 1961, they certainly impress the American visitor as friendly and gracious. There are still certain aspects of the health program apparently closed to foreigners—for example, analysis of costs and expenditures for specific items of service—but most doors one knocks on are opened. There is obviously a great deal that the Russians can learn from the West by exchanges, especially in improvement of the technical content of hospital and medical service. It is equally clear that the West can learn a good deal from the Soviet Union about the organization of an integrated and comprehensive health service available to everyone. Such two-way lessons can have value only if they are applied against the social and cultural backgrounds of our different societies.

NOTES

[1] Sir A. Newsholme and J. A. Kingsbury, *Red Medicine: Socialized Health in Soviet Russia.* New York: 1933.

H. E. Sigerist, *Socialized Medicine in the Soviet Union.* New York: W. W. Norton, 1937.

H. E. Sigerist, *Medicine and Health in the Soviet Union.* New York: Citadel Press, 1947.

J. Wortis, *Soviet Psychiatry.* Baltimore: Williams and Wilkins, 1950.

T. F. Fox, "The Health Service in the Soviet Union." *The Listener* (London: British Broadcasting Corporation), December 16, 1954, pp. 1,049-1,050.

D. M. Baltzan, "An Introduction to Medicine in Russia." *Canadian Medical Association Journal*, Vol. LXXVI, February 1, 1957, pp. 242-243.

I. V. Davydovskii, "Questions of Organization and Planning of Medical Science: A Prospective Plan for the Important Problems of Medical Science, 1959-1965." *Vestnik Akademii Nauk USSR*, Vol. 13, 1958, pp. 46-61. (Translated from the Russian at the National Institutes of Health, Bethesda, Maryland.)

U.S. Public Health Service, *Report of the United States Public Health Mission to the Union of Soviet Socialist Republics.* Washington, D.C.: U.S. Government Printing Office, 1959.

L. Baumgartner, "What about Soviet Medicine and Public Health?" *American Journal of Public Health*, Vol. XLIX, May 1959, pp. 590-600.

K. V. Maystrakh, *The Organization of Public Health in the USSR.* (Main Inspection in Medical Literature, Ministry of Health, USSR.) Washington, D.C.: U.S. Public Health Service, 1959. (Translated from the Russian by the U.S. Joint Publications Research Service.)

G. F. Konstantinov (ed.), *Public Health Administration in the USSR: A Statistical Handbook.* (Division of Medical Statistics, Ministry of Health, USSR.) Washington, D.C.: U.S. Public Health Service, 1959. (Translated from the Russian by the U.S. Joint Publications Research Service.)

World Health Organization, *Public Health Administration in the USSR.* Copenhagen: WHO Regional Office for Europe, 1961.

M. C. Kaser, *Notes on Public Health Administration in the USSR.* (Based on G. A. Batkis and L. G. Lekarev, Theory and Organization of Soviet Public Health.) Oxford, England: processed document, 1961.

H. Schulz and S. P. Dunn, "S. V. Kurashov on Improvement of Medical Care." *I.C.R.S. Medical Reports* (Fordham University Press), April-June 1961, pp. 23-27.

M. S. Sokolovsky, *The Moscow City Sanitary-Epidemiological Stations.* Moscow: processed document, 1961.

N. Kaplan, "Research Administration and the Administrator: U.S.S.R. and U.S." *Administrative Science Quarterly*, Spring 1961, pp. 51-72.

A. Plichet, "Les Etudiants de Medecine en U.R.S.S." *La Presse Medicale*, Vol. LXIX, May 20, 1961, p. 1,105.

G. E. Ostroverkhov, "Higher Medical Education in the U.S.S.R." *Journal of Medical Education*, Vol. XXXVI, September 1961, pp. 986-995.

Part Four

Specific Health Programs

Chapter XVI
Health Programs for Certain Illnesses Around the World

In all countries, organized health services are frequently focused on the treatment or prevention of certain diseases that are communicable or hazardous in other ways to populations, or which are seriously disabling and expensive to treat. Tuberculosis and mental disorder have been the most extensive objects of such social action, but numerous other diseases have summoned a great variety of special programs in both industrialized and developing countries.

A worldwide review of these disease-specific health programs was one section of a general study of the relationships between preventive and curative health service administration in all countries. This study was done for the World Health Organization in 1953-1955 and served as a "working document" for the Technical Discussions of the Tenth World Health Assembly (1957). This chapter is drawn from this monograph, "Medical Care in Relation to Public Health (A Study of Relationships between Preventive and Curative Health Services throughout the World)," an unpublished World Health Organization document (Geneva, December 7, 1956, pp. 138-179), reprinted here by permission. While many changes have, of course, occurred in the intervening years, the administratively "vertical" disease-specific program is still a feature of many ministries of health, and sometimes other agencies of central government. At the same time, there are movements everywhere to integrate these specialized campaigns into comprehensive health service programs at the local area level.

In all countries, medical care programs have developed for the treatment of special diseases which constitute particularly serious social and economic burdens. On the whole, the diseases commanding such special organizational efforts are prolonged, seriously disabling, and expensive to treat. Because they are usually beyond the economic resources of the average individual afflicted, social measures have been necessary. Moreover, for some of these diseases, direct hazards are created to the population if a case is untreated. This has created a sense of urgency which has usually led to governmental action long before attention has been directed toward prevention of the disease.

It has been commonplace, therefore, for curative services for these serious expensive diseases to develop quite independently of overall preventive health services. In later years, however, the relationships have sometimes come to be appreciated and administrative responsibility has been unified. Even when responsibility for curative programs is vested in the national health authority, however, there are great differences among nations in the degree of integration between curative and preventive activities for a particular disease.

The principal diseases for which special organized programs are found are tuberculosis, mental disorder, treponematoses (including venereal diseases), certain other infectious diseases, dental disease, orthopedic crippling disorders, cancer, and other chronic diseases of the aged. In all these programs there are two sets of relationships which may be explored: (1) relationship between treatment and prevention of the specific disease, and (2) relationship between the specific treatment program and other health services being promoted for the population at large.

Just as certain diseases striking anyone have given rise to special social action, so also have certain population groups, with any disease, been the basis of programs of medical care. The social stimulus is often in a broad field of economic, religious, military, or political activity, in which health services are only incidental. Thus, there are programs of medical care for indigent persons, for special occupational groups, for children and expectant mothers, for students, for soldiers, for military veterans, and for other special groups. Since health service is only part of larger activities for these groups, these medical care programs are often quite independent of the health authority.

TUBERCULOSIS

There is great variety in the organization of preventive and curative services for tuberculosis throughout the world. In no disease is the interdependence of treatment and prevention so clear, for the prevention of spread of the disease depends directly on the treatment and isolation of the individual infectious case. This is possible, on the other hand, only through finding cases in the population, a task requiring public health organization. Yet responsibilities for these various aspects of tuberculosis control may be distributed among several different governmental and voluntary agencies.

Recognition of the great value of sanatorium care with long periods of bed rest as the cure for tuberculosis came in Germany around 1850 and in the United States in the 1880s. It was taken up first by voluntary societies, and these tuberculosis associations or antituberculosis leagues still occupy in many countries a key place in the overall program. Some years later, responsibility in some countries of Europe and America for tuberculosis hospitals was taken over by governmental authorities, but not always by the public health agency. Meanwhile tuberculosis preventive services came frequently to be promoted as part of the public health program.

In the older European countries, where social insurance for medical care was extensively developed, tuberculosis treatment has frequently been a function of insurance societies. Financial protection for the costs of tuberculosis may be part of an overall health insurance program or may be covered by a special adminstration solely for tuberculosis. Actual sanatorium treatment may be given in institutions operated by the insurance societies themselves or else by separate voluntary associations or units of government for which costs are covered by the insurance fund.[1]

Thus, there are at least four types of agency concerned with prevention and treatment of tuberculosis in different countries (1) the national health authority, (2) units of provincial or local government other than the public health department, (3) voluntary tuberculosis societies, and (4) social insurance organizations. On the other hand, there are a variety of measures necessary for the control of tuberculosis, preventive and curative. Preventive activities include the operation of dispensaries for case finding, epidemiological contact tracing, and follow-up of cases; mass chest x-ray surveys for case finding; notification; BCG vaccination campaigns and health education of the public. Curative activities include principally the operation of hospitals and sanatoria for the treatment of cases and rehabilitation of discharged patients. Various components of these preventive or curative services may be carried out by one or more of the four types of agency mentioned, so that the programmatic permutations and combinations of functions among nations are highly complicated.

The dispersion of authorities for the control of tuberculosis is illustrated by the pattern in Greece a few years ago. In 1949 a WHO survey in that country reported:

> At the present time, tuberculosis control is divided between at least six different departments of the Ministry of Hygiene, under two Directors-General. In addition the Ministries of Social Welfare, Marine, National Economy, Labour, Interior, and Justice each have their own small field of tuberculosis control. In the provinces, the tuberculosis programme is nominally under the responsibility of the prefectural Medical Officers of Health. . . .

Beyond this, there were in Greece at the time 102 social insurance funds. The largest of these, the Institute of Social Insurance (IKA) operated its own tuberculosis clinics and sanatoria, spending some twenty-five percent of its funds on this disease. In addition, there were a number of voluntary societies engaged in tuberculosis control activities and subsidized by the central government. Among these was the Hellenic Red Cross Society which conducted an institution for bone and joint tuberculosis in children, maintained several BCG vaccination centers, and operated occupational therapy departments in various governmental sanatoria. The first recommendation of this survey, obviously enough, was "the establishment of a Central Tuberculosis Authority within the framework of the Ministry of Hygiene."

In Turkey, there is a Bureau of Tuberculosis in the Ministry of Hygiene which operates tuberculosis dispensaries and sanatoria throughout the country. The Istanbul Antituberculosis Association and other voluntary societies also own and operate sanatoria and dispensaries. In addition there are sanatoria operated by local municipalities. There is no regional organization for tuberculosis control, and the central Ministry of Hygiene exerts no control over local governmental and voluntary institutions except to receive reports and collate statistics. A WHO observer in 1949 concluded conservatively: "There does not exist that close coordination between all tuberculosis services which is essential if the best use is to be made of the available facilities." It is significant that in 1949 new legislation was being planned in Turkey to place control of all clinics and sanatoria under the Ministry of Hygiene. Brazil is another country with a tuberculosis division in its national Ministry of Health, but exerting very little control over the operations of a great many local voluntary societies. These societies, nevertheless, depend largely on government grants for their work. In 1948, the Brazilian Congress of Phthisiology recommended "cooperation of private with official organizations to act effectively on the disease and its consequences" and stated that "relations between voluntary agencies and government ought to be governed by rules applying to each case."[2]

Voluntary societies carry the major responsibility of all aspects of tuberculosis treatment and prevention in some countries. In Belgium, the Ligue Nationale Belge contre la Tuberculose conducts all the dispensaries and associated preventive work for which it receives regular grants from the government. Curative work is handled by the Association Nationale Belge contre la Tuberculose which receives government grants and in turn pays for services rendered in sanatoria owned by communities and friendly societies, as well as in its own sanatoria. Work of both a preventive and curative nature is done among youth by the Oevre de Preservation de l'Enfance contre la Tuberculose. The Belgian Ministry of Health simply receives reports of cases on which its grants are used, but gives virtually no supervision over the services. In the Netherlands likewise the tuberculosis campaign is in the hands of private organizations although social insurance has developed protection against sanatoria fees and has been covering an increasing number of people. Israel is another country in which the bulk of tuberculosis control, both preventive and curative, is exercised by voluntary organizations and the large Workers Insurance Fund (Kupat Holim). The Ministry of Health has its own special dispensaries and sanatoria but it does not control the parallel activities of other agencies.

In Italy, preventive tuberculosis work is carried out mostly by governmental authorities, while curative work is predominantly under the social insurance institutions and voluntary hospitals. Under the High Commissariat for Public Health there are ninety-one provincial officers who administer tuberculosis clinics. Besides this, the National Institute of Social Welfare (Instituto Nazionale Providenzia Sociale or INPS) supervises various health insurance societies. These organizations operate fifty-eight curative establishments for tuberculosis, with 25,000 beds, and the INPS also obtains care for insurance beneficiaries by contracts with many other hospitals. The Italian Federation for the Antituberculosis Campaign and the Italian Red Cross are voluntary societies also operating sanatoria, preventoria, and clinics of their own.[3]

In Switzerland, there is no special office for tuberculosis control in the Federal Department of Health. The only centralized control is exercised by a voluntary society, the Swiss Association against Tuberculosis which is affiliated with leagues in each of the cantons. This association sets standards for tuberculosis sanatoria and acts as a clearinghouse for subsidies from the cantonal governments. The sanatoria are operated by some 430 local voluntary organizations as well as by cantonal governments and municipalities. Social insurance, covering part of the costs of sanatorium care, is carried separately for tuberculosis by associations receiving federal subsidies under the condition of fulfilling minimum standards. Little is done in the way of preventive work.

In some countries, the voluntary societies engaged in tuberculosis control have had a more flexible role, changing their functions as government has assumed increasing responsibilities. Such is the case in Sweden, where the Royal Medical Board has overall national responsibility for tuberculosis control. The sanatoria are operated by units of local government or special funds and, in each province, the medical officer of health is responsible for central and district clinics. As for the voluntary agencies,

> The Swedish National Association against Tuberculosis, founded in 1904, is aiming to fight against tuberculosis as a national disease in Sweden. The Association's first task was to try new ways to fight tuberculosis and primarily support undertakings which had not yet reached their final shape and received state subsidy. When a new field of action has been tried, found its form, and received state subsidy, the Association's contribution has been reduced or detained. In this way, its work has gradually altered. In the beginning the dispensary work thus

received considerable economic aid from the Association. This has now almost ceased and the Association's principal task during the last years has instead been to organize and support mass radiography examinations and BCG vaccinations. The Association also grants money to scientific research.

In many countries, tuberculosis control activities are only meagerly developed, but administrative authority has been placed squarely in the ministry of health. In Egypt, one section of the central ministry operates all tuberculosis hospitals and dispensaries. Iran's sanatoria are under the Ministry of Health. Activities against tuberculosis are quite limited in Iraq, Lebanon, and Syria but virtually everything done is carried out by the ministry of health or through subsidy of a voluntary group by this ministry. In Ethiopia, little has yet been done but authority is centralized in the Ministry of Health. In Aden, there is a voluntary society for financial assistance to needy families stricken with tuberculosis, but all medical activities are under the Director of Medical Services. Considerable progress has been made in Ceylon, where all tuberculosis work, curative and preventive, is administered by a division of the Ministry of Health.

In the Philippines, the Department of Health contains a Tuberculosis Division which operates tuberculosis clinics and sanatoria. It also subsidizes a large hospital operated by the Philippine Tuberculosis Society in Quezon City. It is interesting that in 1954, the Tuberculosis Division was reorganized and granted wider powers to coordinate a comprehensive program of tuberculosis prevention, treatment, and rehabilitation. Activities in Cuba had been diversified at one time but in 1936 all voluntary agencies and the tuberculosis section of the Ministry of Health were incorporated into the National Tuberculosis Board. While associated with the Ministry of Health, this is a semiautonomous body responsible for all preventive and curative services relating to tuberculosis.

The weakness in many tuberculosis control programs which are coordinated at the highest echelon is the absence of an effective service at a regional or local level, closer to the people. In France, we see on the other hand a highly complicated combination of preventive and curative activities which have been administratively coordinated at the regional or *départemental* level. The sanatoria may be owned by a unit of local government, like a *département* or a commune, by a voluntary association, or by a private individual, but they are subject to overall supervision by the director of health of the department, who is a regional official of the Ministry of Health. The same sort of supervision applies to all tuberculosis clinics (which may likewise have various sponsorships) and other preventive services in the *département*. Thus the regional public health official, who is sometimes assisted by a special phthisiological medical officer, supervises all curative and preventive activities for tuberculosis in his territory. Costs meanwhile are met partly by payments from the social security funds for insured workers, partly by subsidies from the Ministry of Health, and partly from local tax or voluntary sources. Nationally, there is a tuberculosis control section in the Division of Social Hygiene of the Ministry of Health, with ultimate powers to coordinate all preventive and curative activities. The striking feature of the French pattern of tuberculosis control administration is that, despite various sources of financing and various types of ownership of preventive and curative facilities, the functioning of all services is coordinated at the central and regional levels. In Denmark, where particularly outstanding tuberculosis control work has been done, there are regional or county tuberculosis control directors who are responsible for both clinics and sanatoria in their areas.

In New Zealand, with its total population of only less than 2,000,000, coordination of tuberculosis activities is achieved in the Tuberculosis Division of the national Ministry of Health. Administration of tuberculosis sanatoria is actually a responsibility of the regional hospital boards which control all hospitals (except mental) in the country, but the central Tuberculosis Division determines medical policy in the sanatoria. It is able to coordinate these institutions with case finding and preventive activities on the one hand, and rehabilitative and social security benefits on the other. It also maintains liaison with the voluntary Antituberculosis Associations which carry on supportive social services for tuberculosis patients. Locally, the medical officer of health is responsible for case finding, supervision of tuberculosis patients at home, and social welfare activities, while the local tuberculosis hospital director supervises sanatorium treatment and diagnostic services in tuberculosis clinics. The tuberculosis control activities of both these officers are coordinated by the same division in the national Ministry of Health.

The problems of coordination of preventive and curative services for tuberculosis have occupied much attention in Great Britain since the organization of the National Health Service. After the establishment of the British Ministry of Health in 1919, a central medical department for tuberculosis control was set up. Generally speaking, the local health authorities responsible for overall public health services were responsible for tuberculosis clinics and preventive activities as well as for the supervision of sanatoria.[4] With the initiation of the National Health Service in 1948, high priority was accorded to the importance of regional organization of hospitals, and the tuberculosis sanatoria were transferred to the jurisdiction of the regional hospital boards. To maintain coordination the chest clinics were transferred with them to the regional boards. The local medical officers of health have been left only with responsibility for certain case-finding services and for aftercare of discharged tuberculosis cases through nursing visits to the homes.[5] The physician in charge of a tuberculosis clinic, however, usually holds a joint appointment between the regional hospital board and the local authority, and this helps to coordinate the whole program.

Certain advantages are undoubtedly gained by administrative amalgamation of the tuberculosis hospitals with all other hospitals in a region. Well before the National Health Service, in 1943, a distinguished medical committee in Scotland suggested that "a proper distribution of tuberculosis patients (of different stages of the disease) requires a regional scheme (of all hospitals) in the interests of economy and good administration."[6] Under the regional hospital boards, it is reported that the staffing and equipment of the sanatoria are of a higher quality than was true under local authority direction. Chest physicians in certain areas, like Middlesex, hold joint appointments in the sanatoria and the clinics, so that both types of problems can be better appreciated. Through its overall control of beds, the regional hospital board can make adjustments to changing bed needs and can move patients in and out of sanatoria, while following their progress through the clinics. A recent order of the Ministry of Health to make room for certain tuberculosis cases in the general hospitals illustrates the flexibility of the system.

On the other hand, the local medical health officer claims that the present pattern puts primary emphasis on the clinical and treatment aspects of tuberculosis control, as opposed to the social and epidemiological side. He would like to coordinate the operation of chest clinics with other public health clinics and would prefer to control admission to the hospital of tuberculosis cases which he considers the greatest hazard in the community. Since he retains some responsibilities, however, for case finding and home visiting, it is possible to coordinate these activities with parallel activities of the health department, especially in public health nursing. Even the sanitary inspector has functions which have an impact on the control of tuberculosis.[7]

Tuberculosis control is only one illustration of some of the problems that have been created by the vertical division of the British National Health Service into compartments for hospital services, ambulatory medical care, and public health services. A good deal of attention is being directed to achievement of horizontal coordination in local communities through establishment of local or regional coordinating committees. In 1952 the Central Health Services Council issued a report on the problems of cooperation among these three classes of service, the sections of which included one on tuberculosis control. The detailed needs analyzed in this British study apply so well to tuberculosis programs throughout the world that a full quotation is warranted.

(a) General
Local health authorities are responsible for preventive and social work (on tuberculosis); Regional Hospital Boards for institutional treatment; and general practitioners and the tuberculosis officers (appointed jointly by the Regional Hospital Board and the local health authority) for domiciliary treatment.

(b) Prevention
(1) Staff, both medical and nursing, should be shared.
(2) Co-operation is needed in use of mass miniature radiography units and the making of mass miniature radiography surveys. (Mass miniature radiography is a diagnostic service run by Regional Hospital Boards.)
Early diagnosis is essential to the preventive work of local health authorities and consequently there should be co-operation between Regional Hospital Boards and local health authorities in applying mass radiography to groups in which tuberculosis is most likely to be found.
(3) Co-operation is required in arranging for examination of staff, especially those who come into contact with children, and in the tracing of contacts.

(c) Admission to hospital
(1) The local health authority needs information from hospitals about availability of beds and waiting lists.
(2) The hospital needs information (e.g. from health visitors) about home conditions of patients, especially those awaiting admission to or discharge from hospital.
(3) Co-operation is needed between almoner and health visitor in seeing to care of patients' dependents.

(d) Discharge
The local health authority needs notification and information from hospital about condition of discharged patients.

(e) After-care
All after-care work in tuberculosis requires the closest co-operation of the chest physician and the local health authority both in securing adequate home conditions for the patient and his family and in the supervision of his resumption of employment or resettlement.

(f) Domiciliary treatment

Co-operation between hospital and local health authority services in providing home treatment and care for chronic ambulant tuberculosis patients can clear hospital beds for new cases likely to benefit from hospital treatment.[8]

There are doubtless different ways of achieving the integration of services suggested in this British analysis. While complete unification of preventive and curative health services at the local level may be the simplest administrative solution, good results in terms of reduced tuberculosis mortality can be attained in other ways. Experience in the United States gives vivid proof. Because of their beginnings. under voluntary auspices or under special commissions of the state government, tuberculosis sanatoria in most states are administered by agencies other than the state health department. In only about one-fourth of the forty-eight states is the health department in charge of sanatoria, although in practically all states it operates a preventive program of case finding, tuberculosis clinics, and nursing services to follow up discharged patients.[9] Voluntary tuberculosis associations operate everywhere, devoting their programs mostly to preventive work. Hospitalization in almost all states is financed predominantly from general tax funds of the state or local governments. Unlike Europe and elsewhere, social insurance plays no part in supporting the costs of care for tuberculosis. While the United States Public Health Service has a Tuberculosis and Chronic Disease Division for giving technical advice to the states, there is little uniformity among the state programs, nor among localities within a particular state.

Coordination, nevertheless, between curative and preventive services for tuberculosis is achieved through various informal arrangements in local communities. It is commonplace for the local health officer to be a member of the board of directors of the local tuberculosis association and for the state health officer to maintain close liaison with the policy making bodies of the tuberculosis sanatoria. Disharmonies occur, it is true, with regard to admission or discharge of patients, especially when infectious cases leave the sanatorium against medical advice and become a menace in the community. It is unfortunately not usual for physicians on a sanatorium staff to serve in local chest clinics, although they frequently read chest x-ray films from such clinics, or from mass radiographic surveys, sent to them. The taking of routine chest x-rays on all patients admitted to general hospitals has been promoted in the United States by both the health departments and the voluntary tuberculosis associations. One of the new by-products of mass x-ray surveys has been an increas-

ing tendency to look for nontuberculous disease of the chest, like cancer or heart disease, in both miniature and large films. Patients in tuberculosis sanatoria requiring major surgery for nontuberculous disease are sometimes transferred to general hospitals nearby.[10]

Relationships between preventive and curative health service administration for tuberculosis (as, indeed, for other diseases) naturally depend on historical developments and the traditional roles that particular authorities have acquired over the years. Reasonable adjustments can be made to almost any pattern of dividing responsibilities, so long as there is good will among officials involved. In some countries, however, the schemes planned for tuberculosis are seen to place overall responsibility for all aspects under a single public health authority.

Thus, in India, the comprehensive recommendations of the Bhore Commission include an integrated program for tuberculosis control under the central and provincial ministries of health. Tied in with the general network of clinics and hospitals contemplated would be a tuberculosis control service consisting of: (1) a domiciliary service, (2) chest clinics, (3) special tuberculosis hospitals, (4) after-care colonies, (5) homes for incurables, and (6) ancillary welfare services—all to be administered by the central, provincial, and local health officials responsible for overall preventive and curative services.[11] India has, of course, a long way to go before these recommendations can be brought to life, but new activities are in any case following a central plan. Where funds are so limited compared with the need, such overall control is obviously essential. The wisdom of such control is reflected in a recent statement of the government of India at a World Health Assembly:

> While not ignoring the need for modern methods of treatment including chest surgery, it has been found essential that during the next five years whatever bed accommodation could be provided should be in the form of simply designed and cheaply constructed institutions for the isolation of infectious cases. . . . In admitting cases, priority would be given to those for whom domiciliary isolation or treatment is impossible. Simpler forms of treatment would be provided in these institutions and, when advanced surgical aid is necessary, this would be arranged in other centres. . . .[12]

With such a policy, limited funds can be spent most judiciously, a policy not always possible when responsibilities are divided among different governmental and voluntary agencies. Similar overall planning under unified direction is a feature of tuberculosis control in countries under communistic governments. In Poland, soon after the change of government in 1947, a foreign observer reported:

> Coordination between institutions, dispensaries and the central authority is appreciated but is not yet in force. A scheme is being prepared which provides that the Central Tuberculosis Dispensary in each province will control the work of the subsidiary dispensaries of the province. The Central Tuberculosis Provincial Dispensaries will come under the general supervision and direction of the Ministry of Health in Warsaw.

In Roumania, a British observer reported that physicians on the tuberculosis sanatorium staffs are responsible for field work in the chest clinics.[13]

There is undoubtedly a tendency in recent years toward a more integrated approach to tuberculosis control in all countries. To some extent this is reflected in the enactment of comprehensive legislation covering all aspects of the control program, such as in France, Tunisia, Finland, and New Zealand.[14] While early legislation was confined to the contagious disease aspects of tuberculosis, requiring notification, isolation, etc., the newer legislation establishes standards for tuberculosis clinics, sanatoria, and various other facilities.

Since sanatorium care for tuberculosis developed earlier than knowledge and techniques for preventive services, it is natural that it should receive more emphasis in most countries. The first tuberculosis dispensary for epidemiological work was organized in Edinburgh, Scotland, in 1887 but it was not until the 1920s that preventive and case-finding services began to be widely launched. In the opinion of international health experts, more would be accomplished in underdeveloped countries if greater emphasis were placed on preventive and case-finding services, using simple facilities for isolation of open cases (as India is planning to do), rather than spending large sums on relatively elaborate sanatoria. A unified direction of tuberculosis services is, obviously, a great help for such an approach.

Aside from the values of coordination within the tuberculosis sphere, there are various advantages for other health objectives in administration of tuberculosis services by an overall public health agency. Case finding for other diseases, for example, can be carried out in conjunction with mass x-ray surveys. In the French Overseas Territories, the public health program calls for polyvalent mobile teams which will do case finding in rural areas for trypanosomiasis, leprosy, syphilis, and tuberculosis at the same time.[15] In the United States, Chile, and other countries, multiple screening tests for tuberculosis, syphilis, diabetes, hypertension, and other diseases of adult groups have been widely promoted in recent years.

With sanatoria under an overall public health agency, the period of hospitalization can be made useful for other purposes. Patients can be taught elements of general hygiene and nutrition which have value beyond the control of tuberculosis. Outpatient clinics can be attached to a sanatorium for the control of other diseases which may be endemic in the particular area. Physicians, nurses, and others on the sanatorium staff are more likely to give service in community clinics if the sanatoria are not administered by an autonomous agency. On the other hand, if clinical specialists from the sanatoria serve in the chest clinics, a better technical job is likely to be done in therapeutic follow-up measures like pneumothorax procedures. Patients coming to a chest clinic, moreover, can be treated or at least advised on other illnesses that may afflict them.

Admission policy in tuberculosis sanatoria can be geared most successfully to epidemiological considerations if these institutions are under the same wing as the general community health program. Discharge policy and rehabilitation activities also can be better integrated with rehabilitation resources in the community, where such exist. Laboratory tests for the tubercle bacillus can be carried out in a general public health laboratory. Community health education on tuberculosis can be part of the general educational program of the health department. The value of including home visiting service for tuberculosis in the generalized public health nursing program, rather than as an independent activity, is widely appreciated. If general hospitals or general medical care programs for the ambulatory patient are a responsibility of the public health organization, along with tuberculosis control, numerous opportunities are presented for finding cases and facilitating prompt referral to a chest clinic or sanatorium. All these economies in money and efforts can be best achieved if responsibilities for all aspects of tuberculosis are coordinated with a comprehensive organized health service at the local level. Indeed, it may be most convenient for sanatoria to be integrated at a national or regional level with the administration of other hospitals, while dispensaries and preventive services come under a special tuberculosis section, so long as at the local level both curative and preventive activities can be supervised by the generalized health official who is in closest touch with the total health needs of the population.

MENTAL DISORDER

Relationships between curative and preventive services for mental disorder are similar in many ways to the situation for tuberculosis. In virtually all countries, serious mental disease has been assumed to be a matter of public concern, and the care of persons afflicted with it has been provided by governmental authorities. The evolution of the modern concept of the mental hospital as a place for treatment and rehabilitation, rather than for punishment and incarceration, is a tale that has been often told, and the evolution in many countries is still by no means completed.[16] In any event, the mental hygiene movement concerned with prevention of mental disease is much younger and in most countries has not even started. Where it has gotten underway, the sponsorship has usually been quite separate from that of mental hospitals.

In a sense, every social activity and every medical activity has a mental health aspect. The prevention of mental disease depends, in part, on housing, occupation, family income, and many factors beyond specific health services. Yet, there are certain specific preventive activities which psychiatric specialists can offer in an organized form—through mental health clinics, mental health services in the schools and in industry, psychiatric consultation in the courts, etc. Problems of interpersonal relationships, important in mental disease, can be ameliorated by education and psychotherapy. There are problems in the community relating to both the admission to and discharge of patients from mental hospitals. In view of the shortage of qualified psychiatric personnel in all countries, much can obviously be gained by close relationships between the staffs of mental hospitals and the mental health services in the community.

The framework for such working relationships is found in most countries, since mental hospitals are usually under the jurisdiction of the health authority. In practice, however, their management may be isolated from other aspects of the health program. Often the mental hospitals are operated as part of a hospital system and quite unrelated to local public health administration.

Without giving a comprehensive review, the administrative organization of curative and preventive services for mental disorder in a few nations may be mentioned. In Norway, there is a division in the national Health Services Directorate (of the Ministry of Social Affairs) responsible for psychiatric services, mental hygiene, care of the feeble-minded and epileptic, treatment of sex offenders, etc. Parallel with this office are others for community health services, hospitals, and all other aspects of public health reporting to the same Director-General. In France, all except a few mental hospitals are owned and financed by units of central or local government, but they come under the technical supervision of the

director of health of the *département*. This official is also responsible for mental health consultation centers which carry out preventive mental health work, case finding, referrals to institutions, treatment of alcoholics, and posttreatment supervision of discharged mental patients. In Great Britain, the mental hospitals are under the regional hospital boards and, along with them, the mental health clinics. Aftercare of discharged patients, however, is a responsibility of local health authorities, and child guidance clinics are operated by the education authorities (the psychiatrists in charge being provided by the regional hospital boards). In most, though not all, of the provinces of Canada, mental hospitals and community mental health clinics are under the jurisdiction of the department of public health. In Soviet Russia, all psychiatric services are under the Ministry of Health and are coordinated with the general network of hospitals and district health centers. Great stress is placed on care of mental patients through neuropsychiatric clinics, rather than in hospitals. Every effort is made to keep the patient in an active community situation, giving him psychiatric and social aid as necessary.[17]

In Egypt, there is a Department of Mental Diseases, with a Director-General, in the Ministry of Health and parallel with the department administering public health services. This department is in charge of the two large mental hospitals serving the entire country and of a few mental health clinics in Cairo. As in most agricultural countries, the facilities are inadequate. In Syria, the mental hospitals are under the Ministry of Health, but no community mental health services exist except through the private practices of the psychiatrists on a hospital staff. In the Philippines, there is no mental health division in the Ministry of Health, but the nation's only special mental institution, the National Psychopathic Hospital, is administratively under the Bureau of Hospitals in that ministry. On the other hand, community mental health services, especially for children, are being developed independently by the Department of Education and the Social Welfare Commission. The administrative situation in Lebanon is unusual, in that the mental hospitals are operated by various voluntary societies and religious orders from overseas, although they receive government grants. In Beirut, the capital, there are two outpatient clinics giving psychotherapy, but no mental health services have been developed as yet in the country as a whole.

In the United States, responsibilities for the curative and preventive aspects of mental disorder are vested in the state governments, but are widely dispersed as to agency. In only one state are the mental hospitals under the department of public health, while in twenty-two states they are under an autonomous commission, in fifteen states under a department of welfare or of institutions, and in ten states under a separate department of mental health.[18] On the other hand, community mental health activities are most frequently supervised by the department of public health. They are under such sponsorship in twenty-six states, under combined departments of health and welfare in two states, and under the separate agencies controlling mental hospitals in twenty-two states. This administrative separation between curative and preventive services diminishes the effectiveness of both programs, in the opinion of a committee of the National Association for Mental Health which recently studied the question. Regarding community mental health work, this study reported:

> We deplore the lack in many states of extrainstitutional community programs . . . as an integral and important part of the work of mental hospitals and mental hospital systems. Mental health is their business outside as well as inside the hospitals. They have a proper and practical concern with the prevention of mental illness as well as its treatment—and their treatment function should not be confined within hospital walls. A more active participation by the hospitals and hospital doctors in the preventive effort would seem to us highly desirable.[19]

There is good reason to incorporate mental health services and a mental health approach in the general program of the public health agency. Recommendations in this sense were made by the World Health Organization Expert Committee on Mental Health which in 1950 explored the implications for mental health of a generalized community health program.[20] On the other hand, starting from the vantage point of curative mental services, the next meeting of this WHO Expert Committee recommended ways in which the mental hospitals could serve the community at large. This Committee recommends that mental health work should be the concern of a division in the ministry of health. It proposes as the "modern" view one in which

> the medico-social team is responsible for all the mental health problems of the community, considering the psychiatric hospital as one of the many tools for carrying out its works.[21]

The specific recommendation is made that physicians on mental hospital staffs should spend one-third of their time doing preventive mental health work in the community. Implementation of this idea would depend, of course, on adequate medical staffing of the mental hospitals.

The cause of both prevention and treatment of mental disease can undoubtedly be advanced by embodiment of mental health services in the general public health agency. One of the great obstacles to modern psychiatric work is the public fear and suspicion which regard mental disease as peculiar and outside the mainstream of community life. Inclusion of psychiatric services in the general public health program can help to overcome this attitude. Mental hygiene education can be part of the general health education effort. The local health department, especially through public health nurses, can facilitate admission of patients to mental hospitals and follow-up at home after their discharge. Mental health clinics for diagnosis and short-term therapy as well as child guidance clinics can be operated by the local public health agency, in close connection with the schools, law courts, etc. There are mental health aspects to the operation of general hospitals and nursing homes for the chronically ill, for which the health department may have some supervisory authority. Many have advocated psychiatric wards in general hospitals which, if they are established, should be served by psychiatrists from the mental hospitals. There are also problems of mental breakdown in tuberculosis sanatoria and of tuberculosis infection in mental hospitals—both of which can be best handled if administration is under a common department.

The purely managerial and business aspects of mental hospitals have much in common with the administration of general hospitals and sanatoria, so that economies and efficiencies can be enjoyed if they are under the same branch of government. Functions of a public health agency in statistics and laboratory services can be useful in both the preventive and therapeutic mental services. To some extent, factors leading to mental disease may lie in housing, factory organization, and general environmental hygiene—conditions which public health agencies can influence, especially if armed with psychiatric consultation. Such consultation can also be useful in the administration of programs of venereal disease control, child health, medical care for the indigent, and other functions for which the health department may be responsible.[22] It is small wonder that the Bhore Commission of India, in its report of unprecedented scope, recommended the creation of mental health organization for both preventive and curative work "as part of the establishments under the Director-General of Health Services at the Centre and of the Provincial Directors of Health Services."[23]

TREPONEMATOSES AND OTHER INFECTIONS

The control of the acute communicable diseases, through isolation, quarantine, immunization, and other measures has been such a classical part of the public health program that it is sometimes not realized that these activities often include a large measure of medical care.

Treponematoses

Since its earliest recognition in Europe, syphilis has commanded the attention of public authorities and the necessity of combining personal restrictions (to prevent spread of the disease) with personal therapy has been recognized. Since 1790, treatment of syphilis has been compulsory and at public expense in Denmark. Throughout the nineteenth century, however, there was a highly secretive and moralistic attitude toward the disease, and it took the International Conference for the Prophylaxis of Syphilis and Venereal Diseases held in Brussels in 1899 to bring the problem out into the open. A system of antivenereal clinics was set up throughout Denmark in 1906 and soon thereafter all European countries did likewise.[24]

In the United States of America the movement did not take hold until the First World War, when antivenereal disease clinics were set up widely through federal subsidy to the states. After 1935, these programs were greatly expanded.[25] Since the 1920s, venereal disease control, with treatment at public expense, has been a governmental function—with greater or lesser adequacy to meet the needs—in practically all countries. Gonorrhoea and other diseases usually acquired by sexual contact are generally included in the service.

In practically every instance, responsibilities for medical treatment are vested in the public health authorities, national, provincial, or local, though other aspects of the problem, like control or supervision of prostitution, may be a duty of police authorities.[26] In the venereal disease clinic we see perhaps the perfect combination of preventive and curative medicine, for therapy is done on the one hand while, on the other, there is epidemiological investigation to trace contacts and halt the spread of the infection. The degree of compulsion to take treatment, the measures of case finding, the pattern for giving treatment as between public clinics and private medical offices, and other features of the control program differ widely among countries, but everywhere treatment of venereal infection is an integral part of the public health program. Voluntary "social hygiene" associations may carry out education work, private nursing agencies may do epidemiological investigations, hospital laboratories may do serological tests, social insurance agencies (as in Norway) may finance treatments, but the local public health agency nearly always has overall control of both preventive and curative phases.

The control of venereal diseases can obviously be more effective if relationships are maintained with other aspects of a public health and medical care program under the health authority. For example, the prevention of congenital syphilis and gonococcal ophthalmia of the newborn depends in large measure on procedures in a maternal and child health program. Premarital and prenatal serological tests for syphilis require procedures in physician's offices, hospitals, and clinics everywhere. Routine examinations for venereal disease may be done on all hospital admissions, in factories, in the military services—calling for cooperation of other branches of organized health service. Serological tests are done routinely on hospital admissions in Scandinavia and elsewhere. In the United States, application for assistance from the vocational rehabilitation program requires, among other things, a VD blood test. In 1948 to tackle the greatly increased syphilis problem, Poland required serological tests before issuance of food ration cards. The school health services can play an important role in sex hygiene education. In many parts of the world, moreover, syphilis is spread nonvenereally and its control depends on general measures of environmental hygiene and health education. Where the prevalence of the disease is low or where facilities are limited, it may be best to have venereal infection treated in polyclinics rather than in clinics exclusively for the one disease group. On the other hand, a campaign primarily designed to attack venereal disease may have byproducts of value for other health objectives. Patients coming for repeated treatments and follow-up at a venereal disease clinic should get medical examinations which may detect other diseases requiring attention.

The value of a campaign against syphilis, or the other major treponemal disease, yaws, in stimulating the establishment of generalized organization for public health has been shown. In Thailand and Haiti, yaws control programs promoted by the World Health Organization have been designed with this purpose in mind. Like in French West Africa, a campaign against sleeping sickness was the initial effort, around which a program of general prevention and medical care was later built. Similar objectives applied to an intensive attack on endemic and nonvenereal syphilis in Bosnia, Yugoslavia, recently carried out.[27] By contrast, a sweeping campaign against yaws in Western Samoa during 1923-1926 was followed by active recurrence of the disease because it was not associated with the establishment of a permanent public health organization.

Other Infections

Other infectious diseases also present opportunities for coordination of prevention and cure. The very birth of modern public health organization in the effort to prevent epidemic disease was associated with a curative service, in the establishment of the pest-house for the isolation of cases of plague and other contagious diseases. For any disease in which an active or quiescent case may spread infectious material to others, treatment and prevention are obviously inseparable.

Special hospitals for infectious diseases, aside from tuberculosis, are becoming less common but they are still operated in and near large cities. In Great Britain, the "fever hospitals" are under the regional hospital boards, but the local medical officer of health is frequently in a consultative relationship to them. In the United States and Canada, contagious disease hospitals are frequently under the jurisdiction of public health officers.

The development of new forms of prevention, by use of prophylactic drugs against communicable disease, has made it increasingly difficult to separate administrative responsibility for prevention and cure. If contacts of a case of scarlet fever or meningococcal meningitis are given sulfonamide or antibiotic drugs, they may be protected from getting the disease. The use of antibiotics might also prevent cardiac damage in persons with rheumatic fever. The spread of typhoid fever may be limited by active therapy of a carrier of the disease.

The control of trachoma is one aspect of communicable disease in which combined curative and preventive services are frequently carried out under public health auspices. In Egypt, there is an entire network of ophthalmic hospitals under the Ministry of Health treating trachoma, ophthalmitis, and other eye diseases causing an enormous amount of blindness in the Mediterranean region. The effective control of infectious eye disease in that region requires treatment of cases combined with environmental hygiene, especially the elimination of flies. In Israel, under the leadership of the Ministry of Health an attack is being made on trachoma requiring the cooperation of many agencies: case finding through the schools, treatment at clinics of the Workers' Insurance Fund, surgical care and management of serious cases in government hospitals, and transportation of patients by UNICEF (United Nations Children's Fund). The general trachoma control program is linked closely with the school health services, which include such other preventive measures as periodic examinations, immunizations, improvement of nutrition, and health education. Since trachoma and ophthalmitis are largely diseases of children, if the control programs are under broad health agency direction, opportunities are presented for advancing other preventive services.[28]

Since ancient times leprosy has been a dreaded disease commanding special organized attack. In countries at every stage of economic development there are leprosaria for isolating and treating persons with leprosy. From the United States and Canada to Egypt, India, China, or Indonesia, ministries of health provide medical services for leprosy in special hospitals. There used to be a spirit of complete hopelessness about confinement to a leprosarium, but with modern drug therapy there is definite hope that many cases can be cured or, at least, arrested so that the patient may expect to return one day to natural community life. Accordingly, the period of treatment in a leprosarium can be an opportunity for general health promotion, health education, and personal advancement rather than the condemnation to "living death" of ancient times.

Just as curative services for certain infectious diseases can provide an opportunity for prevention, other programs primarily focused on prevention can provide an opportunity for medical care. The campaign for immunization against diphtheria or smallpox may bring to medical attention a child who needs corrective surgery. A premarital examination for venereal infection may reveal a hernia or something else requiring treatment. Even a malaria campaign, in which a team of DDT-sprayers enters a rural village for house spraying, can promote necessary curative medicine, if a nurse or other health auxiliary worker is present to make observations and refer individuals to the hospital or clinic. Such broad health objectives can be gained most readily if a unified health agency is responsible for both preventive and curative services.

CRIPPLING CONDITIONS AND REHABILITATION

Throughout the ages, public sympathy has gone to the cripple, the person with an obvious difficulty or defect in walking. Exploiting this sympathy, seriously disabled persons in all countries have become beggars or looked for public aid in other ways. Social attitudes have been mixed; on the one hand came sympathy and, on the other, suspicion. At the same time, efforts to rehabilitate the disabled person have been numerous.

Background of Rehabilitation Services

In 330 AD, a center was established for the care and education of cripples in Constantinople, under the aegis of a Roman Senator. In the Aztec kingdom that is now Mexico, Montezuma established a center for the care of crippled persons in 1502. Other special centers for the care and education of persons with obvious disabilities in their locomotor systems were set up in Voorburg, Holland, in 1709; in Switzerland in 1780; in Montpelier, France, in 1816; in Birmingham, England, in 1817; in Munich, Germany, in 1835; in Florence, Italy, in 1839; in New York City, U.S.A., in 1863; and in Copenhagen, Denmark, in 1871.[29]

These were isolated events, brought about by the initiative of particular leaders and not becoming a permanent feature of governmental policy. It took the mass destruction of human as well as physical resources of the First World War to make the care of cripples a major item on the agenda of governments, first in Europe and then elsewhere in the world. Attention was first directed to the disabled military veteran, but it soon spread to other disabled persons. Faced with a manpower shortage, when every possible worker was needed for the production effort, society had to take steps to salvage the working capacity of every individual, whether able-bodied or disabled. Soon after the war, the modern concept of rehabilitation was born, based on the recognition that physical treatment of a disability was not enough, but had to be complemented by assistance in psychological, social, educational, and vocational spheres.

Thus in 1917, in Great Britain, "government instructional factories" were set up to employ disabled men, especially those who had seen military service. In 1920, in the United States, state programs of vocational rehabilitation were launched through federal grants to state departments of education. Special medical centers for military veterans with orthopedic disabilities were established in these countries and in France, Germany, Belgium, Holland, and elsewhere. National veterans' organizations were active in promoting such services. In response to demands from them, the International Labour Office issued in 1924 what seems to be the earliest international publication on rehabilitation standards, a manual entitled *Artificial Limbs–Appliances for the Disabled*.[30]

Meanwhile, largely through voluntary societies, increasing attention was being given to the needs of the crippled child. Debilitated, orphaned, and crippled children had long won public sympathy and most large cities in Europe had institutions for their care, supported by charitable and public funds, in the nineteenth century. A notable program was organized in Prussia in 1920, emphasizing integration of preventive and curative services, education, and vocational rehabilitation. National voluntary societies engaged in this work were organized, and in 1921 a number of these banded together to organize the International Society for Crippled Children. In this period, several states in the United States, through their state departments of welfare (concerned with the indigent population), launched state programs of medical and social assistance to the crippled child. In 1935, the Social Security Act was passed in this country, starting a nationwide program, through grants to the states, of medical care for crippled children. In many states, this involved the department of public health in a type of curative health service.

With the Second World War, the rehabilitation idea was given great impetus. With thousands of persons disabled from the war, soldiers and civilians both, the countries of Europe and America gave increasing attention to organized medical services, along with social and vocational services, for disabled persons. From the health point of view, the rehabilitation movement has meant the addition of serious orthopedic disabilities to the disorders which, like tuberculosis or mental disease, command organized public action.

Since the end of the Second World War, there has been widespread growth of the concept and practice of "rehabilitation centers." In these structures, all the skills of medicine, education, social service, and labor administration can be brought together to serve the disabled person, child or adult. Such centers serve also as places of demonstration and training in a country, having an impact on the activities of hospitals, schools, employment offices, and social welfare agencies throughout the country.

What relationship do programs for the crippled bear to the general public health movement? Services for the crippled child, while started often under voluntary auspices can obviously benefit from close association with the maternal and child health program of the public health agency. The task of case finding, arrangements for corrective surgery or other therapy, and follow-up in the home of disabled children or adults can be fostered through the regular clinic services and public health nursing program of the same agency.

Services for Disabled Children and Adults

For obvious social and psychological reasons, rehabilitation services for children have usually developed separately from those for adults in most countries. Programs for the crippled child emanated from humanitarian objectives of voluntary agencies, later coming under governmental health or welfare departments. Programs for the disabled adult grew mainly from industrial needs or from sympathy for the war injured; in government they were part of overall services for workers or for veterans. The resultant picture in any country, therefore, usually has many facets, often scarcely related to each other.

There is hardly a field of health service which has so great an appeal for voluntary, charitable action as the care of the crippled child. Societies for crippled children operate in all the economically advanced countries and in many of the underdeveloped countries. They often maintain special hospitals, like the School for Crippled Children in Helsinki, Finland, or the Crippled Children's Center in Beirut, Lebanon, sponsored by the Lebanese Union for Child Welfare. Voluntary organizations for poliomyelitis or cerebral palsy, led often by the parents of children stricken by these conditions, have done much to organize treatment centers concentrating on rehabilitation of these specific disabilities. On the other hand, there may be a tendency to develop services for certain disabilities out of proper proportion to the overall need. The national health authority is obviously in the best position to give guidance which will keep crippled children's services in reasonable balance.

In Japan, special services for crippled children are administered by the Maternal and Child Health Section of the Ministry of Health and Welfare, which is responsible also for preventive services to children. Hospital beds reserved for orthopedic cases among children are indirectly controlled, with respect to their admission policy, by this section. As the disabled child grows to the age of employability, he is referred to the Vocational Rehabilitation Service for adults, administered by another branch of the same ministry.[31]

Many cases of disability in adults as well as children can be prevented, so that the closest association of the curative orthopedic services with the health department provides an effective stimulus to needed preventive measures. Tuberculosis control and milk pasteurization can reduce tuberculous disease of the bones and joints. Rickets can be prevented by adequate nutrition and sunlight. Accidental injuries can be tackled by safety measures at places of work, in the home, and on the public highway. Proper obstetrical service can reduce birth injuries and cerebral palsy. Prompt diagnosis and treatment can reduce the crippling effects of poliomyelitis. Early

and continued medical care can prevent deformities from osteomyelitis.

Within clinical medicine, interest in rehabilitation of the orthopedically handicapped has been associated with the development of the specialty of physical medicine. This specialty, making use of many auxiliary workers—physiotherapists, occupational therapists, and remedial gymnasts—has promoted the viewpoint of patience and hopefulness in working with seriously disabled persons, individuals who may have been bedridden and socially dependent for years. By painstaking and skilled work, the handicapped person is helped to make maximum use of residual neuromuscular powers so as to become independent in meeting his personal living needs and even holding a job. The difficulty is that a regime of such therapy, requiring many personnel and often months of time, is expensive and beyond the means of the average disabled person. Accordingly, the development of this entire clinical field has necessarily depended on various forms of public financial support.

Rehabilitation services for the adult in Great Britain are particularly well developed. The Ministry of Labour and National Service carries out a nationwide effort to reestablish disabled persons in employment. There are: Industrial Rehabilitation Units, institutions under medical direction giving intensive occupational and psychological therapy; Government Training Centres where job retraining is carried out in scores of occupations; and Remploy Factories, a network of subsidized sheltered workshops from which products are sold on the open market. Underpinning all of this is a national law requiring all employers of twenty persons or more to have three percent of their work force composed of disabled persons, certified as such by the government. This certification, as well as the job placement and related activities, is done by a corps of disablement rehabilitation officers.[32] Strict medical services required are rendered through the National Health Service under the Ministry of Health. These are done primarily through the surgical, orthopedic, and physical medicine departments of hospitals in every region, in addition to which there are special hospitals concentrating on treatment of post-traumatic industrial cases, spastic and paraplegia cases, and even industrial psychoneurosis.[33] Artificial limbs are provided through a special network of "limb centres" started by the Ministry of Pensions (for military veterans) but now integrated with the National Health Service.

In the United States, services for crippled children are under auspices quite separate from those for adults. Even crippled children's services are administered by a variety of agencies among the states. In 1947, it was reported:

> Official state agencies administering services for crippled children include thirty departments of health, ten departments of public welfare, four departments of education, five crippled children's commissions, and three state university medical schools or hospitals. There has been a trend toward transfer of administrative responsibility to health agencies, showing an increasing recognition that the program is one primarily involving the field of medical care.[34]

The impetus to rehabilitation services for disabled adults in the United States since the Second World War came from several sources: the experience of the military medical services, the growth of the state programs of vocational rehabilitation under departments of education, and the rising concern for the disabled stimulated by voluntary agencies. The state programs of vocational rehabilitation have increased in tempo; physical restoration services for "static" defects under these programs are usually rendered by private physicians and in general hospitals, financed by the state departments of education.[35] Special centers for comprehensive rehabilitation services meanwhile have developed under various forms of voluntary auspices. In 1954, there were twenty-three such centers giving comprehensive services for the disabled, thirty-eight centers giving partial services, and plans were underway for giving federal subsidies to help establish more.[36] Outstanding among such centers, which helped to set patterns for elsewhere in the country, are the Kessler Institute for Rehabilitation in New Jersey, the New York University-Bellevue Hospital Rehabilitation Center in New York, and the Kabat-Kaiser Rehabilitation Institute in California.

Most of this expansion of services for the adult crippled in the United States, as elsewhere, has been carried out quite independently of the public health agencies. Here and there, public health officials have been involved in a consultative capacity on the medical aspects of local rehabilitation activities—for example, in South Carolina, California, Maryland, and West Virginia.[37, 38] It has become increasingly felt in the United States of America, however, that to meet the problem, rehabilitation programs require active community organization not only in a few large cities, but in every local community. To organize such concerted efforts requires leadership and this can be provided by the local health officer. The health department can assist in case finding of disabled persons, organization of diagnostic facilities, organization of physical medicine and rehabilitation departments in local hospitals, and in

stimulation of local activities for vocational training and job placement.[39]

Financial support in many countries has come from social insurance funds which pay cash benefits for periods of temporary or permanent disability. Rehabilitation of a disabled person would naturally reduce the drain on the insurance fund. Thus, in Austria, for example, there are a number of special institutes giving a full range of physical medicine services, operated by the "Krankenkassen" (sickness insurance funds).[40] In Italy the Accident Insurance Societies maintain their own rehabilitation centers. In Denmark and Norway, on the other hand, services rendered to beneficiaries of social insurance are paid by the Invalidity Insurance Funds, but they are rendered in rehabilitation centers operated under various sponsorships. In Denmark, there are institutions dealing with various aspects of rehabilitation which are entirely private, others that are under voluntary agencies but subsidized by government, and others that are entirely under government (national or local). In Norway, there are four rehabilitation centers operated by the National Health Service.[41] France has put major emphasis on the rehabilitation of paralytic poliomyelitis. Not only medical rehabilitation but also vocational retraining are among the benefits provided by social insurance to beneficiaries suffering from many types of prolonged illness and for invalidity pensioners, including the provision of prostheses. For victims of employment injury, medical rehabilitation and vocational retraining services are also available under the insurance scheme covering employment injury. Five special centers have been developed, the largest being at Garches.[42] In most European countries where compulsory medical care insurance is the general rule, the cost of orthopedic services for the child or adult is covered by the insurance fund, although the services are often given in special hospitals.

Because rehabilitation needs have been conspicuous for persons receiving public assistance due to a disability, much of the initiative in starting rehabilitation programs has come from social welfare agencies. This is the case in Egypt, where centers for the rehabilitation of the blind and the physically handicapped are being developed by the Ministry of Social Affairs, with no participation by the Ministry of Health. A rehabilitation center for the disabled has been developed at Surakarta, Indonesia, under the leadership of the Ministry of Social Affairs, based on the nucleus of a prosthetic workshop which grew out of the orthopedic surgery department of the hospital in that city. In this center are facilities for medical service, vocational training, and social welfare to assist in resettlement of disabled persons in employment.[43] In Australia, the rehabilitation scheme is a responsibility of the Department of Social Services, with centers in each state for retraining of pensioners and sickness beneficiaries in whom the medical prognosis favors return to employment within two years; this agency is advised by a consultative council for the physically handicapped of the department of public health in each state.

In Canada, the earliest and most outstanding program of rehabilitation was developed for disabled workers by the Workmen's Compensation Board of Ontario. Other programs in that country are under either voluntary societies, like the Western Society for Rehabilitation in British Columbia, or the department of public health, as in Saskatchewan. Several provinces of Canada have taken over financial support for poliomyelitis treatment of all types (acute and postparalytic) as a function of their departments of health. Special tax-supported services for children, crippled from any cause, are also administered by provincial health agencies, aided by national grants. In 1953, the national government appointed in the Department of Labour a coordinator of rehabilitation to encourage coordinated programs in each of the provinces. Special grants for medical aspects of rehabilitation are also made available by the Department of National Health and Welfare, while the Department of Education assists the provinces with grants for vocational training of disabled persons.

Services for Blindness and Deafness

In this review of services for crippled children and adults and their relations to public health organization, "crippling" has been considered in the classical sense of defects of the limbs. In a broader sense, of course, there are other, nonorthopedic forms of crippling—like heart disease, blindness, or deafness. Special institutions for the care and education of the blind and the deaf are to be found all over the world. In almost every metropolitan center of the world are schools for the blind and the deaf originated usually by private agencies but now commonly subsidized by government. In these institutions the problem is mainly educational, so that ministries of education rather than ministries of health are responsible. Even in these teaching institutions, however, there is a role for the public health agency in assuring general preventive services and day-to-day medical care. Today, moreover, certain cases of absolute blindness, when due to corneal opacities, can be rehabilitated through corneal transplant operations. Cases of deafness also can be aided through the fenestration operation and

through modern electronic hearing aids. Such possibilities call for continuous access of these institutions to medical advice.

Prevention of blindness and of deafness, on the other hand, is a customary duty of public health agencies. Both governmental and voluntary agencies have long been concerned with prevention of blindness, through such measures as silver nitrate application in the eyes of newborn babies to prevent gonococcal ophthalmia, sanitary measures to prevent trachoma, accident control in industry to prevent ocular trauma, and visual testing in schools with prescription of eyeglasses to conserve eyesight. The provincial Department of Public Health in Saskatchewan, Canada, administers a special fund for "prevention of blindness," but on the whole these functions are an integral aspect of many public health activities, not segregated in any administrative division.[44] National voluntary societies for the prevention of blindness are active in promoting these measures in many countries.

Prevention of deafness is a somewhat newer activity which has followed from recent technical advances. The development of the audiometer, an instrument for detecting minor hearing impairments which might become more serious, has enabled school authorities to detect children needing attention. New radium methods of treating middle-ear disease permit the arrest of a process which can lead to total deafness. In a few states of the United States conservation of hearing has been made an objective of the public health agency.

Problems of Coordination

Inevitably so many agencies are involved in a complete rehabilitation program that some countries have established interministerial committees to coordinate activities. In Israel, for example, such a committee includes representation from the Ministries of Health, Labor, Social Welfare, Defense, Trade and Industry, Agriculture, and the Central Labor Exchange.[45] In all countries, relationships among the various branches of government and between government and voluntary agencies concerned with rehabilitation are highly complex. Yet each component service must be developed as part of a general vocational training program and medical or surgical services should be part of a general medical and hospital care program. Otherwise the rehabilitation idea is not likely to develop outside of a few relatively spectacular centers.

In economically underdeveloped countries, the resources that should properly be devoted to rehabilitation of the disabled must be smaller than in the more prosperous countries. When enormous problems of preventable disease are unmet, it is obviously unwise to spend on a few crippled persons large sums, which could be used to prevent hundreds from dying. Where all classes of medical personnel are limited, how many can be trained in a field like physiotherapy? Yet there are inevitable social demands for aid to the crippled, which cannot be ignored until a nation reaches the "logical" economic stage for it. Yugoslavia has many serious health problems; yet it is developing a rehabilitation center for demonstration and training purposes. A department of physiotherapy and training center for physiotherapists have been organized, with WHO assistance, in the King Edward Memorial Hospital in Bombay, India. Greece is organizing its workshops for prosthetic appliances. All these activities are valuable in establishing the nucleus of a rehabilitation program, and in promoting the rehabilitation philosophy. When the economic resources of the country become better developed, it will then be better prepared to establish a nationwide program on sound principles. Proper balance, with a view to the future, can be assured best if the medical aspects of rehabilitation services from the beginning are under the supervision of the ministry of health.

Wherever social insurance or public assistance monetary benefits are granted to disabled persons, the need for socially financed rehabilitation services becomes more apparent. Otherwise public funds are paid out over the years, even enforcing a spirit of invalidism and hopelessness in the beneficiary. To overcome this difficulty, rehabilitation services— especially active departments of physical and occupational therapy—need to be incorporated in almost every hospital, or at least in the larger hospitals of a regional network. A spectacular rehabilitation center in the national capital may have inspirational value and serve as a training center for personnel, but the problem cannot be met quantitatively unless the entire hospital system is affected. This calls for action from the ministry of health in most countries, even though financial support for the medical services may come from insurance or other welfare funds. Beyond this, the general community contacts of the public health staff can detect cases of moderate or early illness which should be referred for medical care, so as to prevent regression into complete disability and economic dependency.

The administration of disability insurance (as in most European countries) or public assistance for permanent and total disability (as in North America) is not included in this report. It is evident, however, that effective operation of such programs requires close liaison with the health services both in the sphere of medical certifications of disability and in the assurance of medical rehabilitation services where they can be effective.

CHRONIC DISEASE PROGRAMS

While orthopedic crippling and sensory defects often cause long-term disability, there are other long-term disorders for which special social programs have been organized. These are the so-called chronic degenerative diseases which are usually, though not always, associated with deterioration of metabolic processes and of greatest prevalence in the later years of life. Commonest among these disorders are heart disease, cancer, rheumatism, and diabetes. All these and the other chronic degenerative diseases are characterized by their long duration, by the necessity of the patient to accommodate his life to the disease rather than expecting a complete cure, and by the need for continuing and expensive medical services.

As average longevity has increased with the reduction of epidemic disease in many countries, the attention of governments has been increasingly devoted to methods of treatment or control of chronic diseases. Special institutions have been developed for inpatient care and public health agencies have sought methods of prevention or early treatment. As an illustration, services for cancer may be considered.

Cancer Services

In every country there are facilities for the diagnosis and treatment of cancer through the practicing physician and the general hospital, but specially organized services have been launched in a few countries. It is not surprising that France, with its exceptionally high proportion of persons in the later age groups, should be one such country. To promote cancer control there, sixteen centers have been organized under the authority of the Ministry of Public Health. Each center is under the direction of a board representing the public health authority, the nearest medical school, the social security administration, the local hospital, and various technical specialists. The functions of the centers are: case finding, diagnosis and treatment, hospitalization, education of the public, instruction of physicians, and research. Payment for services may come from social security funds or other sources. The cancer centers devote their efforts not only to direct service but also to improving the quality of cancer diagnostic and treatment services in all the general hospitals around them.

In many countries there are special institutes for

cancer research and teaching, where the most advanced forms of surgical or radiological therapy are available. There are the National Anticancer Institute in Belgium and the Radiological Center in Sweden. In the United States there are the Memorial Hospital Center for Cancer and Allied Diseases in New York and many others. India has the Tata Memorial Cancer Research Hospital at Bombay. Methods of payment for services in these centers, of course, depend on the general framework of medical economics in the country. Canada is exceptional in that some provinces have singled out cancer as a disease for which public responsibility is taken, even when insurance coverage in a voluntary prepayment plan or public assistance status would not otherwise justify it. The most comprehensive program is in Saskatchewan, where all costs for diagnosis and treatment of cancer (surgical and radiological) are met at public expense through the Department of Public Health. In Alberta, as well as Saskatchewan, all cases requiring radiological therapy receive it without charge at cancer clinics operated directly by the government. In all Canadian provinces, cancer diagnostic and educational services, at least, are offered by the provincial government, usually in some relation to the department of health and aided by cancer control grants from the national government.[46] The Ministry of Health of Ceylon contains a cancer control office engaged in epidemiological research and cancer health education.

The cancer detection clinic idea has been actively explored in the United States. Relatively little is known about the primary prevention of cancer, aside from certain relatively uncommon occupational cancers (such as bladder carcinoma in workers with aniline dyes) and recent evidence of the relationship of cigarette smoking to carcinoma of the lung. Short of environmental controls based on such relationships, the early detection of tumors can lead to prompt therapy which may save life. On this theory, clinics under various forms of financial support have been organized throughout the United States where presumably normal adults can obtain a general medical examination designed especially to detect early signs of cancer. If evidence of cancer is found, the treatment is usually a financial responsibility of the individual patient. The experience of such clinics is that a great deal more noncancerous disease is found, requiring treatment, than cancer. At the Cornell University Medical College in New York, for example, evidence of cancer was found in thirteen persons out of each 1,000 examined, but other disorders of significance were found at a rate of approximately 1,500 diagnoses per 1,000 persons.

Motivated originally by the problem of cancer

therapy, this approach has led directly to broad interest in cancer prevention. Under the stimulus of financial grants from the federal government, nearly all the states in the United States have developed cancer control activities under public health agency direction. Several states, such as Connecticut, Massachusetts, and California, have made long-term studies on the epidemiology of cancer to gain clues on possible prevention.[47] On the other hand, public health agencies, despite their preventive orientation, have found themselves engaged in organization of diagnostic and treatment services, including provision of laboratory tissue pathology, operation of special cancer hospitals (New York State), and payment for surgical services rendered to low income persons by private physicians (West Virginia).

Other Chronic Diseases

Partially emanating from cancer control efforts, general interest has developed in the United States in prevention of other types of chronic disease. With evidence of the numerous positive findings of other disorders, incidental to cancer detection examinations, a scheme for general preventive examinations developed, making use of various objective laboratory tests not requiring the immediate presence of a doctor. Technicians collect specimens of urine and blood for examination, take chest x-rays, measure the blood pressure, test vision and hearing, determine body weight and height, and perform other such examinations. If any of the laboratory or x-ray findings are suggestive of possible abnormalities, the individual is referred to his private physician for diagnosis and treatment. These "multiphasic screening" programs are promoted by public health agencies, but they lead directly to the provision of medical care through organized efforts.[48] In a series of such examinations done among longshoremen in California, about two-thirds were found to have one or more positive findings and about one-fifth were shown to have disorders discovered for the first time.[49]

Specific chronic diseases, other than cancer, have led to organized programs in many countries. Cardiovascular disease has become the chief cause of death in most of the industrialized countries and special institutes have been established for research and treatment. The Institute of Cardiology in Mexico City serves as a hospital as well as a research center. The National Heart Institute in Washington, D.C. is one of the component parts of the research program of the United States Public Health Service. Special clinics for diagnosis and treatment of various forms of heart disease are attached to hospitals all over the world. Heart disease is so highly prevalent that financial support is usually from general sources, rather than from earmarked funds, as in the case of cancer. Public health agencies, nevertheless, can render valuable service by coordinating various diagnostic and treatment services available in a community.[50]

Special efforts have also been directed to the treatment of chronic rheumatic diseases. Much work has been done in Holland, where these disorders are particularly prevalent. The new endocrine drugs, combined with physical medicine, have stimulated higher hopes for rehabilitation of persons with severely disabling arthritis. To finance such services, which are long-term and expensive, the Arthritis and Rheumatism Society, a voluntary agency, has been organized in Canada and the United States. An international professional society on rheumatology has been organized to advance knowledge. In Sweden a Royal Commission on the Care of Rheumatic Disease was organized and the Royal Medical Board has stimulated the organization of rheumatism clinics in large general hospitals.[51] Special clinics and rheumatism wards are found in the large teaching hospitals in London, Paris, Buenos Aires, and elsewhere.

The generally rising prevalence of chronic, degenerative diseases is compelling public health agencies everywhere to take increasing interest in the organization of medical care—for present knowledge of most of these diseases yields few preventive approaches beyond the value of early diagnosis and prompt treatment. At the same time, interest is being shown in the possibilities of preventing certain metabolic disorders, like arteriosclerosis, through dietary controls and limitation of obesity. In 1951, a "National Conference on Chronic Disease: Preventive Aspects" was held in Chicago in which present knowledge of preventive potentialities was summarized regarding cancer, cardiovascular disease, chronic arthritis, multiple sclerosis, cerebral palsy, epilepsy, diabetes, blindness, deafness, tuberculosis, syphilis, emotional disorders, occupational diseases, and other long-term disorders. "Primary prevention" requires community action of some type for certain of these diseases, but in every instance "secondary prevention" was said to require arrangements whereby persons affected would have ready access to medical care.[52] Even in the name of preventive medicine, therefore, public health agencies are inevitably becoming concerned with the availability of ordinary medical care.

Institutional Care

In many countries chronic diseases, beyond tuberculosis and mental disorder, are treated in special institutions. Some of these are full-fledged hospitals for chronic disease, such as the Goldwater Memorial Hospital in New York. A much greater number are less technically advanced facilities where the patient receives nursing care, rest, a minimal degree of medical supervision, and general attention to his living needs. These "nursing homes" or "convalescent homes" or "old people's homes" are operated by a variety of agencies, private, voluntary, and governmental. Inevitably such institutions attract a high proportion of aged persons and persons of low income, so that they commonly acquire a somewhat depressed and hopeless atmosphere. Much depends, of course, on the source of financial support. Where funds are ample, such as in facilities supported by social insurance societies in Denmark, the level of service is considerably brighter than in those forced to operate on meager support from public revenues.[53]

With the proportion of aged persons having chronic disease increasing all the time, the importance of these facilities for long-term care is growing. In Great Britain, the problem is complicated by the fact that these institutions come under the supervision of local authorities, while hospitals are under the regional hospital boards. Since there is pressure for beds in the hospitals, there is a tendency to transfer patients with chronic disease as quickly as possible to old people's homes (the term "nursing home" in Britain is applied usually to small general hospitals under private auspices). This shifts the financial burden from the Ministry of Health to the local governmental unit. It is often difficult to draw the line between the patient needing care in a general hospital, an old people's home, or simply in a custodial unit (when his own personal home is inadequate or nonexistent). In some British cities, geriatric annexes to general hospitals have been organized, as well as "halfway houses"—homes for the patient who needs less medical attention but is not quite ready to go home. The whole problem of chronic disease care in Great Britain underscores the necessity for coordinating various governmental authorities at the local level.[54]

In continental Europe, especially in Germany and France, the spa or watering place has for centuries been a cynosure for the patient with a chronic disease, especially hypertension, rheumatism, and skin ailments. These health resorts are often operated by units of local government, but attendance at them is ordinarily financed by the individual privately or through a social insurance fund. The regime of "cure" usually counts heavily on rest, recreation, good diet, psychological diversion, and necessary medical care—as well as the hydrotherapy—and, insofar as these measures strengthen general health and disease resistance, they embody a preventive approach to chronic disease. In the Soviet Union, much use is made also of "rest homes" and various health resorts, operated by the trade unions and the Ministry of Health and financed mainly by social insurance, for general supportive therapy of persons suffering from chronic disease or physical and emotional stress.[55]

In the United States, nursing homes under the auspices of local government or private management have been multiplying rapidly to meet the problems of the aged and chronically ill. With the enactment of Old Age and Survivors Insurance and federal-state public assistance for the aged in 1935, it was hoped that the need for almshouses and custodial homes for the aged and infirm would diminish, as older persons received pensions on which they could support themselves in their own homes. The increased longevity of the population, however, has yielded a large number of persons with chronic ailments requiring some type of institutional care—especially associated with economic pressures making it difficult for young families to provide homes for feeble and aged parents. As a result, it has been necessary to establish governmental standards for protection of patients accommodated in these institutions for the aged and chronically ill. In 1953, such supervisory or inspectional authority in twenty-nine of the forty-eight states was vested in the department of public health, and in nine states it was shared between this agency and the department of welfare.[56] These responsibilities for nursing homes have necessarily involved public health agencies in one aspect of medical care for chronic disease. Inspection by health officials is directed, among other things, to maintenance of proper sanitation, nutrition, and other elements of preventive hygiene.[57] Financial support for these patients comes from a variety of private and governmental sources, but it is often meager and there are difficulties in maintaining a proper standard of care and an attitude of active medical therapy with rehabilitation objectives. In a number of places, such as Pittsburgh (United States) and Montreal (Canada), custodial institutions for the aged and infirm have been revitalized and converted into active geriatric rehabilitation centers through the enthusiasm of leaders in physical medicine.

There are other aspects to chronic disease control, which depend on services rendered in connection with hospitals. The extension of hospital outpatient departments and home care services emanating from hospitals are of special benefit to the chronically ill. Organized home-help services, such as have been highly systematized in Great Britain, are of great use. The rehabilitation movement, which has been

oriented mainly to the orthopedically handicapped, has many contributions to make to persons enfeebled by cardiovascular disease and other systemic disorders. Programs of health insurance, making physician's care for the ambulatory person more readily accessible, are relevant. Various voluntary agencies combating particular diseases, like heart disease, cancer, rheumatism, or diabetes, can provide funds for service and research. Public health agencies are meanwhile seeking preventive attacks on chronic disease. All these aspects of treatment and prevention require coordination in local communities, as well as at the level of the province and nation. A National Conference on Care of the Long-Term Patient was held in the United States in 1954 to consider all these relationships. One of its committees concluded:

> A person's chronic illness is characterized not only by its length but also by the changes which occur in his condition and which dictate changes in his care and treatment. . . . The chronically ill person is likely to need at various times a physician, a dentist, a visiting nurse, a hospital, a home-care program, a homemaker service, rehabilitation services, a medical social worker, etc. Of paramount importance to the long-term patient are social aspects of care— food, housing, financial problems, recreational needs, etc. . . . Coordination is needed because of the importance of providing the proper service at the proper time and since, when it brings about early effective treatment and rehabilitation, it can help prevent permanent disability. Coordination is necessary to prevent fractionation of the patient by different special interests.[58]

To provide this coordination, leadership may be expected from ministries and departments of health. A joint committee of the American Hospital Association, American Public Health Association, American Medical Association, and American Public Welfare Association called for such coordinated efforts in 1947, with recognition of the high degree of community organization demanded by the inherent nature of chronic disease. "The problem of chronic disease presents many aspects," it stated, "prevention, research, medical care in home, hospital, and nursing home, and convalescence and rehabilitation." Equally applicable in all countries would be its further observations:

> Undue emphasis on any one aspect would be unwise, uneconomical, and ineffectual. For example, to concentrate on the provision of medical care without paying serious attention to prevention and research would postpone for many years any basic attack on the problem. On the other hand, it is impossible to focus sole attention on research because of the very urgent need for medical care. Likewise, to provide hospital beds for chronic disease without making nursing home facilities available would result in many beds being occupied by patients who do not

need hospital care. Too great an emphasis on nursing homes would deprive many patients of the specialized hospital care which is necessary for their improvement. Failure to plan adequately for home care or for convalescent care and rehabilitation would defeat the purpose of the program—to maintain and restore the individual as a self-supporting productive member of his community.[59]

DENTAL DISEASE

The inseparability of prevention from treatment in dental health is so obvious that only a few words need be said about this field. Enormous inadequacies in dental care are found in all countries, from the economically poorest to the richest. Even in highly prosperous countries, the shortage of personnel to cope with the problem of dental disease is very great, greater than shortages in any other aspect of medical service. Organized efforts, therefore, have had to be applied within a framework of such inadequate dental manpower that only limited programs are possible.

Only in countries with a completely public system of health service, like Great Britain or Soviet Russia, is dental care provided theoretically to all persons. Even in such countries, however, the shortages of staff render dental care unavailable to many, for priorities must be established on what persons can be served. Hospitals and health centers in the Soviet Union have dental departments attached to them, and much use is made of auxiliary personnel.[60] In Britain, while most dental care is given by individual practitioners, paid for their service by the executive councils on a fee basis, a system of salaried dentists is maintained for treating schoolchildren. The high incomes of individual dental practice have attracted dentists from the school services and made it difficult to meet the needs.[61] This trend, however, has been largely arrested by the introduction of charges for dentures under the National Health Service in 1951 and for conservative dental care of adults in 1952, and by a reduction of dentist's fees. Only recently, these fees have been increased in view of the declining income of dentists under the Service.

Because of personnel shortages, priorities in dental care everywhere have been accorded to children. The first school dental service was organized in Germany (Strasburg and Darmstadt) in 1902.[62] Since then, most industrialized countries have developed special programs of dental care for schoolchildren. Probably the highest level of development of such services is seen in Scandinavia. In Sweden, there is publicly financed complete dental care for all children three to fifteen years of age, supported jointly by the Ministry of Health and the provincial gov-

ernments. Service is given by salaried dentists in clinics, which also serve other age groups at relatively low fees. Training scholarships are provided to attract personnel into dentistry and newly qualified dentists must spend two years initially in the Public Dental Service. The service in Norway is similar, with no charges made for treatment of persons six to eighteen years of age.[63] The intent in these countries is gradually to extend the age levels so that eventually the entire population will be covered by the organized program.

In the United States and Canada, some type of organized dental service is conducted for schoolchildren in most states and provinces. Ordinarily eligibility is limited to children from low income families who declare they cannot afford private care. Sometimes public health authorities employ only dental hygienists who examine teeth, clean them, offer dental health education, and apply topical fluorides—referring children to a dentist privately for fillings, extractions, or other therapy. A few of the industrial medical care programs and voluntary prepayment medical care plans in the United States of America include dental services among their benefits, but the vast majority of voluntary health insurance includes no such provisions. More than any other form of health care, dental care has been found to vary, in the volume of services received, directly and strikingly with family income.[64] Much emphasis is placed in the United States of America on the fluoridation of public water supplies as a measure for reducing the incidence of dental caries.

In the Philippines, dental care as an organized service was started by the Red Cross for schoolchildren. Later the Department of Education took responsibility. In 1950, dental services were included in a WHO/UNICEF rural health demonstration project, as part of a public health program. Dental services have been included in the requirements of labor legislation governing health protection of workers, since 1954.

One of the most significant measures to extend dental care has been the program of services by dental assistants or dental nurses in New Zealand. These auxiliary personnel, working under the direction of fully qualified dentists, do fillings and extractions as well as purely preventive work for schoolchildren.[65] Many other countries are expressing interest in emulating the New Zealand pattern, as a practical approach to extending dental service at much lower social investment than is required when all treatment is done by fully trained dentists.

In the Netherlands, corrective dental care is a benefit of sickness funds, through special regulations which authorize needed services to those who regularly attend a dental clinic twice a year.

There is little question of the need to coordinate and even unify the preventive and therapeutic aspects of dental health service in organized programs. Virtually every treatment service has preventive value for bodily health, if not for oral health alone. Even the final extraction of a tooth may prevent systemic infection. Any program of dental care, therefore, involves indirect disease prevention, as well as the direct prevention of measures like topical fluoride applications and dental prophylaxes. Likewise, purely preventive dental programs, such as those conducted by dental hygienists in American schools, can be most effective if they are associated with arrangements for corrective fillings, extractions, orthodontia, and other therapeutic measures as required.

Too often dental health, being supervised by a separate profession, is regarded as totally unrelated to general health. Yet the interconnections between the teeth and the rest of the body are obvious, and a complete health service must provide for dental care no less than care for conditions which may be more manifestly related to life and death. As provided in the long-term plans of the Bhore Commission for India, a dental clinic belongs in every hospital, and mobile clinics can be used to serve isolated rural populations.[66] There are obvious economies for the patient and the paying agency if dental care is provided in the same facilities and at the same time as the patient receives other forms of medical care.

NOTES

[1] J. B. McDougall, *Tuberculosis: A Global Study in Social Pathology*. Edinburgh: E. & S. Livingstone, 1949.

[2] *Revista Brasileira de Tuberculose e Doencas Toracicas*, 1948.

[3] *Bulletin of the International Social Security Association*, Vol. 4, 1951, p. 52.

[4] C. M. Smith, *National Association of Physical Therapists Bulletin*, Vol. 17, 1954, p. 9.

[5] O. L. Peterson, *A Study of the National Health Service of Great Britain*. New York: Rockefeller Foundation, processed document, 1951.

[6] Nuffield Provincial Hospitals Trust, *Interim Report of Medical Committee of the Scottish Advisory Committee*. Edinburgh: 1943.

[7] W. H. Wattleworth, *National Association of Physical Therapists Bulletin*, Vol. 16, 1953, p. 248.

[8] Central Health Services Council, Ministry of Health (England and Wales), *Report on Co-operation Between Hospital, Local Authority and General Practitioner Services*. London: 1952.

[9] H. Hollingsworth, H. L. Johnston, and A. M. Baney, *Health Program Digest: An Outline of Selected Plans, Programs, and Proposals in the United States*. Washington

D.C.: U.S. Public Health Service, PHS publication No. 191, 1952, p. 73.

[10] W. L. Rathbun and J. C. Walsh, "Hospitals for Tuberculosis." In H. Emerson (ed.), *Administrative Medicine*. New York: Thomas Nelson & Sons, 1951, p. 47.

[11] Health Survey and Development Committee (India), *Report*. New Delhi: 1946, four volumes.

[12] World Health Organization, *Tuberculosis in India: A Programme for Its Control* (Document A6/Technical Discussions/1). 1953.

[13] S. Leff, *Hospital* (London), Vol. 48, 1952, p. 233.

[14] World Health Organization, *International Digest of Health Legislation*. Vol. 3, 1952, p. 419.

[15] World Health Organization, *Tuberculosis Control in the French Overseas Territories* (Document A6/Technical Discussion/6). 1953.

[16] A. Deutsch, *The Mentally Ill in America: A History of Their Care and Treatment from Colonial Times*. New York: Columbia University Press, 1938.

[17] J. Wortis, *Soviet Psychiatry*. Baltimore: 1950, p. 42.

[18] R. G. Fuller, "A Study of Administration of State Psychiatric Services." *Mental Hygiene* (New York), Vol. 38, No. 2, April 1954, pp. 177-235.

[19] *Ibid.*

[20] Expert Committee on Mental Health, World Health Organization, *World Health Organization Technical Report Series 13*. 1951.

[21] Expert Committee on Mental Health, World Health Organization, *World Health Organization Technical Report Series 73*. 1953.

[22] Milbank Memorial Fund, *Epidemiology of Mental Disorders*. New York: 1950.

[23] Health Committee (India), *Report*.

[24] R. Sand, *The Advance to Social Medicine*. London: Staples Press, 1952.

[25] T. Parran, *Shadow on the Land: Syphilis*. New York: Reynal & Hitchcock, 1937.

[26] H. Cavaillon and H. M. E. Martin, *World Legislation on Venereal Disease*, second edition. Paris: 1950.

[27] J. L. Troupin, F. W. Reynolds, and T. Guthe, *Bulletin of the World Health Organization*, Vol. 8, 1953, p. 355.

[28] Ministry of Health (Israel), *The Health Services of Israel*. Jerusalem: 1952, p. 130.

[29] Sand, *Social Medicine*.

[30] International Labour Office, *Artificial Limbs, Appliances for the Disabled*. Geneva: ILO, 1924.

[31] Children's Bureau, Ministry of Health and Welfare (Japan), *Services for Crippled Children in Japan*. Tokyo: 1951.

[32] C. H. Rolphe, *New Statesman and Nation*, Vol. 15, No. 22, August 29, 1953, pp. 176, 200, 227.

[33] J. A. Scott, "Rehabilitation and the Follow-up Services to Prevent Recurrence of Disease." In *Proceedings of the Eighth International Hospital Congress*. London: 1953, p. 310.

[34] A. L. Van Horn, "Crippled Children." In *Social Work Year Book*, 1947. New York: Russell Sage Foundation, 1947, p. 138.

[35] Office of Vocational Rehabilitation (United States), *The Doctor and Vocational Rehabilitation for Civilians*. Washington, D.C.: 1947.

[36] O. C. Hobby, *Statement of the Secretary of Health, Education, and Welfare Before the Subcommittee on Health of the Senate Committee on Labor and Public Welfare*. Washington, D.C.: processed document, 1954.

[37] H. Notkin, "Vocational Rehabilitation and Public Health." *American Journal of Public Health*, Vol. 41, No. 9, September 1951, pp. 1,096-1,100.

[38] M. I. Roemer, "A Case for Reciprocity." *Journal of Rehabilitation*, Vol. 15, No. 5, 1949, pp. 20-23.

[39] A. L. Chapman and J. H. Berber, "Rehabilitation: The Role of the Health Department." *Public Health Reports* (Washington, D.C.), Vol. 66, No. 17, April 27, 1951, pp. 529-534.

[40] H. Sholz, "Organization of Physical Medicine in the Sickness-Insurance Centres of Vienna." *British Journal of Physical Medicine*, Vol. 15, No. 11, November 1952, pp. 247-248.

[41] United Nations, *Modern Methods of Rehabilitation of the Adult Disabled; Report of a Group-Training Course Organized by the United Nations with the Co-operation of the World Health Organization and the International Labour Organisation* (U.N. publication 1952, IV, 19). New York: UN, 1952.

[42] H. A. Rusk, *New York Times*, October 3, 1954.

[43] *Bulletin of the International Social Security Association*, Vol. 6, 1953, p. 482.

[44] E. B. Merrill, "A View of Prevention of Blindness in Relation to Public Health." *Sight-Saving Review*, Vol. 12, No. 2, June 1942, pp. 90-102.

[45] Ministry of Health (Israel), *Health Services*, p. 130.

[46] Bureau of Statistics (Canada), *Health Reference Book 1948*. Ottawa: 1949.

[47] R. F. Kaiser, "Cancer Control in the United States," *Public Health Reports* (Washington, D.C.), Vol. 67, No. 9, September 1952, p. 877.

[48] M. L. Levin, "Detection of Chronic Disease." *Journal of the American Medical Association*. Vol. 146, August 11, 1951, pp. 1,397-1,401.

[49] E. R. Weinerman and others, "Multiphasic Screening of Longshoremen with Organized Medical Follow-Up." *American Journal of Public Health*, Vol. 42, No. 12, December 1952, pp. 1,552-1,567.

[50] J. G. Barrow, "Development of a Cardiac Control Program in Georgia." *American Journal of Public Health*, Vol. 43, No. 5, May 1953, pp. 572-576.

[51] Royal Commission on the Care of Rheumatic Diseases in Sweden (Sweden), *Social Department Official State Paper No. 41*. Stockholm: 1945.

[52] National Conference on Chronic Disease: Preventive Aspects, *Preventive Aspects of Chronic Disease*. Chicago: 1951.

[53] V. L. Ellicot, "Geriatric Care in Denmark and Britain." *Geriatrics*, Vol. 9, No. 1, January 1954, pp. 37-40.

[54] T. McKeown and C. R. Lowe, "A Scheme for the Care of the Aged and Chronic Sick." *British Medical Journal*, No. 4777, July 26, 1952, pp. 207-210.

[55] *Bulletin of the International Social Security Association*, Vol. 6, 1953, p. 486.

[56] National Social Welfare Assembly, National Committee on the Aging, *Standards of Care for Older People in Institutions*. New York: 1953, Vol. 2, p. 30.

[57] M. Ranck and R. R. Cunningham, "The Health Department and Nursing Homes." *Public Health Reports* (Washington, D.C.), Vol. 67, No. 9, September 1952, pp. 829-834.

[58] Commission on Chronic Illness, *National Conference on Care of the Long-Term Patient*. Baltimore: processed document, 1954.

[59] "Planning for the Chronically Ill: Joint Statement of Recommendations by the American Hospital Association, American Medical Association, American Public Health Association, and American Public Welfare Association." *American Journal of Public Health*, Vol. 37, No. 10, October 1947, p. 1,256-1,266.

[60] H. E. Sigerist, *Medicine and Health in the Soviet Union*. New York: Citadel Press, 1947.

[61] *Lancet*, Vol. 262, No. 6712, August 19, 1952, p. 814.

[62] Sand, *Social Medicine*.

[63] Norway, *Act of 28th July 1949*, respecting public dental service, Oslo: 1949.

[64] J. M. Wisan, *Annals of the American Academy of Political and Social Science*, Vol. 273, 1951, p. 131.

[65] J. T. Fulton, *Experiment in Dental Care: Results of New Zealand's Use of School Dental Nurses*. Geneva: World Health Organization, Monograph Series No. 4, 1951.

[66] Health Committee (India), *Report*.

Chapter XVII
Rural Health Programs
of Different Nations

The economic and social handicaps of rural populations, relative to urban, have induced special programs of health service in nearly all countries. Much of the special effort is designed to build up rural resources for health care, to attract various types of health personnel, to build hospitals and health centers. Special measures for assuring financial support are often required; agricultural people are seldom regular wage earners, like industrial workers, to whom the social insurance principle has been readily applied. Other means of financial support, principally general revenues, are usually necessary.

Previous chapters have, inevitably, discussed the special efforts of nations to bring modern health care to rural people. In this chapter, these efforts are briefly reviewed in terms of the problems of facilities, personnel, transportation, and other elements of health service which involve difficult challenges in the rural environment. Presented as a paper at a conference in West Virginia on rural health issues, this text was published as a chapter on "Health Care for Rural People: Solutions Attempted Around the World" in Rural and Appalachian Health *(R. L. Nolan and J. L. Schwartz, editors, Springfield, Illinois: Charles C. Thomas, 1973, pp. 65-78). It is reprinted here by permission.*

Deficiencies in health services among rural populations are found in every country of the world. In the poorest countries to the richest, in the most agricultural and underdeveloped to the most industrialized and highly developed, the rural population tends to receive a lower level of health service in relation to its needs than the urban. This is found both by quantitative measures of services utilized and by estimates of the quality of those services.

Striking evidence for this has recently been produced by a national study in Colombia, South America, where a higher incidence of sickness was found among rural people in household surveys (both interviews and medical examinations) than among urban; yet, there was a lower volume of ambulatory and hospital services received by rural people, even counting the ministrations of nonscientific healers. In the developing countries generally, the village-dweller gets a higher proportion of his limited volume of medical care from traditional healers than does the city-dweller; he also depends more heavily on self-prescribed drugs. In the United States, the mortality rates among rural people are somewhat lower than among urban, but the volume of sickness, especially chronic, is higher; the utilization of ambulatory medical and dental services and of hospitalization is distinctly lower.

To cope with these inequities, almost all countries have undertaken special efforts to compensate for the inherent handicaps of the rural environment. These efforts are nearly always put forth at the national level. It seems to be generally recognized that the solution of rural health care problems must be like the treatment of a systemic disease; the rural symptom is only a manifestation of a systemic disorder, and to alleviate or cure it, actions must be taken to modify the functioning of the total system.

For the sake of brevity, I should like to oversimplify a very diversified array of social actions to cope with rural health care problems, and consider them under eight categories. In practice, actions in each of these spheres are obviously interrelated to actions in the other spheres, and the overall effort is heavily influenced by the general sociopolitical design of the health service system. Yet, it is interesting to observe how much consistency exists in certain types of health care effort even among countries at different points on the political spectrum and at different stages of economic development.

PREVENTION OF DISEASE

The prevention of disease or promotion of health through environmental or mass population measures figures prominently in rural health improvement efforts everywhere. In the developing countries, vector-borne diseases, like malaria or schistosomiasis, are highly prevalent in rural populations and are the object of environmental control campaigns. These are usually launched by central governments, filling in swamps, spraying houses with insecticides, eliminating snails from streams, etc., even when there is a local health agency available for personal health services. Improvements in rural water supplies and excreta disposal systems have been a very slow process and, in the developing countries, have usually depended on provision of equipment and technical aid from central ministries of health.

The most widespread preventive efforts in personal health service have been in the promotion of maternal and child health (MCH). The periodic examination of the expectant woman and the checkup of the small baby, with immunizations, advice on proper feeding, and hygienic counseling are a staple of rural health programs in Latin America, Asia, and Africa, as much as in Europe and North America. In the developing world, both the examinations and advice are typically provided by midwives and other auxiliary personnel, rarely by doctors. Moreover, in these countries, the sharp distinction between prevention and treatment applied in the United States is seldom found in rural programs (though it persists in the larger cities); the sick baby is treated to the extent possible. A common program in rural health centers is the rehydration (through parenteral fluids) of infants dehydrated from gastrointestinal disease. The effectiveness of these MCH programs is reflected by the decline almost everywhere of rural infant mortality rates over the last thirty or forty years, even though they generally remain higher than the urban.

Reduced infant mortality has led in many countries of Asia and Africa, less so in Latin America, to another form of prevention, family planning. With declines in death rates, population growth has accelerated. The large field of population control and family planning cannot be discussed here, except to note that in India, Thailand, Ghana, and elsewhere, contraceptive programs have been incorporated within the rural MCH activities. Insertions of intrauterine devices and male sterilization procedures are performed by doctors, but dispensing of pills and contraceptive instructions of other types are usually carried out by rural nurses or midwives. Chile, under its new Marxist government, seems to be the first Latin American country to incorporate family planning into its national health policy.

GETTING DOCTORS TO RURAL AREAS

Concentrations of doctors in the large cities are worldwide phenomena. To some extent, of course, this is quite reasonable, insofar as cities must be centers for serving large regions with highly specialized care. The resultant shortages of doctors in the small towns serving rural districts are often severe and a variety of corrective actions have been taken.

Most basic has been the expansion everywhere of medical schools, so as to produce a greater national output of doctors. As long as the national supply is deficient, the rural areas with their general cultural handicaps will attract the fewest medical graduates. The most impressive increases in the total output of doctors have occurred in the Soviet Union and other socialist countries. Cuba, for example, has much more than made up for its massive exodus of doctors following the 1959 revolution; it now has over 7,000 doctors for its 8,000,000 people—a ratio (about 1:1,150) equal to that of the Scandinavian countries a few years ago. Nearly all the Latin American countries have achieved improved ratios of doctors over the last thirty years, and the establishment of medical schools in the newly emancipated countries of Africa is doing the same.

After production of doctors, of course, the task is to bring about their distribution in relation to population needs, and various methods have been used. Since about 1935, Mexico has made a period of "social service" in a rural village a condition for earning the medical degree; originally this was for six months and now it is for a year. An increasing number of countries in Latin America and Asia are doing likewise. Indonesia and Turkey have such requirements; Iran achieves this end through a period of service in the Rural Health Corps, as a form of military obligation. Malaysia has recently instituted a two-year rural service requirement in connection with the output of the first graduating class from its own medical school (formerly its doctors had to be trained abroad). The Soviet Union requires three years of service by new medical graduates in a rural health center.

Several states in our country have had "rural medical fellowship" programs since the 1940s, including Virginia and North Carolina. The new graduate serves a year in a rural area of need for each medical school year in which he has received fellowship support. The recently passed Emergency Health Personnel Act of 1970 is the first federal approach to the problem, using military obligation as the device for getting doctors to rural areas; appropriations for implementation of this law are still being awaited.

The tougher task is to hold doctors in rural areas after an initial period. The experience of the mandatory rural service programs, both in the United States and elsewhere, is that when the statutory obligation is fulfilled, the young doctor usually leaves for a city. In the Soviet Union, this tendency is countered by payment of higher salaries for a rural than for a comparable urban position. Similar salary differentials for rural work have recently been introduced in Mexico.

Assuring a satisfactory income is, of course, basic to the solution of the rural doctor problem. Even though earnings are obviously not the whole story, we know that in the United States, country doctor incomes are lower than those in all city-sizes except the multimillion population metropolises. Various schemes have been used to guarantee rural incomes. In the rural municipalities of the Canadian prairie provinces, salaries have been paid to general practitioners by local government since 1917. The Highlands and Islands Scheme of northern Scotland pays salaries to doctors who could not hope to make an adequate income from the sparse population in this region. New Zealand has similar arrangements in isolated localities, administered by the national Ministry of Health. Coal mining communities in West Virginia and other Appalachian states have long supported doctors through salaries paid from local employer-employee prepayment plans. The basic issue of adequate income support for doctors and others in rural health service is, of course, tied up with the general problem of economic support which will be explored below.

Other inducements besides income designed to keep doctors in rural places include provision of housing. Many American towns offer an attractive house at very low rental as an inducement. In the developing countries, government-financed housing is a standard feature of rural assignments for the doctor, along with other health personnel. Office quarters at low rentals have also been offered to doctors by small towns in Canada and the United States; many of these are small health centers built with the assistance of the Sears Roebuck Foundation. The provision of modern rural hospitals, of course, is also an attraction for doctors—a basic premise in the back of the Hill-Burton hospital construction program in this country.

In Great Britain, rural settlement of doctors is encouraged by a national policy of designating certain areas as "overdoctored;" in these areas, typically metropolitan, new doctors are not permitted to settle—at least not under the financial support of the National Health Service. As a result, the doctors going elsewhere will sometimes be channelled to rural communities. There was a somewhat similar policy in West Germany, where the local sickness funds with heavy medical participation used to prohibit new doctors from entering, thereby compelling them to settle in areas of greater need; unfortunately for rural areas, a recent German court decision invalidated this policy in the interest of "free trade" for the medical profession. Tunisia, on the other hand, is a country which has banned new doctors from settling in the busy national capital, Tunis, thereby diverting them to other towns. All such policies as these obviously require national health planning and the exercise of considerable control over the flow of funds to pay for medical care.

ANCILLARY HEALTH MANPOWER

The use of personnel other than doctors to meet health needs has been more extensively applied in rural areas than in cities throughout the world. The well-known "feldsher" of czarist Russia was originally a rural medical replacement for the doctor. After the Revolution, with the great increase in doctor output, there was an intention to eliminate this type of health worker as substandard, but ultimately the feldsher was kept. He, or she, now works in both rural and urban areas as a general medical auxiliary, with wider responsibilities than the nurse; in rural posts the feldsher services villages of a few hundred people—too few to warrant a full-time physician. An important feature of the Soviet manpower model is the freedom of feldshers or nurses to undertake further studies and become doctors—this is one of the reasons that so many Soviet doctors are women.

Many countries have trained special classes of middle-level health personnel for rural service. Ethiopia has its famous Public Health Training College at Gondar, where "health officers" are trained for both curative and preventive work in rural health centers; their curriculum requires three years of study after high school, followed by a year of supervised field work. Community nurses and sanitarians are similarly trained in relatively short periods. Venezuela has its rural program of so-called "simplified medicine," staffed by auxiliary nurses and male medical assistants. In Ceylon, rural posts are staffed by dispensers of common remedies, who are still quaintly called "apothecaries." In Malaysia, the old British term of "hospital assistant" is applied to male health personnel who give the curative service in rural health centers, while nurses and nursing assistants give the preventive service. Throughout Africa the "dresser," a male auxiliary with very little formal schooling, is the most common source of medical care, except for primitive healers, for most of the rural population.

Most of the world's babies are undoubtedly delivered by midwives who have learned their skills simply from observation and experience. Throughout Asia and Africa, less so in Latin America, young village women with grade school education have been given formal training of one or two years to serve as "government midwives." The task everywhere is to win over the rural people to use these trained midwives, rather than the untrained ones with whom they are usually more familiar. The trained midwife, of course, is by no means limited to rural areas of underdeveloped countries. She is the attendant at most childbirths in Great Britain and Holland where the infant and maternal mortality records are, incidentally, better than in the United States.

The hundreds of millions of people in rural China have long depended on herbalists and acupuncturists for their medical care. Under the current Communist government, thousands of young peasants have been trained to offer immunizations, first aid for injuries, scientific drugs for common diseases, and education about personal hygiene. These "barefoot doctors," as they are called, are now the mainstays of rural health care in the People's Republic, working as part of a network of both Western and traditional medicine in each province.

RURAL HOSPITALS AND HEALTH CENTERS

Insofar as local wealth has financed hospital construction, rural populations have always been left behind. This has been true in the wealthy United States no less than in India or Brazil. It took the Hill-Burton Act in our country, with its strong priorities for rural states and the rural regions within every state, to improve the relative hospital bed supply for rural people. Over the last twenty-five years

since this program was started, bed supply has been quite well equalized between rural and urban areas; in fact, the dynamics of patient flow today are such that the greater pressures of bed shortage are being felt in the city hospitals which are serving both urban and rural people.

Hospital construction in the main provincial towns serving rural districts is a standard objective in the ministry of health plans in countries of Latin America, Asia, and Africa. While urban hospitals are often built by voluntary bodies or purely private groups, rural district hospitals nearly always depend on central government; the chief exceptions are the hospitals, usually small, established by foreign religious missions. Throughout Latin America, and also in Iran and Turkey, social security agencies separate from health ministries have built many large well-equipped hospitals; these are limited, however, to their beneficiaries who are nearly always industrial or commercial workers in the main cities.

The rural district hospital outside of Western Europe and North America typically has much responsibility for ambulatory care. Its outpatient department provides the specialty care for the whole district, since private specialists are nonexistent in these areas. In Great Britain, all hospitals come under the control of regional hospital boards which attempt to coordinate the response to needs in both cities and the rural sections around them. Sweden also has a regionalization scheme, under which graded responsibilities are assigned to rural, district, and provincial hospitals. The hospital in Chile is administratively responsible for all official health services, ambulatory and environmental, in its catchment area. This is the pattern also in the Soviet Union.

Probably more important on a world scale than the rural hospital is the rural health center—a facility for ambulatory service, curative and preventive. There are different intensities of staffing. In Mexico, for example, there are the Type A health centers, staffed by several doctors with specialty qualifications and located in the main provincial towns; the Type B centers are staffed by one general medical practitioner aided by nurses and other auxiliaries; the Type C centers in small villages are staffed only by auxiliary personnel, visited occasionally by a supervising doctor. Malaysia and Thailand have their "main health centers," staffed by one doctor and several nurses and auxiliaries, and "subcenters," staffed only by auxiliaries. In Sub-Sahara Africa, the health centers are usually staffed only by dressers and assistant nurses, with doctors found only at district hospitals. Sometimes a health center will contain a few

172

beds for some maternity cases or emergencies, pending referral to a hospital. The smallest rural facilities are sometimes called rural posts or stations, where a single health auxiliary, with a small supply of government-supplied drugs, lives in a village.

Health centers, staffed by a general practitioner and a pediatrician, along with nurses and others, are the standard facility for ambulatory care in the rural areas of the socialist countries of Eastern Europe. In the main cities, where specialists are found, the ambulatory units are considered polyclinics, although generalists also work in them. It is interesting to note that Great Britain, after great initial resistance to the idea by general practitioners, is now rapidly developing health centers for housing family doctors along with public health nurses and social workers; the general practitioner sees the patients on his panel, for which he is still paid by capitation, rather than being a salaried employee. Such health centers are now being built by local health authorities both in large English and Scottish cities and in small towns. A similar movement is starting in New Zealand, even though the general practitioners under this country's national health service are paid by fee-for-service.

On every continent the concept of an orderly network of facilities is developing, with health centers operating as satellites of hospitals. Patients are sent from the health center to the hospital for diagnostic work-ups and treatment; after hospital discharge the patient is referred back to the health center for follow-up care. In the Soviet Union, a regular policy of exchange of positions is carried out between health centers and hospitals, for one or two months per year, so that the doctor in each setting can learn about the problems in the other setting. In the United States, the "neighborhood health centers" for the poor have been largely set up in urban slums, but they probably have important implications for rural areas as well. Private group practice clinics, it may be noted, involve a higher percentage of the total doctors in rural counties than in urban counties, and one can anticipate a wider role for such clinics in the future.

TRANSPORTATION AND COMMUNICATION

A critical aspect of rural health service is the availability of transportation and communication. It is likely that greater benefits have been brought about in rural health care through improved transportation than through enlargement of medical resources in the isolated rural districts.

Most fundamental are paved roads which, of course, serve the general marketing needs of agriculture as well as health services. It is ironic that in various countries of Southeast Asia it took the contingencies of guerilla warfare to produce a network of roads which were long needed anyway for the welfare of rural people; those roads can fortunately facilitate movement of village people to the cities for medical care. On the roads are buses and occasionally taxis for seriously sick patients. Ambulances are also attached to most of the district rural hospitals in Latin America and Asia.

The mobile clinic is widely used in the developing countries as a way of reaching villages distant from a health center. In Malaysia, the hospital assistant makes the rounds of several villages once or twice a month, traveling in a small truck that carries a supply of the common drugs. Latin American mobile clinics usually include a doctor along with a nursing assistant. In Africa, rivers are sometimes used as channels for mobile clinics. A certain romanticism attaches to these patterns, but one must realize that a permanent health post, with an auxiliary worker, is nearly always preferable; a medical consultant can then come by periodically.

Home calls by the doctor are becoming rare in most countries, as the demands on the doctor's time have increased. The public health nurse or home visitor is more often sent to investigate matters in rural districts. Yet in Great Britain, the general practitioner is often proud of his continued willingness to make home calls and thereby become acquainted with the real living conditions of his patient. In Belgium, the social insurance program pays the country doctor not only for the mileage involved in home calls, but also for the time consumed in travel, over and above the fee for the medical service.

For extremely isolated rural people, the airplane ambulance is another important adjustment. In Saskatchewan, Canada, when many roads are blocked by snow through the long winter, the airplanes of the provincial Health Department, notified by telephone or radio, pick up patients and transport them to the main cities; many a nighttime landing has been made on a snow-covered wheat field, illuminated by the headlights of three or four automobiles placed to mark out a runway. The stretches of Siberia have long been served also by airplane ambulances, and in Poland helicopters are used. Australia has its Royal Flying Doctor Service—a voluntary agency aided by government grants. More reliance is placed on radio communication and transport of the patient than on conveyance of the doctor. Communication by television is the latest adjustment to rural health care problems; the patient's picture is televised to an urban consultant who then advises a general practitioner out in the field what should be done. This is now being done between Seattle, Washington, and Alaska.

QUALITY PROMOTION AND MAINTENANCE

The isolation of rural health workers makes it difficult for them to keep up with advances in medical science, quite aside from the poverty of rural resources. Everywhere this problem has been tackled through the principle of regionalization, under which small peripheral rural facilities come under the influence of larger urban units.

Regionalization of services is the model for the rural areas of India, Indonesia, Brazil, Sweden, the Soviet Union, People's China, almost everywhere. The more difficult cases are sent from the peripheral facilities into the central ones, and supervision emanates from the centers outward. Rural health personnel may be brought into the main city for various courses of training. Medical schools, of course, along with other types of professional schools, bear a special responsibility for such continuing education. Sending medical students out to work with rural doctors is not only valuable for the student but also helps to keep the practitioner on his toes.

In the United States, the regionalization idea got its first major boost with the Hill-Burton hospital construction program, mentioned above. But it took the Regional Medical Program (RMP) for Heart Disease, Cancer, and Stroke to extend the idea to a functional level. Except for the recent major cutbacks in federal RMP funds, this program was helping to extend the qualitative influence of urban medical centers to rural localities.

ECONOMIC SUPPORT

Basic to the solution of rural health care problems everywhere is attaining adequate economic support. In many countries, the social insurance device has strengthened the economic base of medical care in the cities, where insured wage earners live. But, most agricultural populations are not brought under the social insurance or social security umbrella for reasons that are economic, administrative, and political. As a result, rural health services have more often depended on support from general national revenues.

In the Scandinavian countries, district doctors are supported in the rural areas by the central government, even though they may also earn fees from the health insurance program. The operating costs of health centers and rural hospitals in the developing countries are met typically from national revenues. In the United States, the special comprehensive health care programs for American Indians, a largely

rural people, are financed by the federal government. The same applies to special family health clinics for migratory or seasonal agricultural workers; formerly all federal, these are now supported by federal grants to the states. In Yugoslavia and Poland, small farmers form health cooperatives for meeting both construction and operational costs of certain rural health centers.

As long as the economic base of rural medical care depends solely on rural people, deficiencies must persist; agriculture simply has lower per capita productivity than industry with its greater use of machine power and technology. Rural health care can reach the level of urban health care only by tapping urban wealth. In most countries this is done through the use of various types of general revenue. The United States today is debating the issue of national health insurance, as a means of greatly extending economic support for the whole population. We know that voluntary health insurance protection is weakest among rural people, so there is no doubt that rural people would be the greatest beneficiaries of such a nationwide program. With such economic underpinning, one could begin to have hope of getting improvements in the health personnel, facilities, and programs that rural areas need.

HEALTH SERVICE PLANNING AND COORDINATION

The cities, in a sense, can take care of themselves medically, even though there may be extravagance in the use of resources. For improvement in rural health care, planning is always needed at the national or regional level. This has been recognized in India, in almost all the countries of Africa, in most Latin American countries, and throughout the socialist world.

Health planning has come somewhat later to the industrialized countries of Western Europe and North America, where free private enterprise has been so strong. Yet in America today, comprehensive health planning (CHP) has now been launched in all the states, since the federal grants of 1966 for this purpose. So far, the CHP programs have accomplished little, but we all know that this is because they have no real authority and very little money. The current period, in my view, is a prelude to planning—a tooling-up period. The action will not really begin until we have a program of nationwide economic support for health services, which will provide the resources and, at the same time, the visible urgency to see that the money is wisely spent.

These eight approaches to solving rural health care problems around the world will doubtless sound familiar. There are very few, among the many specific actions, which have not already been tried somewhere in the United States, though not always with adequate intensity. In West Virginia, with its history of health insurance plans in the mining industry (from the old check-off to the modern United Mine Workers of America Trust Fund program), its especially strong program of vocational rehabilitation services, its rural hospital construction program, its impressive new school of medicine, and its recent legislation on new forms of paramedical personnel, I suspect that the efforts have been more positive than in most states.

The ultimate solution to rural health care problems, however, as one can see everywhere, is not to be found solely within the borders of rural states or provinces. It demands action on a national level both for mobilization of economic support and for allocation of resources in some proportion to need. Along with these moves, which obviously require governmental initiative, people within a state can organize existing manpower and institutions to be better prepared for national developments. Today we see, for example, the clear invitation from Washington to set up "health maintenance organizations" as a sound way to systematize both the financing and delivery of health care. We also see many hints at forthcoming expanded support for training new types of health manpower. These steps will strengthen the groundwork for a national health insurance program, which we all expect in the next decade. With this, the prospects of improving rural health services should become brighter than ever before.

Chapter XVIII
Occupational Health Services
in National Governments

Medical inspection of factories and other measures for protecting the health of industrial workers were developed first in Western Europe, as a response to the ill effects of working environments. Responsibilities were usually vested in ministries of labor rather than ministries of health. As public health agencies have become stronger, however, they have also been assigned responsibilities for protecting the health of workers, especially with respect to their general burden of illness as distinguished from the relatively smaller volume of disorders caused directly by the working environment (occupational diseases and work accidents).

Thus, at different rates and in diverse administrative patterns around the world, the narrow health focus of "factory inspection" has been evolving into a broader focus of general adult health service for workers. The changing role of governments in this evolution is traced in this chapter which was prepared on the headquarters staff of the World Health Organization. It was published as "From Factory Inspection to Adult Health Service: A Review of Governmental Administration of Occupational Health" in the British Journal of Industrial Medicine, *(Vol. 10, July 1953, pp. 179-194, R. I. McCallum, editor) and is reprinted here by permission. It is noteworthy that in the 1970s, the first federal legislation on this problem in the United States, the National Occupational Safety and Health Act of 1971, placed administrative responsibility in the Department of Labor; likewise in Great Britain, with its reorganization of the National Health Service of 1974, factory inspection remains a separate function of the Ministry of Labour.*

In Western Europe, the view seems to be widely held that the protection of the health of workers, by definition and by practical necessity, must be a legal responsibility of ministries or departments of labor. There are good historical reasons for this viewpoint, and considerable practical experience to back it up. In today's world, however, where newly industrializing countries are looking to the West for advice, it is worth examining the assumptions of this principle. Certainly, one does not want to export ideas about social organization and governmental administration which would not apply well in other cultures or, indeed, may not even be properly meeting the current needs of the older industrialized nations themselves.

HISTORICAL DEVELOPMENT

The rise of factory inspection in Great Britain in the early nineteenth century, and later on the European continent, was a reaction to the squalor of contemporary industrial production methods. It reflected the growing humanitarian conscience of the day and was the response of government to the demands of working people for a decent life. Naturally, the primary focus was on the protection of the worker—and more especially the woman and child worker—against the harmful effects of the work itself. Occupational diseases, like lead poisoning and "miner's asthma," had been known for some time, and some effort could reasonably be made toward their prevention. The general environment of the factory could be assured, at least, to meet minimum standards of hygiene.[1]

Here and there, benevolent employers made an effort to provide good working conditions for their workers, independently of legal inducement. These employers, in fact, helped to inspire the enactment of welfare laws. On a wide national scale, however, the police powers of the state had to be invoked, and inspection services had to be developed to compel general compliance with minimum standards. The physical environment of the factory was, of course, only one aspect of the laborer's welfare, of which hours of work, periods of rest, and the status of children and women were others. Departments or divisions of labor welfare were the obvious governmental instrument for exercising this authority to inspect and enforce compliance.

Toward the latter part of the nineteenth century and the early twentieth a new conception entered industrial life, namely, the responsibility of employers for the social consequences of industrial injuries. Behind the first industrial injuries or workmen's compensation acts was a long story of social and legal battle. The eventual effect of the new laws, however, first in Europe and later in the United States, was to induce employers to protect their workers by guarding dangerous machinery, installing safety devices, and introducing various measures to reduce accidents.

The first full-time factory inspectors were appointed under the British Factory Act of 1833, and the pattern spread rapidly. In 1898 the first Medical Inspector of Factories was appointed in recognition of the need for understanding the human reaction to toxic substances, as well as the purely environmental aspects of industrial hygiene. In the United States of America, a few states, in the 1880s, appointed factory inspectors to enforce labor codes but all the states did not have factory inspectors until about 1920; and medical guidance was rarely incorporated in the inspectorate. Whether or not medically guided, factory inspection was obviously oriented toward the removal of specific hazards of the industrial environment which might contribute to occupational diseases or industrial accidents. On the whole, the inspection programs in Europe were undoubtedly effective; the incidence of occupational diseases and industrial accidents—relative to the increasing numbers of persons engaged in industry—was reduced.

In the early twentieth century, under the influence of factory inspection and workmen's compensation laws, employers came to recognize that productivity could be increased and the workers kept better

satisfied by providing some direct medical services at the place of work. Physicians were occasionally appointed for regular service in the larger plants and mines. Such appointments were sometimes related to the need for some general medical care in isolated areas, but more often to the desire of employers to reduce compensation insurance costs by providing prompt first aid and treatment of injuries. Such industrial physicians could also perform medical examinations on job-seekers so as to prevent employment of persons physically unsuitable for the work.

The conception of an industrial health service gradually widened to include not only treatment of injuries and preemployment medical examination, but also general preventive health services, medical care for minor illnesses occurring on the job, counseling of the worker on all health problems, and supervision of the work environment. The aim came to be adjustment of the man to his job and the job to the man. This approach developed in the larger plants which had financial resources for the service, and was not made a legal requirement. Laws came to be passed requiring the availability in plants of minimal first-aid staff and equipment but the engagement of full-time medical staffs, specially trained for the purpose, was a matter for private initiative. While this scale of industrial health service, therefore, has come to cover only a small minority of workers— even in the well developed economies of Western Europe and North America—the theory behind it has taken a firm root in social thinking. In recent years, as we shall see, it has had an impact on health legislation.

This broader conception of health protection of workers is of special importance in relation to the place of supervisory authorities for the workers' health in the structure of government. For, while the theory and practice of industrial health service have been expanding, a similar evolution has taken place in government. The role of public bodies, national and local, in the protection of the health of the general population has gradually broadened. The trend has applied to both preventive and curative medicine. Many governmental agencies are involved in this process, but the most important are the ministries or departments of health in which professional skills in medical-social administration have become increasingly gathered.

It is not surprising, therefore, that as the scope of interest in occupational health has broadened from the narrow sphere of occupational disease and accident prevention to the broad sphere of total health service, public health agencies have been brought closer to the factories and mines. The advantage or disadvantage of this relationship will be considered below, but first it may be helpful to review the current methods of administration of occupational health services in government throughout the world. It may surprise some readers to find that the Western European patterns are by no means universal.

In this review, it is helpful to keep in mind a distinction between the supervisory responsibilities of government, and the direct responsibility for clinical preventive or curative services at the place of work. Our focus here is on the former, and this has importance insofar as it may affect the latter. Just as we have seen the influence of private industrial practices on legislation historically, it is obvious that the legislation and methods of governmental administration will shape the content of health services rendered within the factory, mine, or other place of work.

CURRENT GOVERNMENTAL PRACTICES IN WESTERN EUROPE

The basic patterns of factory inspection developing in the early nineteenth century still prevail in the countries of Western Europe. This is not to imply that governmental activity has remained static. Far from it; the scope of the factory inspectors has steadily widened to include all aspects of the working conditions, but the principal objective remains the enforcement of standards designed to prevent occupational diseases and industrial accidents. Beyond this, the medical inspectors of factories are responsible for supervising enforcement of laws regarding medical examinations of certain groups of workers, maintenance of first-aid boxes or factory dispensaries, and other measures designed to protect workers against specific hazards.

In all countries of Western Europe special efforts have been made to develop preventive and, to some extent, curative medical services within factories even without legislative inducement. As a general rule, these health services have been developed by the larger industries quite independently of the requirements of the factory inspection laws. Occasionally, medical inspectors of factories have participated in the promotion of such services, but usually in a voluntary capacity, as informed professional leaders.

The situation in Norway illustrates the general pattern, although in no two countries are practices exactly alike. The Norwegian Ministry of Labor contains a Directorate of Factory Inspection, first organized in 1892.[2] It has a staff of seven labor inspectors covering the country on a district basis, three inspectors of special problems, and three medical inspectors. They make periodic inspections of plants to enforce legislation designed to prevent occupational diseases and accidents, the principal current law being the Workers Protection Act of 1936, with amendments. Preemployment and periodic medical examinations are required for young workers of fifteen to eighteen years of age, and for workers exposed to silica and to radioactivity. In each of 750 communities there is a local labor inspection committee to help enforce the law. An Institute of Occupational Health is maintained by the Ministry of Labor in Oslo to assist in the diagnosis of occupational disease and to perform relevant laboratory tests.[3]

Apart from the provisions mentioned, governmental authority is not concerned with the organization of general health services in plants, but a voluntary body has been established for this purpose. This is the Industrial Medical Service Council representing the Norwegian Federation of Labor, the Employers' Association, and the Medical Association. This body sets standards for comprehensive in-plant health services which would include preplacement and periodic medical examinations of *all* workers, constant supervision of plant hygiene, first aid and treatment of minor ailments occurring on the job, and referral of workers to personal physicians for diagnosis and treatment of general illness.[4] There is no compulsion in this program, and only a small minority of Norwegian workers is covered, but the services are spreading. Cooperation is encouraged with the local public health services in such practices as tuberculosis case finding and reporting, but there is no official connection with the country's public health framework, national or local.

The other Scandinavian countries have a somewhat similar arrangement. In Sweden, Denmark, and Finland the factory inspectorate is in the Ministry of Social Affairs (rather than a separate ministry of labor), but the functions are essentially the same. In Finland there is an Industrial Medical Association devoted to the voluntary promotion of in-plant medical services, very much as in Norway. Research, training, and specialized services for the detection and control of occupational diseases are given by an independent, but government-supported, Institute of Occupational Health at Helsinki.[5] In Sweden a somewhat similar research institute for occupational health is located within the National Institute of Public Health, achieving in this way some coordination with other health research activities.[6]

Practices in Germany reflect the basic approach in Central Europe. Being one of the oldest and largest industrialized nations, with a strong tradition of governmental control, Germany has a deeply rooted system of factory inspection. In each German state there is a department of labor which contains a factory inspectorate, divided into a medical branch and an engineering branch. The engineering branch enforces regulations on environmental standards in the factories. The medical branch is staffed by "state industrial physicians" whose main duties are to determine if illness is of occupational origin, and, therefore, entitled to workmen's compensation, and the degree of disability, to act as medical consultant on the treatment of occupational disease cases, to help enforce regulations on the prevention of occupational diseases, and to advise the engineering branch on environmental controls. Tabershaw has observed that

> none of the state industrial physicians have any concept that their functions embrace interest in non-occupational disease, in the total health of the worker or in furthering general public health.[7]

Health services developed in some of the larger plants are devoted to giving medical examinations to certain workers exposed to special risks and first aid for occupational injuries and other minor ailments. There is little tendency to go beyond the minimum requirements of the law.

The detailed specifications of the classical factory inspection systems of each European country need not be reviewed. A complicated legal structure has grown up over the years, establishing minimum precautions which must be taken by industry to prevent accidents and certain specified occupational diseases. There are also requirements for first-aid services and supplies which must be available in the plants, for general toilet and washing facilities, for the use of safety devices, and for basic standards of space, lighting, ventilation, etc. The enforcement of these regulations is the duty of the factory inspectorate. With minor exceptions, there is no connection between the factory inspectorate and the general public health program of the region.

The relatively narrow scope of the factory inspection approach has been realized in Europe for some years, especially since occupational accidents and diseases have been reduced. It took the social upheaval of the Second World War, however, to cause a major extension in its scope particularly in the French-speaking countries where the upheavals of war and foreign occupation were so great. This is seen best perhaps in the introduction in Belgium and France of the requirement of a general medical examination of all workers before employment. Largely through the practical demonstrations of health programs in big industrial undertakings, the concept grew that it was to the common benefit of the

industry and the worker not only to prevent accidents and industrial intoxications, but also to assure that a worker was physically and mentally suited to a particular job, a principle commonly applied to young workers and to women for some years.

The Belgian law of 1945 requires that each undertaking is responsible for a medical examination of every worker before employment at the expense of the employer. The examinations are performed by any practitioner chosen by the worker, according to a prescribed form. A radiograph of the chest must be included, and may be performed by the National Institute for the Control of Tuberculosis (a semiautonomous organization working closely with the Ministry of Public Health and Families) or by a qualified private physician. The physicians of the factory inspectorate limit themselves to seeing that the examinations are made. The declared purpose of the procedure is not only to assure suitable job placement but also "to inform workers concerning any disorder or deficiency from which they may be suffering and to indicate institutions which can facilitate treatment."[8]

This wider protection of the worker's health under the ministries of labor is seen more strikingly in France. After a conventional factory medical inspection system which had operated since 1915, France enacted in October 1946, the most far-reaching legislation of any Western European country. For the first time in a Western European country, the provision of a systematic medical service in every factory, regardless of size, was made compulsory.[9] This service must provide not merely preemployment medical examinations of all workers but annual reexaminations, and more frequent reexaminations of young persons and workers exposed to special hazards. Annual chest radiographs of all workers are required. Emphasis is placed on proper job placement of the individual according to his particular capabilities, rather than exclusion of the unfit. First aid and diagnosis of any illness are provided in the plant, but for medical care the worker is referred to a personal physician. These services are to be rendered by part-time or full-time physicians engaged by the employer. The law specifies one medical hour per month for about every fifteen workers (less for white collar workers and more for workers under special risk), so that a full-time industrial physician is required for about every 2,250 workers.

This program is supervised by the Medical Inspectorate of Labor and Manpower of the French Ministry of Labor and Social Security. The fourteen regional medical officers of this agency must approve of the medical arrangements made by all employers in their region, and it is their duty to help to organize the services required by the 1946 law. They promote the grouping of small plants which, together, can engage the full-time services of a physician. They also carry out the usual duties of medical inspectors of factories in other countries, such as examination of specific cases of occupational disease for compensation claims, evaluation of environmental hazards, and enforcement—with the general factory inspectors—of regulations. Up to the present time, the new industrial medical service is far from complete, but progress is rapid. By January 1950, approximately fifty percent of the workers covered by the legislation were being provided with medical services through programs in 2,411 companies and 522 intercompany groups. The inspection staff has been unable to keep up with the task of reviewing and approving these services. There is no connection with the public health services except in special instances, such as the impressive coordinated program at Nancy, or the arrangement at Toulouse for nurses from the public health staff to serve in a local factory.

In all European countries, the organization of preventive services in the plants is, of course, influenced by the laws providing financial compensation to workers for industrial injuries and diseases. Large insurance companies may even provide this protection, as they naturally have a financial interest in keeping the accident rate at a minimum. In Italy, for example, there is a National Organization for Accident Prevention which not only conducts general educational campaigns, but actually operates medical clinics in the large plants, providing first aid and minor medical services.[10] The compensation laws have had the salutary effect of inducing employers to prevent accidents or reduce disability resulting from them. At the same time, however, they have tended to concentrate action so much on compensatable conditions that too little attention has been given to the larger health problems of the worker.

Discussion of industrial health services in Great Britain has been delayed because, in the current debates and self-examination of the problem in that country, there are reflected some of the fundamental organizational problems that may eventually be encountered by all countries. With the organization of the British National Health Service, bringing virtually all health care, curative and preventive, under government control, authorities were faced with questions of administrative efficiency and with the necessity to spend the available health funds with maximum effectiveness.

As in continental Europe, factory inspection under the Ministry of Labour and National Service is fo-

cused primarily on the prevention of occupational diseases and accidents. There are some fifteen regional medical inspectors of factories who are experts in the investigation of occupational disease and related environmental hazards. Spread throughout the country are some 1,700 appointed factory doctors—almost all part-time general practitioners—whose duty is to make medical examinations of young workers and workers exposed to special risks, and to investigate cases of occupational disease which are notifiable. The appointed factory doctors are paid by employers on the basis of the number of examinations they make, but they are administratively responsible to the medical inspectors of factories. There are approximately 1,300 full-time and part-time industrial medical officers, employed by private and nationalized industries for general in-plant health services. They are assisted by about 4,000 industrial nurses of whom about 2,600 are state registered. The in-plant health services as in other countries are principally in the larger plants, except for a few special cooperative projects, like the Slough Industrial Health Service near London.[11]

With the pressure on medical manpower under the National Health Service, and with the complexities of comprehensive health administration, many questions have been raised about the soundness of this general system. In 1949 a Committee of Enquiry on Industrial Health Services was appointed by the Prime Minister, under the chairmanship of Mr. Justice Dale. This report (known as the Dale Report) concluded that industrial health services of a preventive nature were valuable, that they were not available under the National Health Service, and that present patterns should be continued substantially without change. Reaction to these conclusions from many quarters was cool—not because there was lack of appreciation of the positive value of a good industrial health service, but rather because there was widespread feeling of a need for some closer administrative coordination with the National Health Service. Debate on this question has been active. In a symposium held at the Royal Sanitary Institute Congress in 1952 several new approaches were suggested. That receiving most attention was made by I. G. Davies.[12] He suggested that supervisory responsibility for industrial health services at the community level should be under the local medical officer of health, who would be aided in carrying out these duties by the appointed factory doctors. Technical advice and consultation on the complex problems of occupational diseases would remain the responsibility of the regional medical inspectors of factories. Thus at the higher levels, the Ministry of Labour and National Service would retain its responsibilities, but at the community level—where health service has its direct impact on people—the Ministry of Health could exercise appropriate supervision and integration of industrial health service with the total health program.

The debate and the proposals in Great Britain have particular significance internationally, because they are the first, or at least the major, instance in Western Europe in which the separation of the factory inspection system from the public health framework of a country has been challenged. This basic issue of relationships between labor and health ministries in the supervision of the worker's health is latent in almost all countries, and it has become sharper as the scope and dignity of public health have increased. In the rest of the world, outside of Western Europe, the respective responsibilities of these two agencies of government are much more fluid, and consequently the pattern of administration of occupational health supervision is taking different shapes.

NORTH AMERICA

As in many aspects of social welfare, the assumption of governmental responsibility for the worker's health came later in the United States than in Europe. Virtually all responsibilities for health and welfare belonged to the states, and supervision of the conditions in factories by an inspection system was not started until the end of the nineteenth century. New Jersey and Wisconsin were the pioneers in 1883. Factory inspection programs in state departments of labor developed slowly in the early twentieth century, modeled after the European practices, but in the American climate of laissez-faire liberalism with minimum government control, they were not very strong. The inspectors were rarely trained in engineering or chemistry or other appropriate fields. In only one state was medical guidance sought, in New York State, where in 1907 a single medical inspector of factories was appointed, but the idea did not spread.

There was obviously a gap to be filled in the development of a scientific program of industrial hygiene which could tackle both the environmental and the medical aspects of occupational diseases. In 1914, the United States Public Health Service attempted to fill this gap by establishing the Office of Industrial Hygiene and Sanitation, primarily for research purposes. Similar research activities were undertaken in the departments of labor of New York and Ohio, but on the whole the state and local public health agencies were not strong enough to do this work. As in Europe, here and there private industry developed preventive and, more often, curative

programs, especially in isolated areas and in large plants. The First World War gave this practice an impetus in the interest of reducing insurance rates. Then came the depression in 1929, and in 1935 a new opportunity was presented to the nation's public health agencies with the passage of the Social Security Act.[13] Under this law larger funds were made available for public health services than ever before through the device of federal grants-in-aid to the states. The Public Health Service administered these grants and, having now had twenty years of experience in industrial health research, it used them to help the states develop industrial hygiene units in the state departments of health. The idea grew rapidly, so that today every state public health agency, except four, and several large city health departments contain specialized staffs for promoting the health protection of workers.

The functions of these public health units in industrial hygiene are very different from those of factory inspectorates. They are not inspecting agencies engaged in the enforcement of laws. They are primarily advisory technical bodies, devoted to the promotion within their states of sound hygienic practices within industry. It is not that they lack enforcement powers, as is sometimes believed, for all public health agencies have general powers to require correction of hazards to health.[14] It is rather that, in the American culture, health authorities are convinced they can achieve better long-term results by a process of education, demonstration, and persuasion than by the enforcement of laws. While the effectiveness of these industrial hygiene units differs markedly among the states, they have developed a nationwide network of consultant services which has helped to reduce the incidence of occupational diseases to an extremely low level.

These developments have a far greater significance, however, than the integration of industrial hygiene services in the American public health system. An opportunity has been provided for bringing to bear the broad field of preventive health services, embodied in the modern public health movement, upon the workers in industry. The need of industry and the community as a whole is a healthy worker, and not merely a worker free from occupational poisoning or injury. The importance of this has become increasingly recognized as studies of sickness absenteeism in the United States have shown that, on the average, only about five or six percent of sickness absenteeism can be traced directly to conditions arising from work.[15] The overwhelming bulk of illness relates to nonoccupational causes. Its reduction, therefore, not to mention the achievement of health, calls for a generalized health program, such as can be promoted by the community public health agency. This concept was stated clearly several years ago by Bloomfield:

> It would seem, therefore, that if we are to improve the general health status of the most important and numerous group in our population, it will be necessary to control not only unhealthful conditions in the working environment, but also to give consideration to such factors as proper living conditions, nutrition, elimination of strain and hurry, communicable diseases—in fact, a general adult health program for all workers. In order to promote a broad and effective industrial health program of this type, it will be necessary to integrate it closely with existing public health activities.[16]

Under the wing of the public health agency, industrial health responsibilities of government in America are increasingly taking the form of an "adult health service." The factory is being used as a channel through which general public health programs are promoted, very much as the schools are a channel for protection of the general health of children. Services are rendered for workers in the control of tuberculosis and venereal disease, immunization against infectious diseases, nutrition, general health education, detection of chronic disorders, environmental sanitation, mental hygiene, dental care, maternal and child health, and medical rehabilitation. Beyond this, industry is encouraged to develop systematic in-plant services.[17] Not that this ideal integration is achieved everywhere, but this is the direction for which the framework has been laid. Health departments still have a long way to go in persuading industry to provide regular in-plant health service programs, especially in small plants.[18]

As might be expected, there has been some dispute between labor and public health agencies in the United States, particularly in the investigation of environmental hazards contributing to occupational diseases. The agreement, in general, however, has been for the factory inspection services to concentrate mainly on accident prevention, while the public health industrial hygiene units deal with the risks of occupational disease and the promotion of general preventive medical services in the plants. When legal action must be taken to enforce correction of an environmental hazard, it is usually, though not always, handled by the labor department. In some states, like California, very close working relationships have developed between the labor and health agencies, under which each not only respects the jurisdiction of the other, but also agrees actively to advance the program of the other by consultation and by referring problems to each other.[19]

In Canada, essentially the same pattern is found as in the United States, with even more authority for the protection of workers against unhygienic working conditions vested in provincial departments of public health.[20] Factory inspection is conducted by the provincial departments of labor or their counterparts, but regulations regarding specific industrial health hazards, including compulsory periodic medical examinations, are issued by provincial ministers of health. In the Dominion Ministry of National Health and Welfare and in each provincial department of health, there are industrial hygiene divisions which investigate occupational health problems and actively promote the organization of general health services at working places.

SOUTH AMERICA

Industrialization in South America is relatively recent and legislation protecting labor did not begin to be passed until well into the twentieth century. The dominant pattern originally was exclusive responsibility for industrial health service in the national labor agencies following the patterns of European nations (Spain, Portugal, and France) with which Latin America was culturally tied. With the "good neighbor" policy of President Roosevelt, the influence of the United States grew, and since about 1940 increasing responsibility for occupational health administration has been assigned to the public health authorities.

In Brazil, the Ministry of Labor, Industry, and Commerce has a Division of Industrial Hygiene and Safety, which engages some twenty-five physicians. These men investigate occupational health hazards, and they also perform medical examinations of workers in certain plants. Owners of large plants (over 500 workers) in isolated places are obliged by law to provide their own medical staff for emergency medical care. The National Department of Health in Brazil has had no official responsibilities in occupational health, except that its training institute includes a three-month course for doctors in industrial hygiene. Plans are underway, however, to organize an industrial health unit in the National Department of Health which would emphasize preventive services.[21]

The Argentine, the second largest country in South America, places a great deal of responsibility for occupational health in its health agencies. The Ministry of Public Health has an Office of Industrial Medicine which advises employers and trade unions on industrial health problems.[22] Physicians in this office also examine workers to determine the degree of disability of industrial injuries, a task done on behalf of the National Social Welfare Institute which administers the social security program. The Ministry of Labor has a Bureau of Occupational Hygiene and Safety which, on the request of trade unions, investigates hazardous conditions and can compel correction, but it does not carry out routine or systematic factory inspection. The Health Ministry's Office of Industrial Medicine also conducts such surveys and advises employers generally on hygienic practices. In addition, it offers training courses for physicians and engineers in occupational health. At the provincial level, little is done in governmental industrial hygiene, except in Santa Fe province where the Health Department contains an active division of Occupational Hygiene and Safety.

The dispersion of authorities for various aspects of industrial hygiene among different ministries is a feature of several countries in South America. The situation in Chile has been summarized by Bloomfield.

> The Ministry of Labour has the right to maintain an Industrial Hygiene Section within its Department of Labour, while the Ministry of Health has authorization for a Department of Industrial Hygiene in the National Department of Health. The Bureau of Labour Accidents is empowered to carry on an advisory industrial hygiene and safety programme among its insured. The Worker's Compulsory Insurance Fund, through its Institute of Labour Medicine, also functions in this field. The Department of Mines and Petroleum has responsibility for the health and safety of workers in mining and allied industries. And, finally, even the municipalities have broad authority in many phases of industrial hygiene.[23]

This dispersion of responsibilities is, above all, a sign of influences to broaden the scope of occupational health service. In the 1930s many social welfare measures were introduced in Chile. As a feature of its social security program, Chile was among the first nations to require a periodic medical examination of all workers, under the "Preventive Medicine Law" of 1938. These examinations are designed mainly to detect tuberculosis, syphilis, and heart disease and, while they are administered by the social security authorities, they obviously advance the occupational health program. In 1952, Chile enacted one of the most significant health laws not only in South America but in the world, its Medical Fusion Act. This sets up a National Health Service in which all governmental health services, including industrial hygiene and the medical provisions of social security, are brought under the unified direction of the Ministry of Health. They are to be administered regionally by public health officers, who will be responsible for all categories of health service in their regions.

Predominant responsibility for supervising industrial hygiene in Mexico, Peru, Bolivia, and Colombia has rested with the ministries of labor, but under the influence of the health program of the Institute of Inter-American Affairs changes are occurring. The primary emphasis of labor agency administration has often been to assure first aid and medical care following injury, rather than the provision of general preventive health services. Administration of the social security laws providing disability payments, and especially compensation for industrial injuries, have occupied major attention. The cooperative *Servicios* developed between the ministries of health and the Institute of Inter-American Affairs (I.I.A.A.), however, have begun to organize industrial hygiene divisions with a broad orientation. These divisions, which will eventually be absorbed in the health ministries, promote activities for the prevention of both accidents and occupational diseases, as well as general programs of tuberculosis and venereal disease control, nutrition, immunizations, health education, and general community sanitation in and around factories. Such activities have been expanding particularly in Peru and Colombia. They are in planning stages in Mexico and Venezuela. In Bolivia, similar programs are being developed by the I.I.A.A. even with the Ministry of Labor.[24]

In South America, as elsewhere, the most advanced work is often done by private industry, especially in isolated areas where the law requires the employer to organize health services. In some of the isolated mines of the Andes there is no community organization whatever for health purposes except that which the company can provide.[25] In this type of situation, occupational health service becomes synonymous with total public health and medical care. There is always a danger of paternalism in activities of this type in the "company town," which the workers dislike. In order to avoid this tendency and to win the support of the workers, the law in Brazil and Mexico requires formation of joint labor-management committees on safety and health. Encouragement of such committees is the policy of the Institute of Inter-American Affairs.

On the whole in South America, there is a distinct tendency toward increasing participation of public health agencies in the supervision of the health of workers. With this trend, there is a broadening of the scope of an industrial health service from concentration on accident prevention and treatment of compensatable disabilities toward an overall preventive health service, complemented by medical care for general illness.

SOUTHERN ASIA AND AFRICA

In Egypt a law was passed in 1904 requiring permits for the opening of "objectionable, unhealthy, and dangerous establishments." It was administered by a Department of Permits with a large staff of inspectors for investigating the physical aspects of all industrial installations. This department was placed in various ministries at different times, and in 1948, as the country's public health program was gaining strength, it was incorporated into the Ministry of Health. In 1939, a Ministry of Social Affairs was established and within it a Department of Labor. In 1944 this department was given responsibility for routine inspection of factories to detect health hazards. Recently it engaged three full-time doctors and a small staff of sanitary inspectors in order to develop a program to prevent occupational disease. Meanwhile the Department of Permits in the health ministry, with a much larger field staff, does similar work.[26]

As in most economically underdeveloped countries, the great problem in Egypt is the hygienic conditions in thousands of very small shops. Employers of 100 workers or more are required to provide first aid and minor medical services at the plant, a responsibility usually dispatched by maintenance of a small dispensary staffed by a male attendant with occasional visits by a physician. To supervise health conditions in the small shops, however, a large field staff is required, keeping in close touch with rapidly changing situations. The public health staff of some 700 physicians, engineers, and sanitary inspectors distributed in regional teams throughout Egypt could provide a skeletal framework for doing this task, if some special training were provided and skilled consultant services were available. Industrial accident rates are high, but by far the greatest health problems of the Egyptian worker are the endemic diseases arising from his total living environment—problems for the public health authorities.

In the other Arab countries, governmental activity in industrial hygiene is extremely limited. In Iran, for example, there are labor laws regarding child labor, hours of work, preemployment medical examinations, working conditions, etc., administered by the Ministry of Labor, but they are not well enforced. The Ministry of Health has been developing interest in the field, as reflected by a recent request for advice from this ministry to the World Health Organization for technical assistance in the formulation of an occupational health program. Actually the most effective supervision at the present time is given by a semiautonomous insurance society, the Worker's Fund. Under the influence of this agency, which handles social security activities, the larger industries provide a limited dispensary service for first aid and minor medical care, usually given by a medical aide.[27]

A somewhat similar situation is found in Turkey, where the most effective controls over health services in industry are rendered by an independent insurance fund, the Worker's Insurance Institute. Legislation in Turkey, since 1930, actually calls upon the Ministry of Health to inspect work places for hygienic conditions and to enforce certain standards. Among these is the requirement that employers of 100 workers or more provide certain in-plant medical services, and that in plants of over 500 workers hospital beds be provided. Turkey is so predominantly agricultural, however, and the limited resources of the public health authorities had to be spread so thinly over vast rural regions, that little attention could be given to the health problems of industry. In 1941, regulations on hygienic conditions in factories were issued by the Ministry of Health and the Ministry of Economics, but enforcement was meager. Then in 1946 an act was passed providing compensation for industrial accidents and occupational diseases, and giving maternity leave. This was made the responsibility of a newly organized Worker's Insurance Institute, under the general supervision of the Ministry of Labor which had been set up in 1945. The Institute collects insurance funds and exercises considerable authority over health conditions in factories and mines with insured workers. Employers who pay insurance premiums are exempted from providing the medical facilities required under the 1930 law, since the Worker's Insurance Institute is now supposed to provide these services instead.[28] A factory inspection system was also recently established under the Ministry of Labor.

The establishment of independent institutes, with power to collect money and to spend it, is a common approach to achieving stability for a welfare program in countries where government is subject to rapidly changing fortunes. This device has the effect, however, of setting up a state within a state, and possibly weakening the hand of government by depriving it of funds and responsibilities. As industrialization develops in Turkey, the workers in the cities are becoming unionized and make increasing demands for welfare services. These demands are surely sound, but the way that government responds to them, in these relatively early stages of industrialization, will shape the pattern of all health administration in years ahead.

In the colonial countries of Africa, little is done by government in occupational health supervision which is equivalent to the practices in industrialized countries. The private plantations or estates may, however, provide medical services for their workers and follow basic hygienic practices on housing, sanitation, etc., in fulfillment of the requirements of government charters. Regulations on hygienic standards in labor camps may be issued by the medical directorate, as in Nigeria.[29] Occasional surveys of the health of workers may be made by the health authorities, like the x-ray studies for silicosis in the mines of the Belgian Congo.[30] Factory inspectorates do not exist and any inspection is a responsibility of the medical department in the colonial government.

In the Union of South Africa factory inspection is organized under the Ministry of Labor and the public health agencies have few responsibilities in the industrial sphere.[31] In India there is likewise a factory inspectorate under the Ministry of Labour, but, by force of circumstances, the public health authorities have become involved in the supervision of hygienic conditions in plants.

There is a great shortage of factory inspectors in India and working conditions in some industries are primitive. There is a medical inspector of factories in the Ministry of Labour at New Delhi, but in most provinces the practice has developed of appointing the public health officers as "ex officio factory inspectors" giving them the right to enter plants and to recommend to the chief inspector of factories the enforcement of corrective measures. The regular factory inspectors look to the health officer for guidance and assistance on hygienic questions. It is interesting to observe that this arrangement did not appeal to a foreign industrial medicine authority whose advice was sought in 1946. The Annual Report of the Public Health Commissioner with the Government of India states that this consultant:

> has questioned whether the medical inspection of the factories should be left in the hands of public health officers or whether it should be done by medical men serving under the Chief Inspector of Factories, as in Great Britain. The Committee adopted a note on the desirability of instituting a Medical Inspectorate of Mines and Factories in India.[32]

This illustrates well the influence of the older nations, in spite of the efforts of more recently industrialized countries to adjust administrative patterns to local resources and needs.

Some large establishments in India, like the Tata Industries, have set up their own occupational health and medical care programs which go beyond the requirements of law. As elsewhere in the world, such enlightened managements have advanced the general recognition of needs for occupational health services.[33] The training of medical specialists is being met in some degree by courses at the All-India Institute of Hygiene and Tropical Medicine, under the Ministry of Health. It is significant perhaps that in many countries, where administrative responsibilities rest with labor authorities, training in occupational health is offered by the health authorities. If nothing else, this would indicate the basic identity of industrial medicine with the other fields of social medicine and public health, for which health ministries are responsible.

WESTERN PACIFIC REGION

The industrialization of Japan since 1860 has been associated with the development of a factory inspection system in the Ministry of Labor. The public health authorities have confined their activities to the control of communicable diseases, environmental sanitation, and other traditional spheres. A remarkable network of over 700 health centers for general preventive services has been developed in Japan in the last few years, but their functions do not, as yet, include health supervision of work places.[34] In 1947, Japan enacted a law requiring preemployment medical examinations of all workers, reflecting a broadening approach to occupational health.

In Australia, industrial hygiene has been developed as a function of the public health agencies. Health services are organized under each of the six state governments, and each state health department contains a division of industrial hygiene. There is also a factory inspection system under the state departments of labor, to which the industrial hygiene divisions are advisory on technical health questions. In addition, these divisions conduct industrial health surveys, give direct advice to industry on the correction of hazards, operate clinics for occupational diseases, and promote the organization of generalized in-plant health services. At the Commonwealth level, in the School of Public Health at the University of Sydney, there is an Industrial Hygiene Unit, with training, research, and advisory functions. In Queensland, the Department of Health and Home Affairs is responsible for overall factory inspection as well as technical services in industrial hygiene.[35]

The governmental pattern in New Zealand is similar. Factory inspection and enforcement of standards are carried out under the Department of Labour and Employment, but the health aspects of industry are supervised by the Department of Health. There are four regional medical officers for industrial hygiene, who advise on health hazards and promote medical service organization in the plants. They are assisted by nurses, who help to set up industrial nursing programs. The regional staff work closely with the factory inspectorate, the local public health officers, and the part-time industrial physicians. They also conduct research into toxic processes, and they train physicians and sanitary inspectors in occupational health.[36]

Practices in Indonesia illustrate the approach to occupational health of a nation which has been overwhelmingly agricultural and has only recently gained its independence in governmental affairs. Faced with enormous problems of disease and with dire lack of medical personnel and facilities, the new government is setting out to develop an integrated health service, based on health centers from which both preventive and curative services are given. Among the functions of the public health staff at all levels is the supervision of factory hygiene. Leimana regards this as a component part of the sanitary control of the environment.[37] Substantially the same practice is followed in the Philippine Republic where sanitary inspection of factories and advice on the correction of occupational disease hazards is a function of the Department of Health.[38]

The Hawaiian Islands, being a territory of the United States, naturally adopt the American pattern of having an Industrial Hygiene Division in the Board of Health. This division investigates occupational disease hazards and advises on their correction; it receives reports of cases of occupational disease coming before the Workmen's Compensation Division, a practice carried out in many American states. Hawaii is primarily agricultural and a dominant feature of the economy is the large sugar or pineapple plantation. For many years, workers and their families on these plantations have received medical care through a system of salaried physicians and nurses giving complete services, preventive and curative. Since these enterprises have been unionized, the medical programs, formerly operated entirely by management, are now jointly controlled through collective bargaining.[39,40]

In colonial or formerly colonial countries generally, plantation medical systems are a major source of health service, preventive and curative, for the agricultural population. It is customary for these programs to come under some surveillance from the ministry of health, especially when the law requires that growers provide certain minimum services. This is so in countries like Ceylon or Malaya with their large tea or rubber estates. The health problems of agricultural production are, of course, very different from those in factories, but these programs are, nevertheless, providing occupational health services in a rural setting. Supervision by public health authorities permits the country-wide application of uniform standards, which are especially important for the control of communicable diseases in tropical areas.

NORTHERN ASIA AND EASTERN EUROPE

An important event in the development of health services in the Union of Soviet Socialist Republics was the institution of a complete system of public medical services. Health protection of workers is a function of the Ministry or Commissariat of Health, carried out as part of the general system of state-supervised curative and preventive services.

Since 1933 the Commissariat of Health has contained an Office of Safety and Hygiene responsible for factory inspection. Engineers are in charge of this work, checking on all new installations and enforcing standards of ventilation, lighting, and so on. This environmental control is coordinated with the system of industrial medical services by the regional public health officer. In all plants there is a medical clinic of some type, connected administratively with the regional system of polyclinics and hospitals for the general population. When a plant has 1,000 workers or more, one or more full-time physicians are employed; for smaller plants a nurse is engaged. Any medical care needed is given within the resources of the clinic, whether the illness is of occupational origin or not; where necessary the patient is referred to a regional health center or hospital. Since the whole system is supervised by the public health officer, general preventive services are applied to the workers through the factory. The entire medical and safety system is controlled, within each plant containing fifty workers or more, by a committee for protection of work, representing the workers. Problems of occupational disease are tackled through research and consultant service given by a network of some forty institutes of labor hygiene, under the national public health system.[41,42]

The countries of Eastern Europe, coming under the same social system have gradually adopted a similar framework for protecting the health of workers. In 1951, Czechoslovakia reorganized all its health services, formerly dispersed among several governmental and voluntary agencies, under the Ministry of Health. In Yugoslavia, the unified pattern is substantially followed. Each of the component republics has a department of health in which one or more physicians serve as "sanitary inspectors for industrial hygiene." There are also labor inspectors who enforce the general welfare provisions in industry, but the public health authorities are responsible for the prevention of occupational diseases, special supervision of apprentices and women workers, and surveillance over medical services in the plants. The workers receive all types of medical care through the factory clinics or *ambulanta* which are financed by the government as part of the general public medical system. A large factory will have its own clinic, while a group of small factories may be served jointly by one. These clinics provide preemployment examinations and other preventive work, but they have not yet developed skills at job placement evaluations. Extra services like dental care, not provided in the state program, may be given at the initiative and expense of the individual factory.[43]

In China, since 1949, there has been an intensification of health services for industrial workers. Previously, all health questions relating to industry were the responsibility of labor authorities. Today each industry is required to provide certain health services for the workers, according to standards set by the Ministry of Health. General medical services for all conditions are given through the plant clinic.[44]

SUMMARY

While this review of the structure of governmental activities in occupational health throughout the world is by no means complete, it may be adequate to demonstrate that widely differing patterns are found, and that the system commonplace in Western Europe is by no means universal. Such a statement could not have been made before about 1930, but in the last twenty-five years a marked change has occurred in the scope and objectives of occupational health work. In Western Europe, where a century of experience has crystallized certain patterns of public administration rather rigidly, this broadening viewpoint has expressed itself differently from other countries, where the whole structure of social services has been more fluid.

The focus of labor authorities on the prevention of occupational diseases and industrial accidents has played an invaluable role historically, but it fails to meet current needs. The restrictions of this focus, in relation to total sickness absenteeism, have been mentioned. Further deficiencies are illustrated in the customary requirements for notification of occupational diseases under labor regulations. Such notification is usually tied to the requirements of workmen's compensation legislation, which tend to lag considerably behind the changing hazards of modern industry. From the health viewpoint, any ailment that is conceivably related to working condi-

tions, and hence preventable, should be notifiable. Again, the limitation of preemployment examinations in so many labor codes to young persons and workers exposed to special risks may satisfy certain welfare conceptions, but it fails to recognize that the prevalence of serious, chronic disease—while not compensatable—is progressively greater in the older worker.

The broadening viewpoint in occupational health can be simply described. It has become increasingly recognized that the protection of the worker's health, both for his sake personally and for the sake of economic productivity, requires concern for his total health and for his physical and mental adaptability to his job. This is a great extension beyond the earlier objectives of avoiding occupational diseases and accidents. The latter purposes remain important and, indeed, call for the application of a vast body of technical knowledge but—considering the total health needs of the worker—they encompass only a small fraction of the problem. The size of this fraction will, of course, vary in different industries and in different countries. Mining in siliceous rock, in a country where preventive measures for the control of silicosis are inadequate, will obviously yield a higher proportionate burden of occupational disease and injury than work in a country where vigorous preventive measures are being enforced or in an industry with fewer inherent hazards. Taking industry as a whole, however, it has probably always been true that purely occupational disease and accident constitute only a minority fraction of the worker's burden of ill health, albeit a preventable fraction. As preventive measures are instituted this fraciton obviously becomes smaller, so that in the economically advanced countries—despite the increased exposure of man to chemicals and machines—the fraction of human disability caused by direct occupational influences drops to only one-tenth or one-twentieth of the total.

The occupational hygienist of the old school, one might say, has been working himself out of a job, in the same way as does the tropical hygienist who has wiped out malaria. But a job remains, if he widens his horizon to encompass the general health needs of the worker. In practical terms, this widening has occurred in stages. A first stage is related to the attainment of industrial efficiency, and a second stage to the achievement of general community health and well-being. In the former stage, the preemployment and then the preplacement medical examination are introduced. An effort is made to fit the worker to the job and, likewise, through environmental controls, to fit the job to the worker. In the latter stage, the above activities remain but, in addition, the factory is regarded as one phase of community life through which measures of value to general health may be applied. These measures may, indeed, advance productivity, but even if they do not do this directly, they are justified as means to improved community health.

We have seen how this broadening horizon has been expressed in Western Europe through gradual extension of the scope of laws governing factory inspection, through the organization of voluntary societies for promotion of better in-plant medical services, and through the direct initiative of enlightened employers. The preemployment medical examination and the periodic reexamination have become widely accepted as desirable. A special influence has been exerted by government beyond its supervisory role when government has become employer. Thus, in the nationalized industries of Great Britain, France, and other countries, particularly comprehensive occupational health programs have been organized. The trend has been reflected in the work of the various research institutes in occupational health like those in Finland and Yugoslavia, where investigations are made in "industrial physiology," to determine the optimal conditions (human and environmental) for working efficiency.

The trend is also shown in the activities of international bodies. The scope of the conventions and recommendations of the International Labour Organization has significantly changed over the last thirty years. The earlier actions were devoted to promoting protective measures in particular trades or in the use of particular chemicals, like lead or phosphorus. The ILO obviously reflected the interests of national ministries of labor. The more recent actions have concerned general medical examination of young persons, general labor inspection, and the safeguarding of maternity.[45] Under consideration now is a new proposed convention on "Protection of the Health of Workers in Places of Employment." While this instrument does not go so far as to call for the establishment of medical services and general preventive measures in plants, it calls for a wide range of preventive medical examinations. In the World Health Organization, organized in 1948, concern for occupational health has been directed toward aspects other than occupational diseases and injuries.[46]

In other continents the broadening objectives of occupational health work have taken the forms found in Western Europe but, in addition, they have found another expression. This has been the increasing tendency to consider the health protection of workers as a branch of general public health work under the direct supervision of the overall public health agency. This change has served to direct attention not only to the task of eliminating occupational hazards, but to promote the general health of workers through the convenient approach of the factory—just as the child's health is promoted through the school. This shifting of official responsibility, as we have seen, is found on every continent in greater or lesser degree.

It cannot be claimed that public health agency administration of occupational health inevitably means this broad approach. In some measure the trend may be due to other reasons, such as the fact that the health ministries are the major resources for skilled personnel in social medicine. In certain instances public health administration may for the moment yield a program no wider in scope than traditional factory inspection. What is important, however, is that public health administration provides the natural framework for a broader approach—one in which it will easily grow—since the public health agency is, by definition, devoted to advancing the total health of the community. It is less likely to have its aims limited by considerations of injury compensation laws or even the needs of productive efficiency.

CONCLUSIONS AND DISCUSSION

Developments in social medicine come in response to social needs, but the development of occupational health within public health administration can help to meet needs beyond those that have provided the immediate stimulus. One of the most pressing needs in modern public health is the development of preventive programs for the adult population, other than maternity services. As communicable diseases are reduced, especially in childhood, the larger disease problems faced by a society tend to become the chronic, degenerative disorders of adult life: cardiovascular disease, cancer, diabetes, and arthritis, as well as mental disorders. It is difficult to tackle these afflictions on a public health basis, but one of the best approaches currently available is through assurance of early diagnosis and prompt treatment. Multiple screening tests given through the place of work are an important method of early diagnosis, and arrangements for prompt treatment can be made through an industrial medical care program. Insofar as nutrition or personal living habits may provide a key to the prevention of arteriosclerosis, hypertension, or other chronic diseases, health education through the factory may be effective. In a word, the work place can be an excellent locale for the promotion of an adult health service, both preventive and curative.

It is also important to consider the administrative relationship of occupational health and of general community health administration. The individual with his family is the common denominator to all health services, but a full understanding of their problems calls for knowledge from many different sources, and effective action requires authority in many spheres. For these reasons, sound application of both preventive and curative health services demands coordination of many different organized programs at the local level. The local public health officer is the obvious instrument for such coordination, but this is possible for the employed adult only if this officer has authority within the walls of the work place. The need for unified health administration at the local level has become increasingly recognized by public health leaders throughout the world.[47] It is undoubtedly at the root of the current debates on occupational health administration in relation to the National Health Service in Great Britain. In the underdeveloped countries, even less can the economies support the extravagance of overlapping or uncoordinated medical-social administration.

It should be stressed that coordination of occupational health and public health services at the local level does not necessarily imply a change in authority at the national level. A ministry of education or ministry of commerce may and does delegate certain authorities to the local public health officer, and there is no reason why a ministry of labor cannot do the same thing.

In most countries the control of nuisances created in the community by industry, through river or atmospheric pollution, rests with the public health authorities, even when control of the internal factory environment lies with the labor authorities. In urban life, this problem can take on large proportions, and it should be more effectively handled if the agency responsible for general community sanitation has free access to the interiors of factories.

All countries possess, or are developing, a network of local health administrations to cover their entire population. These local health departments are close to the people, working with community groups on all questions affecting health. They are in an excellent position to keep in touch with local industries in their area—not on the infrequent basis that is inevitable when a national ministry has only a handful of medical inspectors of factories distributed regionally over a large area, but frequently and regularly. In other words, the local health department can provide the community "family doctor" in close contact with the work place, to be aided by the specialist or consultant at the regional or national level when difficult technical problems arise.

This approach has special value in underde-

veloped countries where the preponderance of employment is in agriculture or in small shops. The organization of small-plant occupational health services on a cooperative basis is widely recognized as the solution to a difficult problem, and the local public health staff is admirably suited to organize such services. Not that the health officer or public health nurse could render the direct clinical services required in the plants—a point on which there is sometimes misinterpretation—but they could promote and organize such programs. The practicability of this idea has been demonstrated in several communities in the United States and New Zealand, although the need is doubtless greater in less prosperous countries.

Finally, one may ask how much therapeutic medicine should properly be provided in a health program centered at the place of work? Obviously the answer will differ in different social systems, depending on the overall national arrangement for medical care. Where most medical service is procured through independent physicians—either paid privately as in America or by insurance as in Western Europe—the tendency is for in-plant health services to be limited to prevention and care of minor illnesses, while most therapy is left to the personal physician. In societies where most medical services are rendered through a public system—as in the communist nations and in many underdeveloped and formerly colonial countries—complete medical services are often rendered through the enterprise (factory or plantation). In either case, there is a need for coordination of preventive services and therapy, if only in the interests of economy for the latter. Social security systems have recognized this need, through their efforts to promote industrial safety and hygiene programs in most European countries. Likewise, when the health ministry has responsibility for administration of medical care programs, its officers have a natural incentive to promote preventive health services in industry, and they have the opportunity to coordinate preventive and curative services.

If trends toward the organization of public medical services continue throughout the world, we may reach a time when most medical care will be given through health centers in each community. If this is done, such centers should be closely associated with all factories and work places, having on their staffs physicians and nurses who would be seconded to industry to provide preventive medical services and on-the-spot care in the plants. The latter services might be financed by the industry or by the government, depending on the general economic system. The important point is that the *services* should be coordinated, so that the physician and nurse, seeing the worker in the plant, would be in close professional touch with the physician in the health center who treats him when he is sick. Similar coordination with the hospital is essential. Such comprehensive, integrated service for the worker and his family would only be possible if all community health services—preventive, occupational, hospital, curative care of the ambulant patient—are administered under a single direction. The public health team of today is trained in the skills of health administration, preventive medicine, environmental control, and social organization, which are applicable within the factory walls as well as outside them.

There is no intention here to minimize the importance of the classical activities of industrial hygiene, designed to limit the wastage caused by industrial accidents and occupational diseases. In many underdeveloped countries, which have hardly yet come to recognize their own industrial hazards, this is an important priority. While they are being tackled, however, the whole picture of the worker's health can be kept in mind. One should also keep in mind the need for integration of specialized services in total community health organization.

The necessity of factory inspection remains for various aspects of work which go beyond the strict sphere of health maintenance, such as legislation controlling the employment of children and women, night work, and rest periods. Likewise the general physical arrangements of production processes are important, not only for the sake of accident prevention, but also for the general comfort and morale of the worker. In some countries, the jurisdictional line between the functions of labor and health agencies has been drawn on this basis, with the labor inspectorate covering safety while the health agency covers all other aspects of health. Enforcement of standards in both spheres, however, may be vested with the labor authority.

The labor ministry may claim that there is an advantage in encompassing the problems of the "whole worker"—his wages, hours, working conditions, collective bargaining, as well as his health. The same argument has been made about the "whole child" or the "whole farmer" or the "whole military veteran"—leading to the establishment of independent, vertical health programs for the child, the farmer, or the veteran. It is these demographic groups themselves who suffer most by isolation from the mainstream of skilled professional service and community health activity. Modern medicine and public health are exacting disciplines, requiring special training and skill. Any nation, or certainly any local community, can acheive the best results by

vesting responsibility for these services in a single health agency where the best professional talents are concentrated. In fact, by dispersing authorities, administrative funds are dispersed and it becomes more difficult to attract competent men and women to public health or social medicine.

In any event, energetic cooperation among all governmental authorities concerned with the health of people is essential. Exclusion of public health agencies in certain countries from the occupational health domain is not only due to laws and traditions and to a jealous guarding of prerogatives by labor authorities, but also to lack of initiative by public health agencies, failure to exploit opportunities, and rigid adherence to certain classical paths in public health. But, even without new legislation, there are numerous opportunities for health departments to render useful service to industry and to workers in epidemiological investigations, communicable disease control, sanitation, health education, and even in maternal and child health work.[48] Within existing legal frameworks, therefore, much can be improved, as was pointed out recently by the Joint Committee on Occupational Health of the International Labour Organization and the World Health Organization.[49] As experience in cooperation is gained, laws and practices may be changed to provide the administrative foundation for completing the evolution from factory inspection to adult health service.

NOTES

[1] L. Teleky, *History of Factory and Mine Hygiene.* New York: Columbia University Press, 1948, pp. 3-74.

[2] H. Natvig, "The Industrial Health Service in an Individual Country (Norway)." First European Seminar on Occupational Health, Leyden, Geneva: World Health Organization, 1952.

[3] World Health Organization, "Information on Occupational Health in Some European Countries (1952)." First European Seminar on Occupational Health, Leyden, Geneva: WHO, 1952.

[4] A. Bruusgaard. *Journal of the Irish Medical Association,* Vol. 30, 1972, p. 32.

[5] L. Noro. *Archives of Industrial Hygiene,* Vol. 4, 1952, p. 597.

[6] S. Forssman. *Archives of Industrial Hygiene,* Vol. 4, 1952, p. 597.

[7] I. R. Tabershaw. *Archives of Industrial Hygiene,* Vol. 3, p. 298.

[8] World Health Organization, "Public Health Services in Belgium (1951)." Geneva: Travelling Study Group on Public Health Administration in Europe, 1951.

[9] J. Bousser and J. J. Gillon. *International Labour Review,* Vol. 65, 1952, p. 184.

[10] G. A. Canaperia. *Scientia Medica Italica,* Vol. 1, 1950, p. 180.

[11] Dale Report, *Report of a Committee of Enquiry on*

Industrial Health Services, Cmd. 8170. London: H.M.S.O., 1951.

[12] I. G. Davies, R. S. F. Schilling, and A. L. Banks. *Journal of the Royal Sanitary Institute*, Vol. 72, 1952, pp. 528, 534, and 540.

[13] M. C. Klem, M. F. McKievar, and W. J. Lear, *Industrial Health and Medical Programs*. Public Health Service Publication No. 15., Washington, D.C.: Government Printing Office, 1950, pp. 321-344.

[14] V. M. Trasko, *Industrial Health Legislation: A Compilation of State Laws and Regulations*. Washington, D.C.: U.S. Public Health Service, 1950.

[15] M. N. Newquist, *Medical Service in Industry and Workmen's Compensation Laws*. Chicago: American College of Surgeons, 1938, pp. 32-33.

[16] J. J. Bloomfield. *American Journal of Public Health*, Vol. 28, 1938, p. 1,388.

[17] M. I. Roemer. *Industrial Hygiene Newsletter*, Vol. 8, No. 9, September 1948, p. 6.

[18] S. E. Miller, "Organization of Occupational Health Services in Small Plants." First European Seminar on Occupational Health, Leyden. Geneva: World Health Organization, 1952.

[19] California State Department of Health, "Plan of Integration and Definition of Responsibilities of the Department of Industrial Relations and of Public Health with Respect to the Health and Safety of Industrial Workers in California." 1952.

[20] International Labour Office, *Protection of the Health of Workers in Places of Employment*, Report VIII (1). Geneva: ILO, 1951, pp. 62-64.

[21] J. J. Bloomfield, *Industrial Hygiene Problems in Brazil*. Washington, D.C.: Institute of Inter-American Affairs, 1950.

[22] E. Escarra, *Occupational Health in Argentina*. Geneva: World Health Organization, 1952.

[23] J. J. Bloomfield, "Industrial Hygiene Problems in Bolivia, Peru and Chile." *Public Health Bulletin* (Washington, D.C.), No. 301, 1948, p. 74.

[24] J. J. Bloomfield, *Recent Developments in Industrial Hygiene in Latin America*. Geneva: World Health Organization, 1952.

[25] J. T. Diaz. *Medical Bulletin*, (New York), Vol. 11, 1951, p. 178.

[26] A. Bruusgaard, *Occupational Health Survey of Egypt*. Geneva: World Health Organization, 1952.

[27] L. Lewis, *Report on Preliminary Industrial Health Survey of Iran*. Geneva: World Health Organization, 1952.

[28] L. M. Petrie, *Health Problems of Industrially Employed People in Turkey*. Geneva: World Health Organization, 1952.

[29] Nigeria: Department of Medical Services, *Annual Report of the Medical Services for the Year 1948*. Lagos: Government Printer, 1950.

[30] Belgian Congo, Direction Générale des Services Médicaux, *Rapport Annuel*. 1950.

[31] E. H. Cluver, *Public Health in South Africa*, fifth edition. South Africa: Central News Agency, 1948, pp. 337-349.

[32] "Annual Report of the Public Health Commissioner with the Government of India for 1946." New Delhi: Government of India Press, p. 54.

[33] H. P. Dastur, *Industrial Health Service in India*. Geneva: World Health Organization, 1952.

[34] Japanese Ministry of Health and Welfare, *A Brief Report on Public Health Administration in Japan*. 1952.

[35] C. J. Cummings, G. Smith, and J. C. G. Hadley, *Public Health* (London), Vol. 66, 1952, p. 21.

[36] J. Brown. *Journal for Industrial Nurses* (Manchester), Vol. 2, 1950, p. 188.

[37] J. Leimana, *The Upbuilding of Public Health in Indonesia*. Indonesia: Ministry of Health, 1952.

[38] Philippine Republic, Department of Health, *Annual Report of the Secretary of Health 1950-51*. Manila: 1952.

[39] H. Doyle. Reported in *Industrial Health Monthly*, (Washington, D.C.), Vol. 11, 1951, p. 133.

[40] W. B. Patterson. *Industrial Medicine and Surgery*, Vol. 19, 1950, p. 343.

[41] "La Prévention des Accidents et la Protection de la Santé des Travailleurs en U.R.S.S." *Travail et Securité*, (Paris), Vol. 2, 1950, p. 159.

[42] H. E. Sigerist, *Medicine and Health in the Soviet Union*. New York: Citadel Press, 1947.

[43] L. J. Goldwater, *Industrial Hygiene and Occupational Medicine in Yugoslavia*. Geneva: World Health Organization, 1952.

[44] C. K. Chu. Personal communication, 1952.

[45] H. A. De Boer, *Trends in Occupational Health Legislation*. Geneva: World Health Organization, 1952.

[46] M. I. Roemer and O. L. Da Costa. *Archives of Industrial Hygiene*, Vol. 7, 1953, p. 111.

[47] J. M. Mackintosh. *Chronicle of the World Health Organization*, Vol. 6, 1952, pp. 180, 219.

[48] H. K. Abrams. *Occupational Health*, Vol. 12, 1952, p. 23.

[49] World Health Organization, Joint Committee on Occupational Health of the International Labour Organization and the World Health Organization, "Report of Second Session (1953)." Geneva: World Health Organization, 1953.

Chapter XIX
Work Injury Benefits in Relation to National Health Insurance Systems

In most countries applying social insurance principles, protection of workers against the economic and health effects of work-connected injuries has antedated the development of insurance programs for meeting the costs of general illness or disability. Thus, when general health insurance has been established, problems tend to arise on how the older program of workmen's compensation for industrial injuries should articulate with it.

It appears that five different forms of administrative relationship between these two types of social insurance program can be identified. These are briefly discussed in this chapter, as illustrated in the practices applied in fourteen countries. This chapter was published as "Workmen's Compensation and National Health Insurance Programs Abroad" in the American Journal of Public Health *(Vol. 55, February 1965, pp. 209-214) and is reprinted here by permission.[1]*

When William F. Ogburn in 1922 propounded the theory of cultural lag as an explanation of the mechanism of social change, he used the development of workmen's compensation laws in the United States as the initial "case" on which to test his hypothesis. He found a lag of roughly fifty years, between about 1860 and 1910, from the time that work injuries had become a massive and serious problem to the time that social adaptations were made in the form of state workmen's compensation laws.[2]

This lag had also occurred in Europe, where the first workmen's compensation law for cash disability benefits and for medical care in work-connected injuries had been enacted in Germany in 1884. Significant industrialization and a major toll of work accidents and deaths had, of course, prevailed for many years before that date. By 1905, however, every Western European country, except Spain and Portugal, had passed similar laws, and in the next forty years (that is, to about the end of World War II), practically every country in the world with some degree of industrialization followed suit. The an-

thropologist's "cultural diffusion" obviously applies not only to water jugs and wooden plows, but also to forms of social organization such as medical care programs. Indeed, some of this diffusion has been so rapid that today many economically underdeveloped countries, with only embryonic industrial activity and little in the way of medical resources for the general population, already have legislation for work injury compensation on the books.

Strangely enough, we seem to have come to a time, on the world level, when organized medical services for work injuries and, to a lesser extent, occupational diseases have become rather highly developed, and the prominent cultural lag applies to all the rest of medical care needs. Not that medical care programs under workmen's compensation are everywhere adequate, but relative to the care of nonoccupational illness, they tend to be a top priority service. Whatever may be the deficiencies in the general medical care of populations, special provisions are usually made to assure that the worker, injured on the job, receives necessary medical treatment and often rehabilitation.

This high priority status for work injury medical care programs almost everywhere in the world poses a key question, namely, what is the relation between workmen's compensation medical services and the provision of national health insurance programs in various countries?

Surveying the world scene, one can detect a complex variety of relationships in this field. There seem to be five levels of relationships, depending on the nature of the workmen's compensation program, on the one hand, and the structure of general health insurance provisions, on the other. We could not hope to review all nations of the world in this paper, but I have selected fourteen for brief consideration, because they represent the principal types of relationships. In the following analysis, one should keep in mind that we are discussing the medical care provisions, and not the cash compensation benefits, of work injury legislation.[3]

SEPARATE AND PREDOMINANTLY PRIVATE ARRANGEMENTS

The United States, as we know, has autonomous state programs for medical care of work injuries, in which the insurance is carried mainly by commercial companies. Injured workers are treated in regular community hospitals by privately practicing physicians, and the costs are paid—to varying extents—by the insurance companies. Relationships to governmental health insurance programs are not a salient question because such programs do not exist to any significant degree. The temporary disability insurance programs in four states and the whole voluntary insurance movement bear certain indirect relationships to compensation medical care—oriented principally to avoiding duplication of benefits.

Brazil illustrates a country in which a great deal of general health insurance has developed under government for certain occupational groups, but where nonetheless medical care for work injury remains predominantly a separate private system. There are seven major programs of general health insurance, operated by governmentally chartered *institutos,* and offering medical care of varying scope to about 16,000,000 persons or twenty-five percent of the Brazilian population. Services are provided in general governmental or voluntary hospitals, as well as in special facilities operated by the *institutos* themselves.[4]

Medical care for work injuries, on the other hand, is a benefit of all employed persons in Brazil, including many not covered by the *instituto* programs. The insurance is carried predominantly by private insurance companies, although sometimes an *instituto* may be used. The necessary medical service is typically provided by private physicians in private hospitals, without any relation to the overall health insurance programs. While efforts have been made to integrate the work injury program with the general health insurance systems, resistance against this from insurance companies and from physicians—who receive special fees—has been effective.

SEPARATE ARRANGEMENTS WITHIN GOVERNMENT

Several countries have developed extensive programs of health insurance covering a major proportion of the national population, while side-by-side are separate governmental arrangements for medical care of work injuries. Even within this definition, however, there are variations.

In Canada, for example, there has evolved in the last five years a program of insurance for general hospital care, covering nearly the whole population, under federal-provincial agreements. Medical care for compensatable work injuries, however, is specifically excluded from benefits under these statutes, since it is covered by separate provincial laws. Government agencies, rather than commercial companies carry the insurance, and the medical care provided to injured workers is supervised by these agencies. In Ontario and several other provinces these agencies operate rehabilitation centers to handle the difficult cases after local resources have been exhausted.[5]

Chile is another country with a program of public medical care for a substantial proportion of its national population. The "National Health Service," as it is called, provides general medical care to about sixty percent of the people—if one takes an average of various estimates—through a network of government-operated hospitals and health centers. These facilities are generally crowded, however, and the quality of care rendered is often perfunctory. This program is administered through thirteen health zones, coming under the Ministry of Health.

Quite independent of the National Health Service (NHS) and supervised by the Ministry of Labor is the program of medical care for work injuries. The major responsible agency is the Work Accident Fund, which operates its own network of special traumatological hospitals. In addition, this fund supervises the medical care provided in company-owned industrial hospitals and in private hospitals for those workers who are insured through commercial insurance companies. The whole pattern is complicated, but it provides more generous care for work injury cases than is usually available for ordinary illness under the National Health Service. Possible unification between the NHS and workmen's compensation has been discussed, but at present the programs are independent of each other.

Another such pattern of separate programs for work injuries and general illness, both under the wing of government, is found in Japan. The general health insurance program in that country is very complex, involving two major systems coming under the direction of the National Ministry of Health and Welfare—one based on occupational categories and the other on place of residence. Both systems administer benefits through local insurance societies, which usually have contracts with private medical personnel and facilities but sometimes operate their own resources.

Entirely independent of these systems is the medical care program for work injuries, administered by the Ministry of Labor. Under this, each employer is directly responsible for the cost of medical care to an injured worker up to 1,000 yen, after which the national work injury insurance fund takes over. The care may be rendered by ordinary private personnel and facilities, reimbursed by the insurance fund, or it may be given in special governmental hospitals and dispensaries.

SEMIINTEGRATED PROGRAMS

Another pattern of relationships is found in countries of western continental Europe, where there is a unified health insurance system for general and occupational illness alike, but with a different scale of benefits for cases of work injury.

Thus, in France, the overall system of health insurance is administered by a network of local funds, coming under a hierachy of regional offices heading up in the National Ministry of Labor. Medical services are rendered by private physicians, paid by the patient, who is then reimbursed by his insurance fund at a rate up to about eighty percent of an approved fee schedule; hospitalization may be covered completely or not, depending on the income level of the patient.

For work injuries, the same administrative network is responsible and the same doctors and hospitals are used. The worker, however, is not required to advance the costs of care and seek reimbursement later; instead, the insurance fund makes payment directly to the doctor at a rate of 100 percent. There are no special personnel and facilities for work injuries and no balance of fees to be paid by the worker.

In Norway, substantially the same semiintegrated pattern prevails. Ordinary illness is insured through a network of local funds coming under the Ministry of Social Affairs. Out-of-hospital medical costs are covered on an indemnification basis, ranging from sixty to 100 percent of charges; hospital care is ordinarily fully financed by government. For work injuries, however, the protection is always at 100 percent of charges, for both physician and hospital services.

Israel illustrates a modification of this pattern with its large voluntary health insurance program that covers some ninety percent of industrial workers— the "Kupat Holim" or Sickness Fund of the National Labor Federation. Most general medical care of workers and their dependents is provided by the hospitals and polyclinics operated directly by this agency. These same personnel and facilities also provide care for work injuries. Insurance for work injuries is carried by a governmental unit, the National Insurance Institute, which pays cash benefits directly and simply reimburses the voluntary Sickness Fund for the costs of care to the work-related cases.

INTEGRATED PARTIAL COVERAGE PROGRAMS

Still other countries demonstrate a pattern in which general health insurance coverage of the population is rather limited, but within it the integration with work injury protection is complete. As the coverage of overall health insurance in these countries is extended, one may expect that the work injury program will move hand-in-hand with it.

Thus, in Mexico, the majority of industrial workers are provided general medical care through the *Instituto Mexicano de Seguro Social*, (IMSS), which operates a great network of its own hospitals and health centers. Persons covered by the IMSS and another similar agency constitute only about fourteen percent of the national population. The quantity and quality of medical care these persons receive, however, is undoubtedly higher than that received by the rest of the population. Within the program, moreover, medical and hospital care for work injuries is provided in exactly the same way as for other illness. The only special provision is an arrangement for subsidy of the IMSS by supplementary contributions of employers, designed to meet the costs of industrial injury compensation.

Similar arrangements prevail in various countries of Asia and Africa, where industrialization is relatively recent and where work injury compensation and general health insurance have been started at about the same time. In India, for example, the proportion of the national population encompassed under general health insurance (enacted only in 1948) is very small, probably under four percent. Insurance in effect only in selected regions, in defined occupations, in firms with over twenty employees, and for workers earning less than 400 rupees per month. Medical services are provided through special insurance facilities, general governmental facilities, or private resources that are reimbursed. Within the limitations of population coverage, however, the provision of medical care for work injuries is identical, and there is not even any subsidy of the program by special employer contributions, beyond those made for the care of general illness.

FULLY INTEGRATED
NATIONAL HEALTH PROGRAMS

Finally, we come to countries which have developed comprehensive national programs of medical care, covering virtually 100 percent of their populations, in which the care of work injuries is handled in exactly the same way as any other illness or accident.

Best known to American public health people is probably the British National Health Service, which since 1948 has provided almost complete medical care to every resident of the United Kingdom. Except for a small amount of cost sharing on drugs and certain prosthetic appliances, all services are publicly financed—about ninety percent through general revenues and ten percent through social insurance. Day-to-day general physician's care is given by doctors in their own offices, while specialist and hospital services are provided through regionalized hospital systems.[6]

For work injuries, the Ministry of Pensions and National Insurance collects contributions (from both employer and worker) and administers cash benefits. Necessary medical care, however, is given entirely through the National Health Service. There is no special subsidy to the Ministry of Health for these services. Within the National Health Service, there are indeed special facilities concentrating on the rehabilitation of injured workers, but these facilities are open to the worker injured on or off the job.

Another British Commonwealth country, New Zealand, developed a national health service with universal population coverage ten years before England and Wales. The benefits are not so extensive, but they are available to everyone whether or not he has paid a social insurance contribution. As in Britain, medical care for work injuries is provided under the national system. Only the cash benefits, which are insured through private commercial carriers, are separately administered. Necessary prosthetic appliances, not fully provided under the general health insurance program, are available without charge for the rehabilitation of the injured worker.

In the Soviet Union, general medical care is avail-

able to the whole population through a network of health stations, polyclinics, and hospitals staffed by salaried governmental personnel. The system is financed wholly by general revenues and, since the government is also the employer, there are no special "employer contributions." Cash benefits for work injuries are administered by trade union bodies, but all health services are controlled by the Ministry of Health. As part of the overall health service program, there is special emphasis on the care of industrial workers, with facilities for general medical care located at the factories and collective farms. The services of these units are available for the care of work-connected and ordinary illness alike.[7]

In Yugoslavia, the general medical care program is less well developed than in the Soviet Union, but there is also full integration between the work injury program and the rest of health service. While cash benefits are administered by a network of social insurance institutes, necessary medical care of work injuries is provided through the general system of polyclinics and hospitals, administered by the ministries of health in each of the six Yugoslavian republics.

While these accounts of work injury compensation and general health insurance programs in fourteen countries have been necessarily brief, they may be sufficient to indicate the variety of patterns found throughout the world. The work injury programs have usually antedated the general health insurance programs. Moreover, the concept of employer responsibility has led to special schemes of financing, in contrast to the broadly based support of care for general illness or injury. Another complicating factor is the frequent involvement of private commercial carriers in work injury insurance, in contrast to various nonprofit or public agencies handling general health insurance. Altogether, these elements may explain the separate administrative arrangements that prevail in many countries for the protection of workers against occupational versus other illness risks.

Nevertheless, we may note how in a number of countries there has evolved an integration—partial or complete—between the work injury program and the rest of the health service system. This integration appears to be most complete in those countries where the overall national medical care system is most comprehensively developed on a publicly financed basis. Where there is less than complete service in the general health insurance system, then the high social priority for medical care of work injuries seems to protect the independent administrative position of this program.

This is not to imply that all work injury medical

care programs are first-rate. On the contrary, there is enormous room for improvement almost everywhere, especially by way of the extension of rehabilitation services and, in certain countries, the reduction of middleman profits. But in most countries, one can conclude that the worker injured on the job has a better chance of getting adequate medical care than the worker with nonoccupational illness or the non-worker with any ailment. So long as national systems of general medical care have serious inadequacies, this special priority position for workmen's compensation medical care will probably prevail. As comprehensive systems of general medical care develop throughout the world, one may expect that the autonomous programs for the care of industrially injured workers will gradually become absorbed within them.

NOTES

[1] This chapter was presented as a paper before a Joint Session of the American Industrial Hygiene Association, the Industrial Medical Association, and the Occupational Health and Medical Care Sections of the American Public Health Association at the Ninety-First Annual Meeting in Kansas City, Mo., November 13, 1963.

[2] William F. Ogburn, *Social Change with Respect to Culture and Original Nature.* New York: Huebsch, 1922, pp. 213-236.

[3] For invaluable assistance in providing the factual data on which much of this chapter is based, grateful acknowledgment is made to Mr. Daniel S. Gerig of the U.S. Social Security Administration. Extensive information on workmen's compensation and health insurance systems is summarized in a report prepared under Mr. Gerig's direction, "Social Security Programs throughout the World." Washington, D.C.: Government Printing Office, 1961.

[4] See chapter 7.

[5] University of Toronto, Department of Public Health Administration, *Workmen's Compensation in Ontario.* Toronto: The University, 1955.

[6] Almont Lindsay, *Socialized Medicine in England and Wales: The National Health Service 1948-61.* Chapel Hill: University of North Carolina Press, 1962.

[7] World Health Organization, *Health Services in the U.S.S.R.* Geneva: WHO, 1960.

Chapter XX
General Practitioner Services under Eight Social Insurance Systems

The provision of medical care under systems of social security has followed a variety of organizational patterns in different nations. The variations depend largely on the relationships between the responsible public authority and the actual providers of service (physicians, hospitals, pharmacies, etc.). When the social security agency makes agreements with independent providers to render services to eligible persons under specified conditions, the pattern may be described as "indirect;" when the agency offers services directly through providers that it employs or controls, the pattern may be described as "direct." Within each of these main patterns, various subgroups are discernable, according to methods of remuneration and the setting of the professional work.

In 1967 the International Labour Office (a specialized agency of the United Nations) sponsored a study of these various administrative arrangements in a sample of eight countries, selected to represent different types of system and different parts of the world. These countries were Belgium, Canada, Ecuador, India, West Germany, Great Britain, Poland, and Tunisia. Documentation was provided by social security experts from each of the countries, and analysis was made of all the components of medical care—the services of general physicians, specialists, hospitals, drugs, dental care, etc.

This chapter is based largely on one chapter from the final monograph (The Organization of Medical Care under Social Security. *Geneva: International Labour Office, 1969). It was presented as a paper at a public health convention,[1] and published as "General Physician Services under Eight National Patterns" in the* American Journal of Public Health, *(Vol. 60, October 1970, pp. 1,893-1,899); it is reprinted here by permission.*

In every system that provides personal health services, the general physician plays a keystone role. He is typically the point of primary contact for the patient, and from his decisions emanate various other health services including drugs, specialist care, diagnostic tests, hospitalization, or other modalities. It is he who theoretically (if not always actually) coordinates the care of patients through the multiple components in complex health service systems.

The way in which the general physician plays this role, however, shows amazing variety among countries. An occasion for studying these varied methods was presented by an invitation from the International Labour Office (ILO), United Nations, to analyze the organization of medical care under the social security programs of eight countries. The countries were selected by the ILO to represent a range of mechanisms of social security, as well as different regions of the world. Rather lengthy structured questionnaires were submitted to national social security experts in each country, so that information could be collected along relatively uniform lines. The findings of this total study have been published in an official ILO monograph, and presented here is only a summary and interpretation of findings on that sector of medical care involving the services of general physicians.

TYPES OF PATTERN

The following are the countries (in alphabetical order) whose patterns of medical care were studied: Belgium, Canada, Ecuador, Germany (West), Great Britain, India, Poland, and Tunisia. In each of these countries there is actually a variety of patterns by which general physician services are provided within different organized settings, of which social security is only one. The approach here, however, will be to discuss the pattern that is most widely prevalent under the social security laws.

To find some order or meaning to the eight different national patterns, it was found possible to classify them into two general types. One type is that in which the governmental social security authorities enter into arrangements with various independent providers of service—physicians, hospitals, dentists, pharmacists, and the like—to furnish services for designated beneficiaries. This was called the "indirect pattern," and under it are various subtypes, depending on the nature of the financial arrangements. The other type is that in which the authorities provide the health services directly themselves, engaging physicians or others as employees, and usually building their own facilities. This was called the "direct pattern" and it also entailed certain subtypes.

Of course, it is dangerous to generalize from only eight cases, except that we know the eight countries studied are similar to many others on the same continents. Accordingly, it appears that the pattern of general physician services in a country, under social security systems, is largely influenced by two sets of forces: the level of economic development and the degree of centralized authority in the national political structure.

The patterns by which general physician services are furnished and paid for under social security laws may be set along a range from highly individualistic to highly collectivistic. If this is done for the eight countries under study, we find that there are four countries using mainly the indirect pattern and four using mainly the direct pattern. The indirect pattern is found to be associated with higher levels of economic development and more decentralized political structures, while the direct pattern is associated with the converse. The principal characteristics of each national pattern may be summarized.

INDIRECT PATTERN COUNTRIES

In Belgium, the private practice of medicine is so firmly entrenched that general physicians have no direct contractual or financial relationships with social security authorities at all. Instead, the patient, who has free choice of doctors, pays personally for his services; then he seeks reimbursement from his mutual benefit fund for seventy-five percent of the fee, according to an official fee schedule which has been negotiated with the Belgian Medical Federation.

The twenty-five percent cost sharing is intended to discourage unnecessary utilization and to lighten the financial drain on the benefit societies which carry the insurance, under a compulsory law. Sometimes doctor's fees are higher, however, than the official schedule, so that the patient's reimbursement becomes less than seventy-five percent. It is obvious that organizational influences on medical performance, under this pattern, are virtually absent.

In Canada, there is a mixture of systems among the different provinces, but in Saskatchewan, where social insurance for general physician's care has been operating the longest, the most common pattern is straight payment of fees by a fiscal intermediary which, in turn, collects the full costs from the government. This involves no cost sharing or reimbursement to the patient. There is free choice of doctor, and he is always paid an established fee. Surveillance is limited to determination that the specified service was, in fact, rendered and correctly identified.

In Germany, the degree of collective responsibility, within the medical profession, for general physician services under a budgeted outlay is somewhat greater. The sickness fund, to which the patient must belong, pays fixed quarterly per capita sums to various associations of doctors. These associations pay the individual doctor his fees, after critical review of claims, according to various rules. If the money in any quarter-year is not enough to meet the charges, however, all doctors must accept a proportionate reduction of their fees. Thus incentives are created in the profession to prevent superfluous or improper medical care.

Great Britain applies a payment method for general physicians' care which, while under the indirect pattern, places still greater responsibility upon the profession to meet medical demands within a fixed expenditure. General physicians are in private practice, but each is paid fixed monthly amounts in accordance with the number of persons who have chosen him for care. The size of a general doctor's panel may change from month to month, and the capitation payments vary by a special formula, but it is evident that the doctor earns no more for extra units of service to a patient. Thus self-discipline is built into each individual medical practice.

There are numerous ramifications to each of these four types of indirect pattern by which general physician services under social security are organized. In all of them, the doctors own and operate their own private offices, but the relationships to patients and to the social security agencies vary. The doctor in each pattern has economic incentives to satisfy his patients, but the incentives toward maximizing medical acts—about which the patient is seldom sophisticated—differ. The pattern in these four countries for specialist medical services, it may be noted, is usually different; the specialist is often, though not always, affiliated with a hospital and may be paid a salary for the greater part of his time.

It may also be noted that all four countries with the indirect pattern are highly industrialized. In these countries, the tradition of an independent medical profession, in small private enterprises, is old and strong. When social security programs were enacted, the political realities led the authorities to enter into contracts with the existing corps of private general practitioners.

DIRECT PATTERN COUNTRIES

In countries using the direct pattern for general physician services under social security, the setting is quite different. In these countries, the world of private medical practice has typically been quite restricted because of the prevailing poverty of the population. The social insurance mechanism created effective demand for a class of people—mainly industrial workers—who without it would hardly have constituted a market for private medical practitioners at all. Local government, moreover, tends to be weak, and political power tends to be quite centralized.

Under the circumstances, the social security agencies have been politically free to establish the most economical pattern for general physician services. This has meant engagement of doctors as employees, paying for the time that they work within facilities staffed and equipped by the agency. As in other forms of "industrialization," the incentives for diligent work take forms that are very different from those affecting the small private craftsman.

In Ecuador, only about five percent of the population is enrolled under social security, and they are concentrated in the main cities. The most common arrangement is by part-time medical salaries, for two or four hours per day, the doctor spending the balance of his time in private practice. The patient goes to the health center nearest his home and is seen by the doctor on duty, with little "free choice." Laboratory, x-ray, and consultation services are generally available on the premises, which are owned and operated by the social security agency. Medical

performance is supervised by a hierarchical professional structure.

In Tunisia, the financial resources of the principal social security agency were too meager to permit construction of its own facilities. Instead, the agency entered into arrangements with the Ministry of Health to use its health centers and hospitals; there, doctors whose salaries are paid by the social security agency see the covered beneficiaries. This integrated use of facilities is believed to be more economical, and it also assists the Ministry of Health, dependent on lean general revenues, in the task of maintaining services for the general noninsured population. Interestingly, there is a second social security scheme for government employees in Tunisia, using the older French indirect pattern of free choice of private doctor with partial reimbursement of the patient. In recent years an increasing proportion of these beneficiaries have chosen to use the governmental facilities for their care, where—despite the deprivation of free choice of doctor—they are relieved of any cost-sharing burden and are treated by an organized team of medical personnel.

India represents another form of integration of general physician services for social security beneficiaries with health care for the general population. Since only about three percent of that large country's population is covered by the scheme, the decision of the social security agency was to pay the state ministries of health for providing general medical services to beneficiaries through established health centers, wherever feasible. In areas with concentrations of insured workers, however, the medical staffing of these centers was markedly increased. These general physicians are on full-time salary under the regular civil service system of the Ministry of Health.

In two large Indian cities, Bombay and Calcutta, however, the market for private medical patients was so great that sufficient doctors could not be attracted into the governmental services. Therefore, other arrangements had to be made for serving beneficiaries with primary general practitioner care. The British indirect pattern was adopted, and insured persons must choose a private physician who is then paid a flat per capita monthly amount. Most of these private offices are very meagerly equipped, and social security administrators claim that the quality of services is poorer, complaints are more numerous, and costs are higher than in the health centers.

Poland differs from the other three countries that use the direct pattern of general physician services in being more highly developed economically, yet not so industrialized as the four countries that apply the indirect pattern. Before 1946, it followed the

German model, with private physicians paid on a fee basis for serving certain insured workers. After Poland's postwar reconstruction under a socialist government, social security coverage was extended to about seventy percent of the population. These persons are served for general physician care by the full-time salaried medical staff of the Ministry of Health, employed in a network of health centers and hospitals. Every Polish physician is obligated to work seven hours a day in the public service; beyond this, however, he may still engage in private practice. Persons who are noninsured—mainly small farmers—may still be served by the same network of facilities, but they must pay for the services.

SOME COMPARISONS

While extremely abbreviated, these accounts of eight national patterns for providing general physician services under social security programs may be enough to show the great variety of ways in which this task is approached. In an anthropological sense, they may demonstrate how different economic and political settings generate different patterns of medical care organization. Conversely, the student of social medicine may say, "Tell me how doctors are working and being paid, and I will tell you about the economic and political culture of the country."

Aside from these interesting intellectual pursuits, the critical social policy question is: What are the consequences of the different patterns of organization? Ultimately we would like to know which of the patterns is most effective in saving lives and reducing disability. Even short of this ultimate question, it would be useful for purposes of national health planning to know which pattern uses a given volume of resources (personnel and facilities) most efficiently to yield the highest rate of medical services—such as general physician contacts per 1,000 persons per year—at a given cost.

The research problems presented in attempting to answer such questions of international comparison are quite overwhelming. The variables affecting the health status of a population, aside from the medical care system, are multitudinous. Likewise, the cultural characteristics of a people, as well as mundane matters like transportation or communication, have enormous influence on the rates of utilization of medical services, regardless of the system. The most serious comparative studies undertaken so far on medical care utilization—those by Dr. Kerr L. White and his collaborators—have not yet been able to attribute the differentials found to the features of the medical care system, as distinguished from the other socioeconomic and cultural variables.[2]

At this point, therefore, comparisons among national patterns must be confined to much more modest commentaries on certain operational aspects of the systems, rather than their outcomes or achievement of goals. Based on information provided to the ILO by expert observers from the eight countries reviewed, a few such comments may be offered with respect to general physician services.

Although it may sound "pollyannish," in all countries—regardless of system—there seems to be a high level of satisfaction by insured persons with their particular pattern. There is quantitative evidence for this from household surveys in the indirect pattern countries, like Germany and Great Britain, and from obvious public clamor for extension of the direct pattern programs in Ecuador, India, and Tunisia. Perhaps the critical factor is the financial protection of a social security system, under which people are largely satisfied with almost any organizational pattern of physician's care. Moreover, the health care pattern, except for that in Poland, has always been largely built upon that which prevailed before enactment of the social security laws—that is, the pattern to which most people were accustomed.

In the industrialized countries with capitalist economies, the indirect pattern tends to be attractive to both patients and doctors. Free choice of private physician meets the psychological needs of most patients and satisfies the entrepreneurial interests of most doctors. The fee-for-service payment method tends to create incentives for a relatively high volume of service since, beyond the initial contact, utilization is decided mainly by the doctor. Even the capitation payment method does not discourage service, although it encourages referrals from general practitioners to specialists.

The quality of general physician services under the indirect pattern, on the other hand, has led to serious questions in all countries using it. Usually practicing alone, the general physician does not have the benefit of convenient consultation from colleagues or much assistance of technical aides; in several countries he usually lacks the stimulus of any hospital affiliation. The financial incentives of the fee pattern may lead to unnecessary services or may discourage appropriate referrals to specialists. Where costs can be compared in the same country, as in India and to a small extent in Ecuador, the indirect pattern is found to be more expensive per person covered than the direct pattern. Equitable geographic distribution of doctors, in relation to the ecology of people, is difficult to achieve when each physician is a free agent—even though some inducements toward rural settlement have been offered by official regulations in Germany and Great

Britain. Efforts at some controls over quality and costs entail a great deal of bureaucratic paperwork under the indirect pattern, and a certain controversial tension between physicians and social security authorities is the normal state of affairs in these countries.

The direct pattern of general physician services also has its problems, although many of them are attributable to the poverty of resources in countries where it is applied more than to the pattern itself. Health centers or polyclinics may be frugally staffed, so that there is not enough time per patient. The very size of a medical facility may lead to a certain impersonality, and the patient does not easily develop a continuing relationship with one general physician. An organized framework naturally deprives the doctor of some of his independence, and it may lower his morale.

Nevertheless, the organized arrangements of the direct pattern give the general physician access to more ancillary personnel and equipment than would be likely in a private office. Being in close contact with other colleagues, he is more likely to be on his toes, and yet he may seek consultation readily. Professional supervision is built into day-to-day work. Some health centers apply medical audits or other quality surveillance methods similar to those used in hospitals. The young doctor's time can be used to full capacity early in his career, without the wastage of waiting for patients in a private office. Rural populations can be served more readily by assigning doctors—sometimes with higher salaries—to rural facilities. Demands on the doctor's time for clerical or other simple tasks are less, since other personnel are on hand. The salary method of remuneration also reduces much of the paperwork. The costs per person served are lower, presumably due to the economies of scale, the rationalization of equipment and auxiliary personnel, and the reduction of unnecessary services.

DISCUSSION

These comments are based on the observations of social security experts in the eight countries studied. Firm statistical data to back them up are not available. It is conceivable that the direct pattern has been more generally applied in the developing and the socialist countries simply because it is less expensive, regardless of other consequences. It may also be argued that the direct pattern has been established and retained in countries because it has been effective in reducing mortality rates and satisfying the people. The wealthier industrialized and capitalist countries are evidently willing to spend more, both absolutely and relatively (i.e., as a percentage of national income), on personal health services than are the poorer developing and socialist countries, if one can cautiously interpret the findings of the World Health Organization study of this difficult question.[3] In other words, some rich countries are presumably willing to be extravagant with their health service dollars in order to retain the indirect pattern of physician's care.

International comparisons of this sort are so beset with problems that one may be able to draw firmer conclusions from comparative studies within one country. Programs like the Health Insurance Plan of Greater New York or the Kaiser-Permanente Health Plan illustrate the essential characteristics of the direct pattern of physician's care within our own borders; these have been compared with the more widely prevalent indirect pattern, suggesting both higher quality and lower costs for the former.[4] Such findings add strength to the nonquantified observations made by various national social security experts in other countries.

Other evidence of the overall advantages of the direct pattern is suggested by a view of the worldwide trends. In virtually all countries, rich and poor, one can observe an increasing tendency for physicians—both general practitioners and specialists—to work in organized frameworks. This is quite evident throughout the United States in the development of general hospitals, group practice clinics, special health centers, and both public and voluntary health service programs of many types. In Latin America, the extension of social security and public health programs has brought increasing proportions—well over two-thirds—of doctors under the direct pattern of medical work. In Africa, this pattern is the rule, except for private practitioners in the capital cities, and often even they have part-time salaried employment. In the socialist countries, most recently Cuba, almost 100 percent of doctors give service through the direct pattern. In Great Britain and Western Europe, the general physician remain still largely a private practioner under the indirect pattern, but the proportion of total physicians engaged in specialties—coming mainly under organized hospital employment—is steadily rising. In India and other Asian countries, except People's China, about half the physicians are still principally in private practice, but this proportion is declining as governmental and other organized services are expanding.

Thus, the global trends suggest that the direct pattern of physician's care is found to serve social needs more effectively than the indirect pattern. With rates of utilization of medical care rising, as they seem to be everywhere, the demands can be met only by greater mobilization of the services of nurses, aides, and other auxiliary health personnel. This requires organized health service frameworks. The collectivization of costs for increasing proportions of the population, moreover, leads to mounting pressures for economy and efficiency.

Much more careful research would be needed to demonstrate the ultimate consequences of different patterns for providing general physician services, and indeed all components of medical care, uninfluenced by other social or demographic variables. Until then, the presumptive evidence suggests that, while there are many subtleties at play, the net advantages are greater for the direct pattern of service.

NOTES

[1] Ninety-Seventh Annual Meeting of the American Public Health Association, Philadelphia, Pennsylvania, November 11, 1969.

[2] Kerr L. White and June H. Murnaghan, *International Comparisons of Medical Care Utilization: A Feasibility Study*. Washington, D.C.: National Center for Health Statistics, Series 2, No. 33, June 1969.

[3] Brian Abel-Smith, *An International Study of Health Expenditure*. Geneva: World Health Organization, Public Health Paper No. 32, 1967.

[4] Sam Shapiro, "End Result Measurements of Quality of Medical Care." *Milbank Memorial Fund Quarterly*, Vol. 45, April 1967, pp. 7-30.

Chapter XXI
Allied Health Manpower in Developing and Socialist Countries

All nations have been making increasing use of allied or paramedical health manpower, working in various relationships to physicians—with them, under supervision, or independently. As the demands for health service everywhere have risen, the training programs for these allied health personnel have become more developed and their scopes of function have evolved along several lines.

In this chapter an overview of this movement is taken, as it is seen in the developing and socialist countries. In these countries, where rural populations are so large and their needs generally so inadequately met, the allied health worker has special importance. Four basic types of allied health manpower may be distinguished, and their principal characteristics are summarized in this chapter which was published as "The Role of Allied Health Manpower in Developing and Socialist Countries" in the Journal of Allied Health *(Vol. 3, Summer 1974, pp. 77-85). The article is reprinted here by permission.[1]*

INTRODUCTION

The use of health manpower throughout the world follows such a bewildering diversity of patterns that, in the hope of achieving some clarity, these remarks will be confined to practices (1) involving allied health personnel, and (2) in the developing and certain socialist countries. Even with these restrictions, the subject is quite complex, since policies vary with the socio-political structure of different countries, and they are undergoing changes continually as science advances and as social expectations or demands for medical care keep rising everywhere.

Although I have had the opportunity to study something of the health services of forty-one countries, on all the continents, I feel far from certain about how to analyze the policies and practices involving allied health manpower. First, however, allow me to define these "allied" personnel as those associated in some way with the mission of doctors of medicine, but not being doctors themselves. Even doctors, with their august tradition going back to

Hippocrates or earlier to Imhotep in Egypt, are not so easy to define—as the World Health Organization has recently shown through its struggles in 1972 to define the word "physician" in a way that would have universal international acceptance.

Let me assume, nevertheless, that in all countries there is a type of health worker who has had a maximum period of formal training, on the basis of principles now defined everywhere as "science," and that he is considered to be a physician. In relation to him, and engaged in various tasks of rendering health service to the people, I believe we can distinguish at least four basic types of allied health personnel: (1) traditional healers, (2) paramedical health workers, (3) elementary doctor substitutes, and (4) trained primary health practitioners.

While the lines between these categories are not always sharp, and though personnel in one category may over the years evolve into another, we may look briefly at each of these types of allied health personnel, as seen in the developing and socialist countries.

TRADITIONAL HEALERS

The modern carry-over of preliterate civilization is the traditional healer, who takes many different forms. In general, he holds himself forth as capable of treating all ailments, of any degree of severity, but the methods differ. A large proportion of the world's population—those in the rural areas of Africa, Asia, Latin America, and elsewhere—still depend mainly on traditional healers to serve their health needs.

The oldest type of traditional healer invokes magic or supernatural forces to cure disease. The "witch doctors" of Africa, applying "voodoo" or similar powers, are of this type, as are many of the *curanderos* of Latin America. In a sense, we see the same concepts in the faith healing (Christian Science, for example) of the industrialized nations, for the line between magic and religion is not so sharp.

Another type of traditional healer has formulated, over the centuries, a body of empirical knowledge based on physical processes. He has learned about benefits gained—or believed to be gained—from certain diets, from various herbs, from processes like heat or exercise. In the older civilizations of Asia, these healers have developed a large body of knowledge which has been codified and is taught in formal schools. Ayurvedic medicine in India has its own theory of disease, much like that of the four body humors of ancient Greece, and treatment is based on attempting to achieve equilibrium in the system by use of various natural drugs. "Serpasil," a well-known antihypertensive drug in all countries, is actually a product of Ayurvedic medicine. The government of India maintains several Ayurvedic teaching centers, but there is no attempt to integrate this type of healing with that of modern scientific medicine.

The Chinese traditional doctor, of whom we hear so much in recent years, is also in this category. He has developed an elaborate pharmacopoeia from plants and animal parts, which is designed to treat diseases believed to be caused by an excess of *yin* or *yang*—the two vital forces of the universe believed to be flowing in each body. Another component of traditional Chinese medicine is acupuncture or insertion of needles at various points in the body, designed to open up channels believed to connect various organs. There is an enormous literature in this field, which was viewed with almost universal skepticism by Western doctors until recent demonstrations of the effectiveness of acupuncture as anesthesia. The current Chinese government is attempting to subject the practice of both traditional herbalism and acupuncture to scientific testing, to determine which features are demonstrably effective.

In the meantime, the government is encouraging the integration of traditional and modern medicine in everyday care of patients, including services in hospitals.

A third form of health personnel that may be considered among the traditional healers, although this may be a distortion, is the charlatan or medical imposter. In many developing countries, there are health science students who have failed or dropped out of their schools. To make a living, they go to some isolated village and set themselves up as "doctors." They use or misuse modern drugs, but they also apply remedies concocted themselves, based perhaps on some of the local traditions. Some of these healers may have served at one time as auxiliaries in an organized health program, but they left to engage in this more lucrative type of role.

This is a much oversimplified account of traditional healing, but it may clarify the general idea. There is sometimes overlap among the three subtypes mentioned, especially between the magical and empirical healers. In general, traditional healers work with patients on a one-to-one basis, and are not part of an organized health care system. They make no use of hospitals, and often have no quarters of any sort, treating patients in their own homes. They live in the villages and are widely used by rural people because they are close at hand, inexpensive, and may show great understanding of the patient's feelings. Often they are really part-time healers, being mainly engaged in agriculture or something else. They are a reflection of human demand for health service, which has not been met in some other scientific or systematic way.

PARAMEDICAL HEALTH WORKERS

The paramedical health worker is very different—a product of the complexities of modern scientific medicine. He is the allied health person who works at the side of the doctor, strictly under his supervision, carrying out delegated functions. In the industrialized nations, the numbers and types of paramedical health personnel have grown very rapidly, but even in the developing countries their importance is great.

Probably the most numerous of the paramedical workers is the nurse, who has evolved from the religious sister tending the sick in hospitals. The story of Florence Nightingale who, after helping wounded British soldiers in the Crimean War, returned to London to start the first formal school of nursing in 1860, is well known. The objective soon became to attract well-educated young ladies into the field, instead of unschooled poor girls or "wayward women" who had previously done the dirty work in hospitals. As a result, nursing has gradually elevated its educational standards, requiring several years of training after high school graduation and now, in America, often university graduation.

One of the great fallacies of international health policy, in my opinion, has been the attempted diffusion of this European and North American concept of professional nursing to the developing countries. The point is that high school graduation (variously defined) is a relatively rare achievement in Asia, Africa, and Latin America—especially for women. Most young women who have gone this far, typically in the small middle class, and wish to go further in their education, will choose the university or some other pursuit, rather than nursing. As a result, the supply of what Westerners call fully qualified or graduate nurses is very low in almost all the developing countries. In Latin America, for example, where the ratio of doctors to population has been improving but is still less than half of that in the United States, there are approximately only 0.33 graduate nurses per doctor; in the U.S., it is the other way around and there are about 2.0 nurses per doctor. Hence, relative to population, there are only one-sixth as many graduate nurses in Latin America as in North America.

To meet the massive needs for nursing care, therefore, the developing countries have had to train various forms of nursing auxiliaries. Typically there are three or four times as many auxiliaries produced as graduate nurses. These are young women from the villages or the poor districts of the cities who have typically had very limited schooling—perhaps four to six years of elementary school, so that they can read and write. Then they are given a course of practical training that may last from two or three months up to a year, and are called "nursing auxiliaries" or "assistant nurses" or the like. Theoretically they work in hospitals, health centers, or small health stations under the supervision of a graduate nurse or a doctor.

I say "theoretically," because the reality is reflected by what I saw in Venezuela a few years ago. In a small village at a health station, the only person on hand was a young nursing auxiliary, born in that village, who had received three months of training after six years of elementary school. She was supposed to be working under the supervision of a doctor, but he came around only once a week or so; in between she made all the decisions on medical care. Meanwhile her much better educated middle class sisters, so to speak, who were graduate nurses, worked exclusively in the big city hospitals, at the elbow of the doctor. They did nothing except on specific medical instructions. In a word, one type of nurse was vastly overeducated, the other vastly undereducated for her functions—a moral inequity that can be understood only in terms of social class values as between rural proletariat and urban middle class populations.

If Latin American and other developing countries invested in the training of village girls to be reasonably qualified health workers what they invest in the training of middle class daughters to be graduate professional nurses, handmaidens to the doctor, the rural people of this world would be getting much better health care. This approach seems to be taken in socialist Cuba where, since the Revolution, there has been an increase of schools producing graduate nurses from six to thirteen, but for schools giving a one-year course to turn out auxiliary nurses the increase has been from zero to fifty-eight.

There are many other types of paramedical personnel who assist the doctor, although in the developing countries their functions are seldom as clearly articulated with the doctor's role as in the United States. The pharmacist, for example, is the outgrowth of the medieval apothecary, who compounded remedies and sold them directly to the people. It was well into the nineteenth century before pharmacists came to fill a paramedical role—that is, compounding and dispensing drugs on the prescription of doctors. They may still, of course, dispense drugs not requiring a prescription under law directly to the patient, but so may any grocery store.

My point is that in the developing countries, where doctors are so few in the rural areas and where drug control laws are weak or nonexistent, the pharmacist dispenses most of his medications directly to patients who come and seek help. As in Arthur Laurent's "West Side Story," he is the "Doc" who serves the poor. Moreover, most of the operators of stores that sell drugs, along with other things, are not trained pharmacists. They have learned a little about drugs, in relation to common symptoms, by observation or apprenticeship. Because of competition for paying patients between pharmacists and doctors, most of the few private doctors in small towns of Asia or Africa dispense their own prescriptions. In the larger health centers operated by government, a "dispenser" (essentially an auxiliary pharmacist) is commonly on the staff.

The laboratory or x-ray technician is probably the most incorruptible type of paramedical worker, since he is an assistant only for diagnosis and can hardly help the patient therapeutically by himself. But in this category too, the influence of the industrialized countries has not always been beneficial. Various quality standards emanating from Europe and America have raised educational requirements so high that there are seldom enough of these technicians to staff the hospitals or health centers. Fortunately, the ministries of health of the developing continents have usually gone ahead and trained young men and women to do this technical work without university education. The training is nearly always in patient care institutions, rather than schools or colleges.

When I worked in the Canadian prairie province of Saskatchewan in the 1950s, we had a corresponding problem in staffing small rural hospitals with technicians. The university-qualified laboratory or x-ray technicians (now often called "technologists" to signify a higher status) wouldn't go to the rural districts. So in the provincial Ministry of Public Health we had to set up our own one-year course for training "combined technicians," capable of doing simple laboratory and x-ray work, to staff the rural hospitals. A similar course of action was taken for producing "combined rehabilitation therapists," who could do useful work in physical therapy and occupational therapy, without going through the two separate university regimes required by licensure law for each of these fields.

ELEMENTARY DOCTOR SUBSTITUTES

In contrast to these paramedical workers who, at least theoretically, are intended to assist the doctor and to work under his direct orders, there is a third type of allied health worker which I am calling the "elementary doctor substitute." These personnel are intended to cope with many of the problems of diagnosing and treating the sick by themselves—referring to doctors only those cases that they think they cannot handle. Because they have this relatively broad role, and because fully trained doctors in nearly all countries concentrate in the cities, these elementary doctor substitutes are typically devoted to the care of rural populations.

It is very difficult, despite my efforts at classification, to give an accurate account of these elementary doctor substitutes in the developing countries. In nineteenth century Russia under the czars, when this was surely a rural, underdeveloped country, the "feldsher" was probably the classical illustration, but over the years and especially since the socialist Revolution of 1917, his role has changed. Dr. Victor Sidel's 1968 report on "Feldshers and Feldsherism" is undoubtedly the best American account of the changing role of this type of health worker.[2] It boils down to this: In czarist Russia, when there were few doctors to serve the rural people, the feldsher was an elementary doctor substitute considered "good enough for the peasants;" he had very limited train-

ing but wide responsibilities. When the Soviet system of socialized health services was developed, with a massive output of physicians, the feldsher's role gradually changed to serving as a member of a health team, working under definite medical supervision. There have been many ups and downs in this evolution, however, and in the rural areas of the Soviet Union the feldsher's role is still more independent than in the cities. The entire definition of the feldsher's role in the Soviet health system continues to be in flux, and more will be said of this below.

In the European colonies of Africa, the elementary doctor substitute was used extensively. The only fully trained physicians were the white men from the ruling country, and they served mainly in cities. (Exceptions were medical missionaries, like Albert Schweitzer, setting up their hospitals in the hinterland.) When rural health posts were established, they were staffed by male medical assistants or "dressers," who had learned about some surgical techniques and later about commonly used drugs by assisting doctors in the hospitals. Their training was seldom formalized, however. After independence was gained by the African countries following World War II, the former colonial medical systems of the British, French, Belgians, and others were largely carried over.

The principal change of policy after national independence has been to provide more systematic training to the dressers or medical assistants designated by other names like *officiers de santé* (health officers). They have been taught about preventive service also and they give immunizations, advice on environmental sanitation, and some health education. They have learned to give certain medications for fevers, diarrheas, respiratory disorders, etc. But the basic education of these health workers is so limited that their treatment of disease is bound to be essentially symptomatic. There are so few doctors available in Africa that they have little supervision, and if a patient's sickness persists he is sent to a hospital—usually distant and only if transportation is available.

The Latin American auxiliary nurse, mentioned earlier, while theoretically a paramedical worker, in practice serves as an elementary doctor substitute in many rural areas. These are typically young village women. In some of the Latin American countries, men who were originally trained as sanitary inspectors (environmentalists) may be given a bit of medical orientation and sent out to staff isolated rural posts in the same way.

The newly developed "barefoot doctors" of the People's Republic of China must really be placed in

206

this category of elementary doctor substitutes. Despite the sensational achievements in development of these personnel, their educational preparation has necessarily been very limited. The entire movement to train peasants, city workers, and housewives for these part-time medical roles has been a reasonable response to gigantic health needs, all the more remarkable for its rapidity and the large numbers of these health workers trained. But we must regard this, in my opinion, as a transitional approach in China—necessary to meet an overwhelming need mainly in rural areas—which will eventually be replaced by preparation of more systematically prepared medical and allied health workers, as the nation develops.

TRAINED PRIMARY HEALTH PRACTITIONERS

Finally there are in many developing countries the better trained primary health practitioners—allied health workers who have usually evolved from the elementary doctor substitutes just reviewed. Their preparation and mode of work have been shaped by different socio-political influences in various countries.

The Soviet feldsher today—in many although not all districts of that large country—probably represents the clearest prototype. The feldsher has a structured program of training of about four years after secondary school (compared with two or three years for nurses and six years for doctors). He or she (about half are men and half women) works as a distinct team member in a system with large numbers of doctors (one to about 400 people—much more than in the U.S.), so that his role is clearly defined as giving ancillary and not definitive medical care. In rural districts, he is expected to spend a high proportion of time on preventive services and to refer all but the simplest cases to physicians. Some feldshers play specialized roles as sanitarians, industrial hygienists, or midwives, but the majority are generalists. In urban polyclinics or hospitals, the feldshers work under the close eye of doctors, but even in rural locations a doctor is within call at any time. Judging from Dr. Sidel's study, this may be a slightly idealized description, since in the Soviet health services, as in our own, personnel do not always do exactly what is officially expected of them. Nevertheless, some of the criticisms which Soviet doctors themselves level at feldshers who exceed their proper role come, I suspect, from the very diligent professional standards of those doctors. Everywhere, one often finds, the severest criticisms of the status quo arise not where conditions are worst but where the observer has the highest expectations.

In Ethiopia, since about 1955, there has been an impressive program training primary health practitioners to a much higher level than the customary African dresser. Located at the mountain city of Gondar, the Haile Selassie Public Health College and Training Center gives a three-year formal course to men who have completed twelve grades of education (primary and secondary schools), and are then appointed to positions as health officers in rural health centers. Their responsibilities combine administrative, public health, and clinical functions. On the clinical level, they serve as primary practitioners, treating the simple ailments and referring difficult cases to a district or provincial hospital. (With relatively few physicians and hospitals available, however, the Ethiopian health officer would inevitably make referrals much less often than the Soviet feldsher.) Meanwhile, it is interesting to note, Ethiopia continues to train and use dressers, who are young men with one year of hospital training after six years of schooling. A school somewhat like the Gondar College was developed in British Fiji some years ago for training "native doctors" of a rudimentary level; it has, however, evolved into a full-dress medical school.

Through a process of evolution from the nineteenth century, the former British colonies and now the British Commonwealth countries have developed training programs for various types of primary health practitioner, short of doctors. In Ceylon where I did a study for WHO twenty-one years ago, they were called "apothecaries" because originally they served in hospitals dispensing drugs. Gradually they were given more training—typically two years after eleven grades of basic schooling. Then they were assigned to rural posts, with full authority to diagnose and treat the sick, referring only the perplexing cases to a hospital.

In Malaysia, which I studied in 1968, the mainstay of primary medical care in the rural areas is called the "hospital assistant." His training is equivalent in length to that of the graduate nurse—three years after high school (eleven or twelve years)—but different in content. He is taught to diagnose, treat with drugs, and do minor surgery, but not preventive work. The latter is done by nurses, graduate or auxiliary levels, who work along with him in a rural health center. Fully trained physicians are theoretically responsible for the whole health center operation, but they visit only about once a week, since each doctor is supposed to supervise three to five health centers. Difficult cases are asked to return to see the doctor at his scheduled visit.

In these British Commonwealth countries, and I am sure in others, there is a manifest delineation of health care responsibilities among allied health workers along sex lines. Personal preventive service, especially for babies and mothers, is often given by women—as various levels of nurse—but diagnosis and treatment of disease, in any patient, is done usually by men. One can hardly doubt that this policy springs from the prejudices of male-dominated societies in which women are not entrusted with critical decisions—like treating the sick. It is also related to the historical origins of many of the doctor substitutes or allied primary health practitioners from the military services. This was true for the Russian feldsher, who was originally a field corpsmen in the czarist armies, no less than for the African dresser or the current American "Medex" from the Vietnam War. When emancipation of women has become a top national priority, as it did in post-Revolutionary Soviet Russia, this policy seems to change. As we know, a substantial majority of physicians and about half of the feldshers in the USSR are women. One sees the same trend today in Cuba where, in sharp contrast to pre-Castro days, fifty percent of the medical students are women.

One important type of allied health worker, whom one might consider either a doctor substitute or a primary health practitioner, is invariably female—the midwife. In this sector of health care, the United States and Canada are really the exceptions of the world, for almost everywhere else, in Europe no less than the developing continents, the major proportion of obstetrical deliveries are done by midwives. In the advanced countries of Western and Eastern Europe, the normal childbirths (about eighty percent of the total) are attended mainly by trained midwives, inside hospitals, and only the complicated or high-risk cases are referred to obstetricians. In the developing countries, midwives, with various levels of training, are responsible for nearly all deliveries in rural areas and for most in the cities. A majority of rural childbirths are still probably attended by untrained midwives, who have learned their skills from observation and tradition, but a rising proportion are being done by trained and government-certified midwives. In Asian and African countries, moreover, there are often minimally trained assistant midwives (one year of training after six grades) in the villages, who are supervised by professional nurse-midwives (three or four years of training after twelve grades) in a district health center or hospital.

There are trained primary health practitioners of other special types, aside from doctors, that time allows us only to mention. The so-called "dental nurse," pioneered in New Zealand in 1920, has now been emulated in about twenty countries; she does no nursing in the usual sense, but rather gives virtually complete dental care to children in the schools with very little supervision from a dentist. There are pediatric assistants, often trained originally as nurses, who give complete care to children in rural areas. For visual problems, there are opticians or, as we call them in the U.S., optometrists, to whom people go for eye care without passing through referral by a doctor. Podiatry is another such allied field, in the civilized cultures of the tight shoe, but not so often seen in the developing countries.

COMMENT

From this sketchy and by no means comprehensive account of allied health workers of four basic types in developing countries, one may offer some general observations:

1. In all countries, the training and the functional role of allied health personnel are undergoing continuous change. The role of personnel who were strictly paramedical aides at one time, like nursing auxiliaries, changes to a role of elementary doctor substitutes under other circumstances. The elementary doctor substitute, with very little training, of one period becomes the trained primary health practitioner of another.

2. The role of allied health workers depends heavily on the supply of physicians in a country. Where they are very few in relation to population, more responsibility is obviously placed on allied health workers. This applies to the elementary doctor substitutes or the primary health practitioners more than to strictly paramedical personnel; the latter (technicians, nurses, physiotherapists, etc.) are most highly developed where the ratio of doctors is also high and specialization has become prominent.

3. The roles of allied health workers depend also a great deal on the system of organization of health services and the whole political structure of a country. In the socialist countries, health services have become predominantly organized under government, with only a very small private sector, but even in the nonsocialist developing countries health care in rural areas is largely under governmental control. Within a governmental framework, greater use tends to be made of allied health workers because they are more readily subject to supervision that way. The socialist countries, like the USSR, China, and Cuba, differ from the others in the greater relative investment they seem to be making in all types of health service—involving training of more doctors as well as more allied health workers. Speedy response to rural needs, by rapid training of large numbers of allied health workers for rural jobs, also seems to be a

special emphasis of the socialist countries in recent years.

4. Attitudes of governmental authorities toward traditional healers are influenced evidently by history as well as politics. In Latin America, where the *curandero* was a product of the Indian culture, the attitude of modern governments, with their Spanish and Catholic roots, has been to replace him. Little or no effort is made to weave the Indian healer into the modern health service system. Likewise in Africa, the witch doctor has no meaning in the official establishment adapted from recent European rule. In India, however, the ancient Ayurvedic doctors, who came from the tradition which now rules India (albeit with British modifications), are still supported by the government. In the People's Republic of China, major efforts are being made to integrate the traditional doctors with the modern health service system.

5. The schedules of education of different types of allied health worker depend very much on the overall educational system. Where high school education is largely confined to the main cities and to the children of middle class or some skilled worker families, limits are placed on the source of personnel for various health manpower roles. Thus, it is the youth from better-off city families who become doctors, dentists, and graduate nurses, and enter other fields requiring high school graduation. The lower level allied health workers, requiring only four or six grades of basic schooling, are recruited mainly from rural, agricultural families.

6. These class distinctions in basic education affect the whole possibility of career ladders in the health field. When auxiliary nurses or dressers are taught some practical functions after a sixth-grade education, they can have no hope of moving along into higher levels of service, without going back to high school—which is seldom feasible. But, when all allied health workers have first completed a high school education, then—if they perform well in the allied worker role—they can move forward to higher levels with further education. Thus, in the USSR, about twenty-five percent of medical students are former feldshers or nurses. Some of the graduates of the Ethiopian Gondar College are now going on to medicine at the new medical school recently established in Addis Ababa. This is a rare occurrence, however, in the nonsocialist countries, marked by rigid class distinctions.

7. Language is another factor exerting a strong influence on the training of allied health manpower. In former colonies of Western powers, even after liberation, the European language is often learned only by the small percentage of young people from the favored classes who move along to high school. The professional schools for doctors and higher levels of allied workers, like graduate nurses, however, teach only in English, French, or one of the European tongues. This alone restricts children of the rural or urban proletariat to the lower auxiliary health roles, with little hope for advancement.

8. The most basic determinant of the role of allied health workers, in my opinion, is the overall philosophy of the nation's health service system, with respect to the rights of the population to obtain medical care. If health service has been made essentially a civil right, available to all without a market price, then allied health workers develop as part of a health care team whose functions are determined by considerations of efficiency, rather than the social pedigree of the patient. In mixed or pluralistic societies, however, where some health care is provided under organized governmental schemes and other care is purchased in the private market, there is, in my view, a different meaning to the role of allied health workers. Whether the policy is explicit or subtle, allied health workers of the doctor substitute or primary practitioner type tend to be used only for lower class patients, while full-fledged physicians with paramedical aides are reserved for the upper crust. This sort of policy, in my view, is a definite hazard in the United States, which can be averted only by developing a national health system, with rationally organized delivery patterns and equal access of all persons to the services.

The rationale of health service teams, with abundant use of allied health workers, is a logic that should be based on the requirements of medical technology and the objective needs of different patients or illnesses. The functioning of these teams should have no relation whatever to the social class of the patient being served. The allegation that the training or use of certain types of allied health workers implies "second class medicine" has meaning only if the social status of the patient influences what these workers do. But if efficient and effective health care delivery is the sole objective, then international experience shows that well-trained allied health workers can greatly hasten the achievement of good health service for everyone in all types of country, developing or industrialized.

NOTES

[1] Paper presented at a session on "Health Manpower Utilization: An International Comparison," sponsored by the New Professional Section, American Public Health Association, 100th Annual Meeting, Atlantic City, New Jersey, November 13, 1972.

[2] Victor W. Sidel, "Feldshers and Feldsherism." *New England Journal of Medicine*, Vol. 278, April 25, 1968, pp. 934-939.

Chapter XXII
World Trends in Organized Ambulatory Services

Historically, health services for the ambulatory patient have been organized throughout the world along several paths: (1) separate dispensaries for treatment of the sick, (2) hospital outpatient departments, (3) specialized preventive clinics under public health agencies, industries, or schools, (4) private group medical practice, and (5) health centers of either preventive or integrated preventive-curative scope. All five of these types of organized service continue to expand throughout the world, in relation to a declining importance of private individualistic medical practice. The trend is toward integrated ambulatory service for both preventive and curative services in health centers. The staffing and scope of health centers vary with the economic development of a country and its prevailing political philosophy. As a result of dialectical dynamics between hospitals and ambulatory care centers, these two types of service are becoming integrated in regionalized networks, increasingly supported by funds from collective sources (both taxation and insurance) and designed through national health planning.

This chapter is based largely on a monograph prepared for the World Health Organization (Evaluation of Community Health Centers. Geneva: WHO, Public Health Paper No. 48, 1972) and was published separately as "Organized Ambulatory Health Service in International Perspective" in the International Journal of Health Services. *(Vol. 1, No. 1, February 1971, pp. 18-27, Greenwood Periodicals, Inc., publisher). It is reprinted here by permission of Baywood Publishing Company.[1]*

From a global perspective on health service, we seem to be entering a period when the major social focus is shifting from hospital care to care of the ambulatory patient. Measured in expenditures, hospitalization still absorbs the largest portion of the health service outlay, but more and more organized social effort is clearly being directed to the improved delivery of out-of-hospital services.

It may help in getting an appreciation of current trends of community health care in the United States, if we take a look at developments in other countries. Everywhere the effort to improve health services is expressed through organization—mobilizing teams of health personnel, equipment, and facilities, so as to provide an enhanced quantity and quality of services. Organization occurs also in

the work of the individual health practitioner, but the impressive trend is toward increasing replacement of independent service—whether it be from a traditional healer or a modern scientific practitioner—by service emanating from various forms of organized framework. In a sense, the organization of persons, things, and processes that has long characterized hospitals is coming to be applied increasingly to ambulatory service. It is this trend toward organization of out-of-hospital care around the world that will be reviewed in this chapter. But first a word of history.

BACKGROUND

The first organization of health service to the noninstitutionalized patient was oriented to the treatment of the poor. In the seventeenth century, doctors of Paris, and later London, established a consultation service to help the poor.[2] This was offered in a building unrelated to any hospital; it was many years before outpatient departments were organized in hospitals. Since drugs were dispensed, these units came to be called "dispensaries." It is worth recalling that in colonial America of the eighteenth century, separate dispensaries were also organized in New York, Philadelphia, and Boston.[3]

It was only in the eighteenth and nineteenth centuries that hospitals began to establish clinics for the ambulatory patient. Like their inpatients, the outpatients were also expected to be poor, since anyone with adequate financial resources was expected to see a private physician for medical care. With the rise of social insurance in Europe, working people of low income were enabled to see private doctors (whose fees were paid by the insurance funds) but these were essentially limited to general practitioners. For specialist care, a hospital outpatient department would have to be consulted, but insured workers did not want to be objects of the charity identified with hospitals. Therefore, the insurance funds organized separate ambulatory centers, defined as "polyclinics," for specialist care. Later, beds for the care of insured and other private patients were added to these polyclinics.[4]

Organized clinics for purely preventive services did not come until the early twentieth century. These were started first by voluntary bodies, and later by official public health agencies, for the welfare of babies, including the distribution of milk to the poor. Special clinics were also organized for tuberculosis and venereal disease. In factories, health stations were organized for first aid to injured workers, and in schools clinics were set up for examinations, immunizations, and first aid of schoolchildren. All these ideas originated in Europe and were soon transplanted to America.[5]

In the sphere of private ambulatory medical care, the idea of organization actually originated in the United States. Here, unlike in Europe, specialist service was not tied to the hospital. In the hospital outpatient department for the poor, a range of specialty services could be provided, but for the private patient consultation with specialists meant visits to several different places. To coordinate the specialties and to bring specialty service to small towns, the private medical clinic or "group practice" idea was launched, starting with the initiative of the Mayo brothers in Rochester, Minnesota in 1887. The idea soon spread in the midwest and western states, more slowly in the urbanized east.[6] In other countries,

group practice of private doctors came later, and in other forms, as we shall see.

With the intent of bringing several streams of development together, another idea took shape in Europe in 1920. In that year the British Consultative Council on Medical and Allied Services, chaired by Lord Dawson of Penn, issued a report advocating a network of "health centers."[7] These were to be located in every neighborhood and were to combine the preventive services of local public health authorities and the primary treatment services of general medical practitioners. They were to be open to everyone, not just the poor, and the preventive and curative services were to be integrated in their day-to-day operations. A few years later, the same concept was proposed by Dr. Hermann Biggs, Health Commissioner of New York State and by Dr. J. L. Pomeroy, Health Officer of Los Angeles County, although the integrated services of these health centers were to be limited to the poor.[8, 9]

The 1920s, however, in the aftermath of World War I, were a period of "back to normalcy" and conservatism. In this climate, the proposals of Lord Dawson, of Drs. Biggs and Pomeroy, and doubtless others, did not fall on fertile ground. The private medical profession was growing stronger and doctors objected to the idea of a facility that might either present serious economic competition or employ them as salaried servants of the state. Therefore, the health center idea soon became restricted to the provision of purely preventive services, leaving treatment to the private doctor—or, for the poor, to the charitable dispensary or hospital outpatient department.[10]

Thus, when the health center concept was first implemented, it was not in Europe or America at all, but in a rural British colony, and it was purely preventive in purpose. In 1926, the village of Kalutura, Ceylon became the site of a small structure staffed to offer health examination of mothers and babies, immunizations, midwifery, health education, and environmental sanitation services.[11] Ambulatory treatment was not provided, on the grounds that this was the function of hospital outpatient departments and that its provision would overwhelm the staff so that preventive services would be neglected. The Rockefeller Foundation played a key role in the pioneering program at Kalutura, and in its health work in other developing countries it stressed the same purely preventive viewpoint. With the massive problems of infectious disease and enormous infant mortality rates of Asia, Africa, and Latin America, this preventive emphasis was quite understandable. When the League of Nations held a European Conference on Rural Hygiene in 1931, its advocacy of "rural health centres" was also restricted to units with an essentially preventive purpose.[12]

It took a social revolution in czarist Russia to achieve broad implementation of the Lord Dawson concept of the health center. Soon after the 1917 Revolution, the health services of the Soviet Union were completely reorganized on the basis of health centers, providing integrated preventive and primary curative services.[13] Under a socialist government, medical entrepreneurship was cast aside, and doctors (along with other health personnel) were engaged on salary by the Ministry of Health. Later, the health centers were placed under the control of hospitals, which served at the hub of regionalized health care modules.[14]

Not until after the worldwide depression of the 1930s and the sufferings of World War II was the concept of the integrated health center, combining preventive and curative goals, widely accepted. One of the most important milestones was the report of the Health Survey and Planning Commission of India, chaired by Sir Joseph Bhore, and published in 1946.[15] Among other things, this monumental study advocated a network of primary health centers for both curative and preventive service to blanket this large country. Similar plans were made after the independence of Indonesia from the Dutch following World War II, and in the nations of the Indochina peninsula after independence from the French.[16]

It is interesting to note that nations coming under the influence of the United States moved to the integrated health center concept somewhat later. In Latin America, the policy of the Institute of Inter-American Affairs, set up by the United States during World War II, was to promote purely preventive functions in health centers, and this did not change to an integrated approach until the mid-1950s.[17] The same preventive focus is seen in the rural health centers of postwar Greece under the aid of the Truman Doctrine.[18] Likewise, in Japan, under the occupation of American military forces, the Ministry of Health established several hundred health centers throughout the nation, but their functions were solely preventive and they were quite unrelated to the system of medical care through private doctors, financed by various insurance plans.[19]

In summary of these historical trends, we can discern at least five main paths along which ambulatory or out-of-hospital services have been organized: (1) the separate dispensary for treatment of the sick, (2) the hospital outpatient department, (3) specialized preventive clinics under public health agencies, industries, or schools, (4) private group medical practice, and (5) health centers of either preventive or integrated preventive-curative scope.

THE CURRENT SCENE

Looking around the world today, we see the continuation of all these types of community health service. The trend is clearly toward expansion of the integrated model, but all the types seem to be growing, at the expense of purely individualistic medical practice.

The separate dispensary or clinic for treatment of the sick is still found in many places. The Latin American social security programs, for example, operate many free-standing clinics for medical care, while preventive services are available only at other facilities operated by ministries of health.[20] There are also numerous special public emergency clinics in these countries, unattached to hospitals and open to everyone. Separate large polyclinics are still found in some Western European cities, and an occasional welfare department in the United States still operates a special dispensary for the poor. On the whole, however, this model is a changing breed.[21] The separate curative facility is widening its scope to include preventive service or is becoming absorbed into the administration of a hospital.

Hospital outpatient departments are generally expanding everywhere. In Europe, as well as in all the developing continents, they are the major locales for provision of ambulatory services by specialists. As specialization of medicine has increased and as general rates of medical care utilization have risen everywhere, the importance of hospital outpatient departments has enlarged.[22] One finds in the more recently constructed hospitals everywhere an enlarging proportion of space devoted to the outpatient clinics, in relation to the wards for inpatients.

Larger hospitals tend to have numerous specialty clinics for medicine, surgery, obstetrics, pediatrics, and so on. Indeed, one of the most widely perceived problems in many countries is the fragmentation of care in these specialized clinics, with no primary physician taking an overview of the patient. This is seen in the large municipal hospitals for the poor in the United States, no less than in the urban hospitals of India or the provinical general hospitals of Malaysia. It is less of a problem in Great Britain or the Soviet Union, where every patient has a primary general practitioner who is ordinarily responsible for referrals to the hospital outpatient department.[23]

In smaller district hospitals of the developing world, the outpatient department is usually nonspecialized and sees patients as they come. Typically, these clinics are overcrowded and under-staffed; patients usually come early in the morning and simply wait their turn, but they may come at any hour of the day or night. In American general hospitals, this is the function of the so-called emergency room. The demands on emergency room services have been steadily mounting in the United States, as people of all income levels are finding it difficult to get an early appointment with a private doctor; hence, the great bulk of emergency room services today are for conditions that are not truly definable as medical or surgical emergencies.[24]

Regarding specialized preventive clinics, they are operated most extensively for babies and expectant mothers and for certain communicable diseases such as tuberculosis or venereal disease. In the wealthier industrialized countries, these are often separate programs under the direction of a public health agency, or, as in Holland, a voluntary agency. In the developing countries, these services are usually part of the general program of a health center, as applies also in the socialist countries. Clinics for industrial workers in factories and for schoolchildren in schools, on the other hand, are common in both the industrialized capitalist countries and in the socialist countries, but seldom in the developing countries. A few countries have put special emphasis on dental clinics in the schools, especially Scandinavian countries, Great Britain, and New Zealand.[25] Special clinics for alcoholism, drug addiction, or general mental illness have also been increasing in the industrialized nations, as these psychosocial problems have become more serious.

The private group medical practice movement has had its greatest vitality in the United States and Canada, where private specialty medicine as a whole has greatest strength.[26] But in other countries, group practice has also grown, though in other forms than the North American. In Great Britain, for example, groups of general practitioners have been forming at an increasing rate.[27] Most of these groups are composed of only two or three doctors, but the pattern has become so common that it is currently estimated that hardly twenty-five percent of British general practitioners remain in purely solo practice. In the last few years, moreover, there has been a marked tendency for general practitioners to move into health centers, operated by local public health authorities; the doctors see their own patients (on their capitation panels) and pay rental to the local government, but they are in close association with the preventive clinics and visiting nurse services of the local health department.[28]

Group practices of both multispecialty and general practitioner types are also found in the Scandinavian countries, West Germany, and Holland; they are infrequent but growing.[29] France has been having a more rapid growth of teams of doctors, paid by salary, under the encouragement of the social security system.[30] These teams actually describe their practices as "centres de santé" (health centers), although they are not operated by units of government. Many of these private health centers also offer preventive maternal and child health services, which in France are a condition for receiving monetary family allowances.

In the United States, the growth of group medical practice in recent years has become increasingly rapid. Defining it as three or more physicians practicing cooperatively with sharing of income, the latest national survey (by the American Association of Medical Clinics) found over 6,000 such group practices, with 39,000 physicians.[31] This is about fifteen percent of active physicians (nonfederal and nonretired), which compares with six percent in 1950. About one-third of these doctors are in single-specialty groups, sixty percent are in multispecialty groups, and the balance (about seven percent) are in small general practice groups. Hardly two percent of all these group practices are affiliated with prepayment plans, although, being larger, these contain about ten percent of the group doctors; these prepaid group practices give greatest attention to preventive service, but it is clear that most American group practice is essentially curative in orientation.

The Health Center

Coming finally to the health center, the development of the concept from a purely preventive to an integrated preventive-curative orientation has been discussed. Today we see both types throughout the world, but the swing is toward the integrated type.

Outside of North America and Western Europe, the health center is probably the place where most people have their greatest contact with scientific health service. In the villages and rural areas of Asia, Africa, and Latin America, the local traditional healer may be the most frequently used resource for curative care, but insofar as scientifically grounded service—preventive or curative—is obtained, the health center is the most common place. In general, health centers serving rural populations tend to have the most integrated approach, while those in the larger cities tend to be more exclusively preventive, on the assumption that a hospital outpatient department is nearby to treat sickness.[32]

The exact range of functions, staffing, and administrative structure of health centers, of course, shows great variety among nations. In the very poorest countries, such as those of Africa, health centers are typically very simple structures staffed only by auxiliary personnel.[33] The African "dresser" or other medical assistant usually has formal training less than that of a diploma nurse in this country; six years of basic schooling followed by two years of hospital training or apprenticeship would be one illustrative pattern (though there are great variations). Yet, at a rural station he is authorized to diagnose and treat, usually with drugs, nearly all the patients who come from a population of 10,000 to 20,000. He gives vaccinations, does minor surgery, and offers advice on environmental sanitation. He is supposed to refer patients who do not recover under his care or who present unusual symptoms to a district hospital, where a physician is located. If the health center is properly staffed, there will also be a midwife and various auxiliary nursing and environmental assistants on hand. Periodically, perhaps monthly or weekly, a physician may come by for supervision or consultation on specific cases. This is the frugal reality of ambulatory health services for African countries, nearly all of which until a few years ago were colonies of European powers, where the supply of doctors approximates one to 50,000 population (most of these few being in the main cities), where schools of medicine, nursing, dentistry, or pharmacy are just getting started.

In developing countries of somewhat greater economic strength, a physician is supposed to be on the health center staff, along with medical aides, nursing assistants, sanitation inspectors, midwives, a drug dispenser, and sometimes a laboratory technician. But vacancies in the medical position are common, and the rest of the staff is then on its own. A frequent pattern has such a health center for 20,000 to 30,000 population, with health posts or subcenters around it, staffed only by auxiliary personnel for about 5,000 population each. This is the model being developed in Syria and other Eastern Mediterranean countries.[34] In Malaysia and other Southeast Asian countries, a similar regionalized network is being evolved, but the population coverage of the "main health centers" is 50,000 to 75,000, with correspondingly larger populations served by each of the subsidiary units.[35]

In Latin American countries, the supply of doctors, nurses, and other health personnel has been rapidly improving, and the standards for health centers are somewhat higher than in Asia or Africa. There are, of course, great variations among these countries, but in the more prosperous of them, such as Chile, Venezuela, Jamaica, or Mexico, almost all rural health centers as well as the urban ones are staffed with doctors, and small health posts get visits from doctors

at least once a week.[36] The male medical assistant, with wide authority to diagnose and treat, is less used than in the former colonies of the East, and more use is made of ambulances to transport rural patients to large health centers or hospitals. In Cuba, since its 1959 Revolution, the distribution and staffing of health centers has been markedly improved.[37]

With respect to professional nurses—the equivalent of the American R.N. or the nurse with a college degree—there is a strange paradox in many countries of Latin America and elsewhere. For many social reasons (the lesser education of young women, the social class structure, attitudes toward manual work) there is a lower supply of professional nurses than of doctors. These well-trained nurses are kept in the main cities, working usually in the hospitals at the side of the doctor. In the rural health centers and health posts, the positions are filled by nursing assistants and nursing auxiliaries with much less training.[38] Yet these rural nursing personnel are only occasionally assisted or supervised by a doctor. Their responsibilities for solving the problems of patients in health centers are actually broader than are the responsibilities of urban hospital nurses, but their backgrounds of knowledge and skills are far less. One can explain these paradoxical inequities only in terms of a value system that places the health of rural people at a lower level than that of city-dwellers.

In the wealthier industrialized countries, the health center has meanings both more restrictive and more comprehensive. In the more restricted sense, the health center of the United States, Japan, or Australia is simply the locale for the preventive services of the local health department. In the broader sense, health centers in these countries provide a wide range of preventive and curative ambulatory services for all the people nearby. This is the pattern in Israel for units sponsored either by the Ministry of Health or the Workers Health Insurance Fund (the Kupat Holim).[39] It is the pattern in the Soviet Union and other socialist countries of Eastern Europe. It is the conception of the new wave of health centers being established in England and Scotland. It is basically the idea in the back of the "neighborhood health centers" launched recently by the U.S. Office of Economic Opportunity in the slum districts of American cities.[40] All these health centers typically have not one but several doctors, often including a number of specialists.

CONCLUSION

In summary of this polyglot picture of organized ambulatory or community-based or out-of-hospital health services around the world, what can one say?

Borrowing from Hegel and Marx, we can see a dialectical process in the provision of health care. The "thesis" was discernable in the founding and growth of hospitals for bed care of the seriously sick. With them came an enormous growth of medical specialization and development of more and more specialized health care programs. The reaction or "antithesis" has come in the application of technical and social organization to ambulatory service. Various types of clinics and health centers attempt to treat the patient while his illness is not yet grave, or better yet, to prevent disease while he is well. Part of this reaction is a renewed emphasis on primary health care, on overall health counseling and guidance of the patient and his family, in contrast to specialized therapy of the case. Part of it is also the intent to avoid hospitalization, which is everywhere more costly than care of the patient who is living at home.

The outcome of this conflict or the "synthesis"—whether we regard it as ideological or material—is, in my view, the theory and practice of regionalization.[41] With this movement, which we see evolving throughout the world, both the hospital-specialist and the ambulatory-generalist services are becoming coordinated into systems. This coordination involves the integration of curative and preventive services for the ambulatory patient and the close working relationship between ambulatory care—whether it be in a dispensary, a health center, or a private medical office—and hospital care. Meanwhile, knowledge and techniques have become so specialized that the effective provision of ambulatory service can no longer be done by the lone practitioner, but demands organized teams of health personnel.

There is a cost dimension to this whole dialectical process which we have not discussed. The path of progress—for the dialectical dynamics are simply a way of explaining social progress—has meant an increasing allocation of resources to the health sector. Both absolutely and relative to total wealth or gross national product, health service costs are rising. This means that the costs can be met for all strata of the population only through the use of collective financing—via tax funds, insurance, or other devices. It means removal of health service increasingly from the entrepreneurial market and establishing it as a social service available equitably to all, in relation to need.

This economic trend is proceeding at different paces in different countries, in relation to their dominant political philosophies.[42] Where the private market and economic individualism are strong, the process is slower than in countries where collectivism is stronger—whether from social reform, social revolution, or social responses to the threat of revolution. In these more collectivistic countries there are, of course, many gradations and we can detect a kind of struggle between individualist and collectivist philosophies. This may be illustrated, for example, in the Egyptian or the Peruvian doctor who is salaried by the state for services in a health center every morning, while he sees patients for private fees in the afternoons.

In countries of all political color, however, the process of collectivization of financing is visible, at some pace, along with the organization of the delivery of health services. This explains, in my view, the rapidly growing interest everywhere in comprehensive health planning—even in free-enterprise America where a few years ago "planning" was a dirty socialistic word.[43, 44] It also explains the mounting concern, as part of planning, for rationalization of the technical process of health care through maximum delegation of duties to auxiliary health personnel. When costs are mounting, derived from the whole population, and clearly visible, there is bound to be rising social concern for the training of appropriate types and adequate numbers of health manpower. Economic waste can be avoided only through a system in which both personnel and equipment are appropriate to their functions, and not more elaborately prepared than is necessary. At the same time quality can be maintained only if these resources are sufficiently well prepared to do the job which society demands.

This delicate balance of goals is the challenge presented today to all institutions engaged in the education of health workers. It is the reason why we are seeing so much fresh questioning today about the proper role of doctors and nurses and many new types of medical assistant. The social expectations of both economy and quality are also the forces in back of the increasing organization of ambulatory, community health services, throughout a world of heterogeneous nations, that this paper has attempted to review.

NOTES

[1] Paper presented at the Conference on Community Health Care, University of North Carolina, Chapel Hill, October 9, 1970.

[2] R. Sand, *The Advance to Social Medicine*. London: Staples Press, 1952.

[3] M. M. Davis and A. R. Warner, *Dispensaries: Their Management and Development*. New York: Macmillan Company, 1918.

[4] A. Newsholme, *Medicine and the State*. London: G. Allen and Urwin, Ltd., 1932.

[5] H. E. Sigerist, *Landmarks in the History of Hygiene*.

London: Oxford University Press, 1956.

⁶ H. E. Sigerist, *American Medicine*. New York: W. W. Norton and Company, Inc., 1935.

⁷ Ministry of Health, Consultative Council on Medical and Allied Services, *Interim Report on the Future of Medical and Allied Services*. London: His Majesty's Stationery Office, 1920.

⁸ M. Terris, "Hermann Biggs' Contribution to the Modern Concept of the Health Center." *Bulletin of the History of Medicine*, Vol. 20, No. 3, 1946, pp. 387-412.

⁹ J. L. Pomeroy, "Health Center Development in Los Angeles County." *Journal of the American Medical Association*, Vol. 93, November 16, 1929, pp. 1,546-1,550.

¹⁰ H. E. Handley, *Health Center Buildings*. New York: Commonwealth Fund, 1948.

¹¹ W. G. Wickremesinghe, *The Premier Health Unit in Ceylon*. Colombo: 1951.

¹² League of Nations Health Organization, European Conference on Rural Hygiene, *Recommendations on the Principles Governing the Organization of Medical Assistance, the Public Health Services and Sanitation in Rural Districts*. Geneva: 1931.

¹³ H. E. Sigerist, *Socialized Medicine in the Soviet Union*. New York: W. W. Norton and Company, Inc., 1938.

¹⁴ M. G. Field, *Soviet Socialized Medicine*. New York: The Free Press, 1967.

¹⁵ Health Survey and Development Committee (India), *Report of the Health Survey and Development Committee*. Delhi: Manager of Publications, 1946.

¹⁶ J. Leimana, *Demonstration or Experiments on Providing Units of Well-Organized Medical and Health Services for a Community or for a Special Group of the Population in Rural Areas of Indonesia*. Geneva: World Health Organization, October 1951.

¹⁷ See chapter 7.

¹⁸ American Friends of Greece, *Health Centers for Greece*: New York: 1944.

¹⁹ Japanese Ministry of Health and Welfare, *A Summary Account of the Development of Health Centers and Their Present Status*. Tokyo: 1952.

²⁰ A. L. Bravo, "Development of Medical Care Services in Latin America." *American Journal of Public Health*, Vol. 48, April 1958, pp. 434-437.

²¹ M. I. Roemer, "General Hospitals in Europe." In J. K. Owen (ed.), *Modern Concepts of Hospital Administration*. Philadelphia: W. B. Saunders Company, 1962, pp. 17-37.

²² See chapter 23.

²³ A. Lindsey, *Socialized Medicine in England and Wales: The National Health Service 1948-1961*. Chapel Hill: University of North Carolina Press, 1962.

²⁴ American Hospital Association, *Outpatient Health Care (A Report and Recommendations of a Conference on Hospital Outpatient Care)*. Chicago: AHA, 1968.

²⁵ D. J. Beck, "Evaluation of Dental Care for Children in New Zealand and the United States." *New Zealand Dental Journal*, Vol. 63, July 1967, pp. 201-211.

²⁶ B. E. Balfe and M. E. McNamara, *Survey of Medical Groups in the United States (1965)*. Chicago: American Medical Association, 1968.

²⁷ British Medical Association, *Report of the Working Party on Primary Medical Care*, Planning Unit Report No. 4 (Margot Jefferys, chairman). London: B.M.A., May 1970, p. 66.

²⁸ M. Curwen and B. Brookes, "Health Centers: Facts and Figures." *Lancet*, No. 7627, November 1, 1969, pp. 945-948.

²⁹ "Group Practice: Views from U.S. and Abroad." *Medical Tribune*, June 22, 1970, pp. 1 and 26.

³⁰ "Evolution des Centres de Santé et Organisation Sociale de la Médecine" (III Congres National des Médecins de Centres de Santé—Soins et Prévention). Supplement to *Centre de Santé*, April 1964.

³¹ "Group Practice Gains Predicted." *American Medical News*, September 14, 1970, pp. 1, 8-9.

³² World Health Organization, *Participation of Health Centres in Ambulatory Care*. Geneva: WHO (unpublished document), February 11, 1959.

³³ Maurice King (ed.), *Medical Care in Developing Countries (A Primer on the Medicine of Poverty and a Symposium from Makerere)*. Nairobi (Kenya): Oxford University Press, 1966.

³⁴ Central Treaty Organization, Subcommittee on Health, *Conference on Teaching Health Centres–Report*. Ankara (Turkey): 1962.

³⁵ L. W. Jayesura, *A Review of the Rural Health Services in West Malaysia*. Kuala Lumpur: Ministry of Health, 1967.

³⁶ M. A. Byer, R. J. Gourlay, and K. L. Standard, "The Role of the Health Centre in an Integrated Health Programme in a Developing Country." *Medical Care* (London), Vol. 4, January-March 1966, pp. 26-29.

³⁷ W. P. Butler, "Cuba's Revolutionary Medicine." *Ramparts*, February 1970.

³⁸ M. I. Roemer. Personal observations in Venezuela, Peru, and other Latin American countries.

³⁹ S. Btesh, *The Health Centre: Its Philosophy and Function*. Jerusalem: Ministry of Health, May 1956.

⁴⁰ J. D. Stoeckle and L. M. Candib, "The Neighborhood Health Center—Reform Ideas of Yesterday and Today." *New England Journal of Medicine*, Vol. 280, June 19, 1969, pp. 1,385-1,391.

⁴¹ H. R. Leavell, "Regionalization of Health Services." Geneva: World Health Organization (unpublished document), 1969.

⁴² B. Abel-Smith, *An International Study of Health Expenditure and Its Relevance for Health Planning*. Geneva: World Health Organization, 1967.

⁴³ Pan American Health Organization, *Health Planning: Problems of Concept and Method*. Washington, D.C.: P.A.H.O., April 1965.

⁴⁴ I. Cater, W. R. Willard, E. I. Sox, and P. G. Rogers, "Comprehensive Health Planning." *American Journal of Public Health*, Vol. 58, June 1968, pp. 1,022-1,038.

Chapter XXIII
National Hospital Systems
in Thirteen Countries

Everywhere in the world, hospitals have come to play an enlarging role in the provision of health service–not only as places for treatment of the seriously sick, but as centers for provision or supervision of all types of health service in a geographic region. Inevitably, therefore, hospitals have come under the increasing influence of government, with respect to both their initial construction and their standards of operation. The forms taken by this public influence, however, differ in relation to the political structure and the stage of economic development of nations.

In 1966 the World Health Organization undertook to study national hospital systems and hospital legislation in a number of countries. The countries were selected to represent different stages of economic development and different points along a political spectrum ranging from localism to centralism in the exercise of public authority. These countries are: Bulgaria, Chile, France, Great Britain, Iran, Israel, Malaysia, the Philippines, Peru, the Soviet Union, Sweden, Togo, and the United States.

This chapter is a summary of the principal features and trends in these thirteen countries, from which data were gathered by field visits, questionnaires, and study of documents in the World Health Organization files and library. In a preliminary form, this appeared as an unpublished WHO document, a working paper for the WHO Expert Committee on Hospital Administration, under the title "Hospital Systems in Different Nations" (Geneva, Ocotber 1967). Later it appeared, in modified form, as one chapter in a WHO publication–R. F. Bridgman and M. I. Roemer, Hospital Legislation and Hospital Systems. *Geneva: WHO, Public Health Paper No. 50, 1973. It is reprinted here by permission.*

GENERAL TRENDS IN HOSPITAL ORGANIZATION

In all nations, hospitals have been established as important resources for the provision of health services. While starting in all cultures as places for the treatment, in bed, of the seriously sick, they have gradually widened their scope of activities. Likewise, they have gradually come to serve broader demographic groups, initially being devoted to military men or to the indigent and now usually serving the whole population.

The methods of establishment of hospitals in various countries have had much in common, but there have also been significant differences; more variable than their origins have been their patterns of administration and operations. In spite of this, one can detect in different nations certain common trends in hospital organization. These seem to be in response to the demands of science and technology which—despite differences in the cultural and political settings of countries—exert certain more or less uniform influences. In all nations, therefore, both the establishment and operation of hospitals appear to be undergoing a rising degree of planning and systematic controls. The precise forms taken by this movement differ greatly among the nations, but the goal everywhere appears to be similar—namely to apply the techniques of medical science in the most efficient manner that is consistent with the national culture.

While the thirteen national hospital systems reviewed here cannot be claimed to be a perfect sample of all the countries of the world, they are believed to be illustrative of the principal patterns along the two conceptual dimensions used: economic development and hospital authority patterns. (See table XXIII.I.) In this chapter an attempt is made to present a composite account of the eight aspects of the subject which were used to define a hospital system, relating these to the cells in the conceptual matrix in which the countries fall. To a limited extent, observations will be drawn from experiences in some countries not included among the thirteen reviewed in detail.

HISTORIC DEVELOPMENT OF HOSPITALS

The earliest hospitals were developed for soldiers of the ancient Roman legions, unless one regards the still earlier Aesculapian temples of healing as equivalent to hospitals. There were also ancient *valetudinaria* for slaves, whose recovery from illness represented a preservation of productive manpower.

The hospitals of today, however, are usually traced to Europe of the Middle Ages when, under the influence of the Christian church, buildings were established for sheltering the sick, the aged, and the destitute. Some of these houses of shelter were associated with monasteries, others with the cathedrals in the large cities. A somewhat similar development occurred with religious inspiration in the Moslem world, though not so directly tied to the Church. The line between church and state in medieval Europe was not so clear as it is today, and many of the early hospitals involved a sharing of responsibilities between secular and clerical authorities.

As hospitals grew in the main cities, and as urban populations increased, the cost of operating these institutions for the sick and the poor also rose. Even while their ownership and control were largely religious, therefore, financial support was solicited from and provided by local government, especially in cities like Paris and London. In the sixteenth century, representatives of the public authorities came to be represented on the boards of directors of hospitals, in order to exert greater influence. Also, city governments began to establish new hospitals themselves. Medical science meanwhile was developing, and the hospital was becoming a place more clearly for the sick, as distinguished from the aged or destitute. It was some years further, however, before hospitals came to serve the self-supporting sick, as distinguished from the indigent sick.

Table XXIII.1 National Hospital Systems by Level of the Nation's Economic Development and Its Hospital Authority Pattern			
National Economic Development	Hospital Authority Pattern		
	Localized	Moderately Centralized	Highly Centralized
Weak	Peru	Philippines	Togo Malaysia
Moderate	Israel	Iran Chile	Bulgaria U.S.S.R.
Strong	United States	France Sweden	England & Wales

Through the seventeenth and eighteenth centuries hospitals expanded under both religious and secular authorities, with increasing importance for the latter. In Latin America, colonized by Spain and Portugal, the pattern of religious sponsorship was carried over with the founding of scores of *beneficencia* hospitals. When wealthy persons died, they often bequeathed valuable properties to the hospital, from which income would be earned. Gradually, as in Europe, rising costs led to governmental subsidy of these facilities, and with this certain controls.

Larger political events, like the French Revolution (1789) or the Mexican Revolution (1910), led to governmental supervision of church activities in civil life. Hospitals formerly under church control were taken over by governments completely, and usually assigned to administration by cities or provinces. The relative balance between church and state, however, varied in different countries. The socialist revolutions of the twentieth century led to sweeping conversion of pluralistic hospital ownership and operation into nationalized networks under a single governmental authority.

In the early nineteenth century a new type of hospital sponsorship emerged: the "voluntary" nonsectarian institution. A group of citizens, often aided by one or two large benefactors, would establish a general hospital without involvement of either church or state. Financial support would be derived from charitable donations, from the payment of fees by patients (now that nonindigent persons began to use hospitals), and later by subsidy from government for the care of the poor. This pattern became especially prominent in England and in the British colonies overseas, including North America, Australia, and India.

In the later nineteenth century, another important socioeconomic development in Europe had great influence on hospitals: the birth of social insurance. This source of relatively stable economic support for medical care of workers and their dependents led to the financial (and therefore technical) strengthening of existing hospitals, and also the establishment of new ones. Now the hospital care of working class families could be paid for by an insurance fund, on a more adequate basis than had been forthcoming from charity or public funds. Many polyclinics were constructed directly by social insurance funds, as well as special hospitals for tuberculosis and occasionally some general hospitals. In Latin America of the twentieth century, many large and impressive general hospitals came to be built by social security programs for insured persons and sometimes their dependents.

Also in the late nineteenth century there were enormous technical developments in medicine which led to the greater appreciation of the hospital as a place of choice for treatment of serious illness, regardless of a person's economic status. With asepsis, vast improvements in surgery, anesthesia, the development of professional nursing, etc., hospitals became centers of medical science as well as of care of the unfortunate sick. Medical schools became increasingly affiliated with large hospitals.

Recognition of the infectiousness of tuberculosis and the possibilities of cure through prolonged bed rest gave rise to the sanatorium. But to be economical these usually had to be large, and the most practical sponsorship was a larger unit of government than the city or commune. Hence, the province or *département* (in Latin America the *departemento*) or state, and sometimes the national government, established these institutions. A similar development applied to asylums for the insane or mental hospitals.

National governments also established hospitals for certain populations of national importance. Military personnel and police usually came first, and hospital barracks of a simple type had been established for them even in earlier centuries. Merchant mariners were provided special hospitals at the main ports of England and in the early postrevolutionary United States of America (1798) by the national authorities. Later in the nineteenth century special hospital systems were developed for railroad workers. In the twentieth century, other servants of the national government, especially in the less well-developed countries, were provided with separate hospitals

Private industry in the late nineteenth and early twentieth centuries also came to recognize the value of medically protected workers. In the main cities, hospital care was available in public or voluntary institutions, but in isolated locations there was nothing. Hence, in mining or lumbering settlements, small hospitals were developed directly by the industrial management and these served both the workers and their families. In the underdeveloped countries of Latin America, Africa, and Asia, such small private industrial hospitals were often established on sugar plantations, tea estates, and other agricultural enterprises, as well as at mines or isolated factories. The workmen's compensation legislation from 1883 onward encouraged the establishment of some of these hospitals, since the employer was compelled anyway to meet the medical costs of industrial injuries.

In colonial territories, the mother country (usually European) tended to duplicate, to some extent, the pattern of hospital organization at home. In the French colonies, the pattern of local governmental hospital boards, subject to clear centralized controls, was applied. As noted, voluntary nonsectarian hospitals were established overseas by the British, church-related hospitals by the Spanish. At the same time, the colonial governments were, of course, much more centralized than the governments at home since local public authorities had no significant role. Hospitals in the African colonies and elsewhere, therefore, were set up by the central governments—first in the colonial capitals and then in the provincial towns. As these colonies have become emancipated as autonomous nations, the strong centralized control of public hospitals has usually been maintained.

Religious missions from Europe and North America have also established hospitals in Africa, Asia, and elsewhere as an aspect of spreading the Christian gospel. These have been constructed from distant charities, but often maintained by local payments and contributions—sometimes even from governments. As countries of Africa and Asia (especially India) have developed their own hospital systems, these mission hospitals have often become incorporated in them.

Finally, in the twentieth century, some hospitals have been established as purely private commercial enterprises. In the main cities throughout the world, there has usually developed (except in the socialist countries) a strong private practice of medicine. Usually with the combined support of these private physicians and wealthy families, "proprietary" hospitals, serving high income or upper middle class families, have been established. These are typically small and very well provided with nursing personnel and modern equipment. They serve only those who can pay relatively high prices, although sometimes they accept injured workmen covered by workmen's compensation programs or other patients covered by social insurance or private insurance.

A special variant of the proprietary facility is the "private society" hospital established in many colonial or formerly colonial countries by well-to-do families from a particular European nation. The Spanish, the British, the French, the German settlers overseas have set up societies which build and operate hospitals for their own members. Sometimes care is provided also to indigent persons of the same national background, but most of the hospitalization is privately paid for. These are nonprofit institutions, but they are not open to the general population, as are other voluntary nonprofit or public institutions.

This brief historical account of the development of hospitals under different sponsorships throughout the world may help set the stage for understanding current patterns of hospital organization in different nations. The relative strengths of the different channels of hospital development vary, of course, among the countries. Likewise in every country there has been an evolution, in which the relative importance of one sector or another in the hospital spectrum has changed in the wake of larger political and economic changes. In the next section, we will examine the current characteristics of this variable spectrum or mixture of hospital ownership or sponsorship around the world.

HOSPITAL OWNERSHIP PATTERNS

With the multiple origins of hospitals just sketched, it is evident that most countries today have a mixture of hospital ownerships. The proportions in the mixture, however, are highly variable, and they are changing every day. The relative distribution of hospital ownership in a country has great importance for the purposes of hospital planning. If the direct responsibility for a hospital lies in private hands—whether religious, nonsectarian and nonprofit, industrial, or purely proprietary—it is obviously more difficult to integrate the operation of that hospital within an overall system than if all hospitals are governmentally owned. On the other hand, many advantages are gained by the sponsorship of local and voluntary hospital bodies—a spirit of initiative and hard work which has been responsible for some of the greatest achievements and innovations in the hospital field. These two philosophies, which are at first sight divergent, are found in a sort of continuous equilibrium throughout the world, and there seems to be evidence that they can be reconciled or blended in various ways.

Recalling the conceptual typology outlined earlier, we can examine briefly the patterns of hospital ownership in countries of different stages of economic development, where differing political philosophies are reflected in their hospital authority patterns. In Peru, the Catholic church is a powerful force and its *beneficencia* hospitals, with local semiautonomous boards, have forty-two percent of the general hospital beds. Along with hospitals under private industry or other proprietary ownership, fifty-six percent of the general hospital beds are in nongovernmental facilities. Israel has somewhat higher economic development, and most of its hospital beds are owned by voluntary insurance societies, other voluntary philanthropic bodies, or private proprietors; only forty-five percent of beds are under sponsorship of any level of government, central or local. In the highly developed countries of North America, both the United States and Canada, local and voluntary entities have greater importance than governmental authorities—for the health and welfare services as well as for other sectors of the economy.

In the United States of America, the majority of beds, about sixty-five percent, are actually owned by national, state, or local governmental authorities, but this is somewhat deceptive since these beds are largely in mental and tuberculosis hospitals serving long-term patients. In general hospitals, which account for ninety-five percent of all hospital *admissions* each year, sixty-seven percent of the beds are nongovernmental—whether voluntary nonprofit, church-supported, or proprietary. In Canada also, despite its national social insurance program for meeting hospital costs of the entire population, the actual ownership of general hospitals is predominantly by voluntary bodies.

Other countries appear to be in a middle range of partially centralized authority over their hospital systems—that is, they have developed considerable central control, while still having much autonomy in local hospital operations. The local autonomy may apply to hospitals under certain forms of nongovernmental sponsorship or it may apply to public hospitals under local levels of government.

The Philippines are at present an economically underdeveloped country in which centralized controls are strong, but only for governmental hospitals which contain less than half of the beds for general illness care. Iran has thirty-two percent of its general hospital beds under private auspices, but of the governmental beds less than half are owned by the central Ministry of Health, the others being distributed among several other governmental agencies. Chile has eighty percent of its beds owned by the national government under fairly strong central control, but twenty percent are owned by private bodies and are quite autonomous.

In the more highly industrialized and urbanized countries, it is *local* government (rather than voluntary body) control of hospitals that explains the "moderately centralized"authority pattern. In Sweden, almost eighty-four percent of the beds are in governmental hospitals, counting both general and special facilities. It is local units of government rather than central, however, that own and operate them. Essentially the same applies in France.

In countries with very highly centralized hospital authority patterns, the ownership is naturally at a corresponding level. An example of a highly rural African country is Togo, where ninety-seven percent of the beds are attached to the Ministry of Health. In Malaysia, while as many as seventeen percent of the beds are nongovernmental, they come under strong governmental influence and eighty-three percent are owned by the *central* level of government.

In the socialist countries, USSR and Bulgaria, virtually 100 percent of the beds are owned by the central ministry of health. In England, with its National Health Service, it is about ninety-six percent. The day-to-day management of these hospitals, nevertheless, is delegated to administrative bodies closer to the scene of operation—in Malaysia to state public health authorities, in the socialist countries to provinces and districts, in England to regional hospital boards. The ultimate powers of decision, however, rest with central ministries of health in these countries for nearly all existent institutions.

From these varying patterns of ownership there follow, of course, many implications for hospital operations. The more centralized ownership countries can maintain greater uniformity in internal hospital practices; the more localized patterns yield greater diversity. In spite of this, it is interesting to observe the flexibilities that tend to emerge even in the hospitals of centralized national cultures, where local imagination or initiative begins to express itself; the national standards tend to set a minimum floor, but not necessarily a ceiling on hospital services. On the other hand, in the more localized cultural settings, many uniformities tend to develop because of the influence of hospital legislation and also of nongovernmental movements for maintaining quality performance.

The long-term trend certainly appears to be toward a greater share of governmental ownership of hospitals on a world level. As medical technology has advanced and become more costly, and as popular expectations have risen along with this, the establishment of hospitals has increasingly required large economic resources, which can only be provided by government. This is particularly true in the less wealthy developing countries. The Philippine Republic is exceptional in its rapid growth of privately owned hospitals in recent years, and the new Iranian policy of encouraging doctor-owned hospitals in provincial towns is a unique experiment. Even these institutions, however, will depend on governmental support for services to many or most of their patients, who are indigent.

Moreover, as observed in the historical review, the economic survival of many religious or other voluntary hospitals has come often to depend on regular governmental subsidies. When such subsidies increase to a major proportion, political forces are set underway which often lead to the complete takeover of the voluntary hospital by public authorities, as happened in France and Mexico after their revolutions, in England after the launching of its National Health Service (1948), and in Chile after its *Servicio Nacional de Salud* (1952). In the socialist countries, of course, such nationalization of all hospitals has been complete.

Indeed, as programs of social financing of hospital services (through social security, private insurance, or general revenues) have advanced, and with them various quid pro quo standards, the line between public and private institutions has become more and more fuzzy. Even in highly individualistic countries, like the United States of America, it has become increasingly common to refer to hospitals as "public utilities" (like water or electrical power systems), whether their ownership is governmental, voluntary nonprofit, or even proprietary.

There are many fine points related to the ownership of hospitals which space does not permit us to discuss. Within the jurisdiction of government, there may be differing sponsoring agencies (for example, ministries of defense, of labor, of interior) which follow policies at great variance with ministries of health. In the hierarchy of central, provincial, and municipal governments, the degree of communication or of delegation of authority may be very different from one country to another. Hospitals developed by private industry or by semiautonomous social security programs may become absorbed into governmental networks (Argentina); on the other hand, hospitals owned by local government may become largely dependent on social security payments for their operation (France or Norway). The ferment in the field is high, and the identity of the original builder and sponsor of a hospital is getting to be less important than it used to be.

HOSPITAL CONSTRUCTION POLICIES

While hospitals over the centuries have been built mainly by the initiative of local individuals or groups, private or governmental, in response to the locally perceived needs, the last fifty years have seen the rise of a new perspective. Improvements in transportation, the advances of medical science, and the rise of the concept of health care as a basic human right have led almost everywhere to the principle of "hospital planning." This principle refers to a deliberate effort to construct hospitals of reasonable size and function at locations appropriate to the ecology of populations. (The phrase "hospital planning" should not be confused with the architectural design of individual hospital buildings, which is also sometimes referred to as "planning.")

In countries of all degrees of localized versus centralized hospital authority, planning is being undertaken. At the localized end of the range, however, the scope and impact of the planning are less extensive. The hospital planning in Peru is effective for governmental hospitals of the Ministry of Health, but not for facilities under other auspices. In Israel each of the main sponsoring organizations has its own planning activities, but they are not integrated with each other.

In the state health departments of the United States of America or the provincial health departments of Canada, there are hospital bureaus which are theoretically responsible for hospital planning throughout their jurisdictions. One must say "theoretically," however, because the enforcement powers of these agencies are limited; they tend to be restricted to those hospitals which are entitled to receive governmental subsidies for construction, but not to other hospitals. Regarding the majority of hospital construction projects, there are sometimes *voluntary* "regional" or "metropolitan" hospital councils which attempt to influence new hospital construction on the basis of persuasion or informal advice to private donors to construction costs. This entire movement for deliberately controlled hospital planning, however, is actively expanding. In a few states of the United States of America, for example, legislation has been passed (New York) or is under consideration (Michigan, Illinois) which would grant the state health department complete authority to approve or disapprove all proposed hospital construction, public or private.[1]

The countries of moderate centralization in hospital policies exert somewhat greater influence in hospital planning. Insofar as hospital beds are owned by governmental agencies in a higher proportion, the impact of governmental planning bodies tends to be stronger.

Both the Philippines and Iran have national planning offices for hospital construction. Five-year plans and seven-year plans for the total economies have included sections on health services and hospitals. In both these developing countries, the major effort is going toward construction in the rural areas, where spontaneous voluntary initiative has always been weakest. In Chile where a larger proportion of total hospital beds are under the central government, almost all new construction has been consistent with an overall hospital master plan.

In the more industrialized countries with stronger local governments, national hospital planning must be carried out in cooperation with the local authorities. Both France and Sweden have national offices of hospital planning, but they work in conjunction with similar commissions or councils at the regional or local governmental level. While the influence of these planning agencies on private hospital construction may be limited, the relatively small proportion of private beds and the modest financial resources for private hospital construction mean that nearly all new hospital projects in recent years have been part of the public system.

In the countries of highly centralized hospital authority, planning is naturally of widest scope. Decisions on virtually all new hospital construction are ultimately made at the national ministry level. This is true even though recommendations may originate at local governmental levels—in the states of Malaysia, the *oblasts* of the USSR, or the regional hospital boards of England. Even if new hospitals are to be launched with purely local funds—as in the collective farms of the Soviet Union—they must be approved at the top, since their future operating costs will have to be met by the national system of health services.

Hospital planning has both a positive and a negative aspect; it means the deliberate launching of new or expanded facilities deemed to be necessary for the population, and also the prohibition of hospital construction deemed not to be sound in the light of medical or economic considerations. The negative aspect is easily enough enforced in the more centralized countries, but not so easily in the more localized countries. The positive aspect, on the other hand, is easy to implement everywhere so far as political authority is concerned, but it often faces economic obstacles. New hospital construction is expensive and the best of plans depend for their execution on the availability of funds from public or private sources.

The financial support of hospital construction, like geographic planning, varies with the authority pattern, but it depends especially also on the economic affluence of the country. In the more localized pattern countries, with their greater diversity of hospital sponsorships, the costs of construction are met by the diverse voluntary, proprietary, or governmental (local, provincial, national) bodies. In Peru or Israel, for example, construction costs would come from voluntary charitable societies, social insurance organizations, private investors, or governmental authorities, depending on the sponsorship. The relative proportion of monies from nongovernmental sources, however, is larger in the United States with its greater general affluence. The economic strength of local government, furthermore, compared with national, is greater, so that more hospital construction funds come from local and state than from national authorities.

In this type of country, moreover, even within a single hospital construction project, the sources of financing may be multiple. National or state (provincial) governments may give construction grants even to voluntary (both religious and nonsectarian) hospitals. Thus a voluntary hospital may be built with funds derived from (1) private philanthropic donations, (2) governmental grants, and (3) loans from a bank which will be amortized over the future years from the earnings for patient care (paid by hospitalization insurance, private fees, governmental payments for the indigent, etc.). A hospital of local government may receive construction subsidies from higher governmental levels and may float public bonds, which will be repaid also through future income for patient care. Hospitals under provincial or national governmental ownership tend to be constructed entirely from governmental revenues.

In the countries with moderately centralized hospital authority patterns, government is the main source of construction funds, but the level differs according to the degree of economic development. In the economically weaker countries (the Philippines, Iran, and Chile) it is almost entirely national government. Included in this must be counted the resources of social security agencies, like that in Iran, which is a national governmental agency even though it is outside the Ministry of Health. In the economically stronger countries (France and Sweden), the major construction costs come from local government. Voluntary hospitals in these countries may also receive construction grants from government, insofar as they will be serving indigent patients in the future.

The countries of central authority patterns, at all stages of economic development, finance their new hospital construction almost exclusively from governmental sources. The revenues come nearly entirely, moreover, from national governments. The mechanism of handling funds is, of course, quite different among countries like Malaysia, the Soviet Union, or England, but the assumption of financial responsibility for hospital construction by the national government is the same in principle.

In all three authority patterns, it is evident that in the less economically developed countries, hospital construction is dependent much more heavily on governmental financing, especially at the national level. The wellsprings of charity in these countries are usually not very abundant, and the relative wealth of the churches, in relation to high modern hospital costs, is not so great as in former centuries. In the more highly developed countries, on the other hand, it is the local level of government that is usually important—except under the most centralized authority patterns (the Soviet Union and England).

Regardless of the strength of hospital planning in a country, or the pattern of financing of its construction, there is a third feature of hospital construction of great importance: the promulgation of physical standards of construction or architectural design. The worldwide trend in this sphere is also clear— namely the increasing imposition of minimum standards by government—national, provincial, or local.

Even in the highly localized pattern countries, laws have been passed specifying minimum standards of physical design. The provision of adequate space per hospital bed; proper water supply and sewage disposal; physical layout to prevent crossinfection; minimal laboratory, x-ray, and surgical equipment; protection against radiation; proper kitchen and laundry facilities; etc. are usually covered by these regulations. Usually, these standards are intended for hospitals of all types of sponsorship, though the application of the rules is likely to be more rigorous in public institutions.

The letter of the law, on these standards, is often more impressive than the practice, since the staffing of public health agencies responsible for inspection and enforcement is typically very limited.

In the moderately centralized authority patterns, there is a substantial difference in the application of construction standards as between the lesser and the more developed economies. In the Philippines, Iran, and Chile the ministry of health staff responsible for hospitals has little if any time for supervising nongovernmental hospital construction, but governmental hospital construction—being done by national authorities—requires no external supervision since the standards are applied by the same ministry as launches the construction. In France and Sweden, on the other hand, the construction of the great majority of hospitals is done by local governmental authorities, so that central government must see to it that physical standards are being met. As for nongovernmental hospital construction, the volume is small and the central authorities can exercise reasonable surveillance.

In the highly centralized hospital systems, the problem of enforcement of construction standards is different. Virtually all hospital construction is financed and executed by a centralized ministry of health, so that the application of standards is automatic, not involving an external "licensing" process. Model architectural plans are used, in large measure, throughout the nation. The major problem is not one of administrative authority, but of the amplitude of funds to construct facilities with high enough physical standards.

The general level of hospital construction standards in all types of country is rising. Physical design is encouraging greater sensitivity to the personal needs of patients (e.g., wards with only four to eight beds, rather than thirty beds), as well as the demands of modern medicine. There is also increasing emphasis on outpatient facilities, as hospitals are evolving into comprehensive centers of health service for ambulatory care and prevention, as well as bed care. Relatively more space is being assigned to supportive diagnostic and therapeutic equipment, to expedite intensive patient care and shorten the average length of stay. A specialty of hospital architecture is being developed in many countries and many of the construction standards are being spread by informal communication and example rather than by official regulation. As new architectural ideas gain currency, they tend to become embodied in manuals of hospital design issued by ministries of health, intended either as mandatory or advisory standards.

LEGAL CONTROLS OVER HOSPITAL OPERATIONS

In all countries, there is some system of external and official controls over the operation of hospitals just as there are controls with respect to hospital construction. The degree of rigor of these controls, however, varies with the political philosophy of the government and its hospital authority system.

In the localized pattern countries, the day-to-day operations of hospitals are subject to very little external surveillance. The governing bodies of *beneficencia* or social security institutions in Peru, or of the Kupat Holim or Hadassah hospitals in Israel exercise the controls without any systematic review by governmental authorities. Even within the governmental hospitals the operational discipline is not very rigorous.

In the United States of America there are laws in all the fifty states specifying minimum standards of hospital operations; these cover subjects such as nursing service, laboratory and x-ray procedures, record systems, operating theater, maternity service, etc. The level of enforcement, however, is relatively modest. Of greater impact perhaps is the influence of a nongovernmental body, the Joint Commission on Accreditation of Hospitals. Since "accreditation" by this body has come to carry great prestige (and is even recognized by governments for certain purposes—such as the treatment of cases under crippled children's programs of the states), most general hospitals attempt to meet its standards, which put great stress on sound organization of the medical staffs. Another localized pattern country of high economic development is the Netherlands; here each of the religiously based voluntary societies exercises supervision over its own hospital operations, as do the local governments with respect to their facilities.

In the weakly developed countries of the moderately centralized hospital authority level, operational controls over nongovernmental hospitals are also virtually nil. Most governmental hospitals, however, being organs of the central ministry of health are subject to day-to-day supervision. In Iran this supervisory responsibility has been delegated to the health officer of the *ostan* (province) and in Chile to the zone health officer, both of these being central government appointees.

In the more economically developed countries at this level (France and Sweden) hospital board decisions are subject to external review, but in different manners. In France, all hospital board actions must be reviewed by the prefect of the *département* (on advice of his public health officials) to be certain that they are consistent with national law and regulations. The prefect, moreover, is a centrally appointed official. Sweden, on the other hand, does not require such operational review by agents of the central government, but all board decisions of public hospitals (with the vast majority of beds) are approvable by the county council (local government) authorities.

In the highly centralized countries, all, or virtually all, the hospitals are part of a national system with a hierarchy of control over hospital operations which flows essentially from top to bottom. Of course, the day-to-day management is delegated to more localized bodies, but the general administrative policies that they follow have been determined at the central level. In a small African country, like Togo, these policies pass directly from the Ministry of Health to the individual hospital. In Malaysia, the central ministry policies are executed by the state chief medical health officers, to whom the hospital medical directors routinely report. In a larger European country, such as England, these policies are mediated through regional hospital boards, appointed by the Minister of Health, and then further delegated to the hospital management committees. In a large socialist country, like the USSR, the policies on hospital operations are delegated from the central Ministry of Health to the republic ministries and thence to the *oblast* health departments; from these agencies the responsibility is delegated to the *oblast* hospitals, where there is a chief physician who, in turn, is responsible for smaller *rayon* hospitals at the next lower level. Thus, while the channels of delegation are numerous, the ultimate determination of hospital administration policy is in the central government.

In practice, of course, there are great flexibilities in day-to-day hospital operations everywhere, even in countries with highly centralized authority patterns. The promulgation of rules from higher levels tends to set minimum standards, but these may be exceeded by energetic leadership within an institution. A great deal depends, of course, on access to money. If the hosptial must depend for all its operating funds on budgetary allotments from a higher authority then there are limits to its freedom of innovation—although within this budget there is always bound to be some leeway. A given dollar or peso may be spent in various ways. When operating funds are derived from local and diverse sources, the flexibilities are greater, but, by the same token, the level of performance may—in some institutions—fall rather low.

In very broad terms one may say that the trend of legal controls over hospital operations seems to be promoting a sort of equilibrium between centralized and localized responsibilities. Increasingly, minimal operating standards are being stipulated at a level above that of the individual hospital, whether that is a nongovernmental body, a local governmental authority, a national governmental agency other than the ministry of health or the central ministry of health itself. At the same time—whether by delegation of authority or primary possession of responsibility—individual hospitals have much freedom in the application of these standards. An increasing volume of communications through professional societies, journals, conferences, etc. is promoting a certain uniformity of practices and elevation of performance norms, quite aside from legal controls. Much influence is also exerted by the major medical centers found in all countries, usually affiliated with schools of medicine, as well as by schools for the formal training of health facility administrators.

INTERNAL HOSPITAL ADMINISTRATION

In this aspect of hospitals there are probably greater variations among different nations than in any other aspect. More than any other feature perhaps, the patterns of internal management of hospitals depend on the overall system of health service organization and financing in the nation.

Countries with a large sector of private medical practice, such as the United States of America or Canada or Australia, tend also to be those with relatively weak central governmental authority over hospitals. In those countries, there is usually much autonomy in the work of physicians. General hospitals of the United States of America, for example, are usually characterized by two lines of internal authority: the medical and the administrative. While theoretically the medical staff comes under the supervision of the hospital board of directors, its latitude for decisions tends to be very wide. Since most general hospital patients are under the private care of an individual physician, he has the greatest legal and moral responsibility for patient care. Limitations and restrictions on his behavior are imposed by an organization of the medical staff itself, and only indirectly by the board of directors. There are usually rather strict limitations to the responsibility of the hospital administrator—who is nearly always a nonmedical man—despite his being the agent of the board of directors.

The composition of the board of directors in these countries is almost always a matter for its own choice. Its membership depends on which group or individual built the hospital originally and who owns it. Once established, the board is usually "self-perpetuating"—that is, the members choose their own successors. They likewise select the administrator and they make the appointments to the medical staff. Except for the general requirements of legal standards on construction and operations, the board is responsible to no higher authority.

This American pattern, however, is quite exceptional in the world scene. In the less economically developed countries with localized authority patterns (Peru and Israel), the internal management of hospitals is not so split between medical and administrative lines. The top executive of the hospital is typically a physician, who is assisted by a business manager or administrative officer. The medical staff members are usually on full-time or part-time salaries and work according to some type of hierarchical framework. Appointments of doctors and other personnel are usually made, however, by local boards rather than a centralized ministry.

In the countries with moderately centralized authority patterns, the internal administration of hospitals is quite variable. The hospitals of the Ministry of Health in Iran, the Philippines, and Chile have no boards of trustees, but rather a bureaucratic structure leading from the medical director of each facility up to a provincial or district health officer and thence to the central ministry. The medical staff consists of salaried civil servants. The numerous voluntary hospitals in those countries, however, usually have a local board of trustees, with a more flexible medical staff receiving individual fees from private patients, as well as some salary for the care of indigent patients. In France the composition of the board of directors of public hospitals (the great majority of total beds) is determined by national law and includes various governmental officials or their designees; daily administration is entrusted to a nonmedical administrator. Sweden, on the other hand, allows each local county council to designate the hospital board of directors. The daily management is assigned to a medical superintendent who is appointed by the county council. In both France and Sweden all personnel in nongovernmental hospitals are appointed simply by their boards of directors.

In the countries of highly centralized pattern, those of weaker economic development (Togo and Malaysia) vest appointment powers at the top in the central Ministry of Health—not only for the hospital director, who is always a physician, but for the entire professional staff. In Malaysian hospitals, there are boards of visitors, but they are solely advisory. An exception is made in the national capital of both Togo and Malaysia for a single large teaching and research hospital, for which a board of trustees functions (but still under the Minister of Health). Throughout these countries, however, the public hospitals providing ninety percent of the patient care are administered essentially as outposts of the central government.

In the more economically advanced countries of the centralized pattern, the internal hospital arrangements in England illustrate one pattern and in the USSR another. The English regional hospital boards appoint the hospital management committees, which take direct charge of each hospital; they also appoint the senior medical staff and the hospital secretary who, in turn, appoint subordinate personnel. Under the hospital management committee the daily operations are carried out through tripartite administration by the hospital secretary, the chief of the medical staff, and the matron. Only if an issue cannot be settled by these three officials is it brought to the management committee for decision.

The Soviet hospitals do not have boards of directors, but rather chief physicians who are appointed by the echelon above them—that is, a *rayon* hospital chief is appointed by the *oblast* hospital chief physician, and he in turn by the *oblast* health department. All other hospital personnel are appointed by the chief physician. He is assisted by various deputies for economic matters, for outpatient services, etc., as well as by advisory committees composed of other hospital personnel; final decisions, however, are his, subject to review by his superiors in the hierarchy.

In all these patterns except the North American, physicians tend to be employees of the hospitals, full-time or part-time. They may have some private practice outside the hospital as well, but insofar as they work in the hospital it is as medical employees. They are legally responsible to the hospital's governing body or chief physician, rather than to the individual patient—except for the relatively small number of patients whom they may serve privately. Because of this close identification of hospital physicians with the administrative authority of the hospital, appointments to the medical staff are usually rather selective. In the more highly developed countries these are usually limited to specialists or consultants, while general practitioners may only work in offices or health centers outside of hospitals. Again the principal exception to this generalization is in North America, where the general hospitals (not the special ones for mental disease or tuberculosis) are typically "open staff"—that is, permitting almost any licensed physician to join the staff and admit private patients. In Soviet hospitals there is also a policy of assigning general physicians or pediatricians to certain responsibilities on the hospital wards, though they are primarily attached to polyclinics. Likewise, in English hospitals, general practitioners may have certain limited access to laboratory or x-ray services through the hospital outpatient clinic.

On a world level one can detect a certain movement toward a more balanced relationship between physicians inside and outside the hospital walls. Since the hospital is increasingly recognized as a center of postgraduate medical education and research, there is a recent tendency in Europe (both Western and Eastern) to let down the barriers and permit access of extramural practitioners to the stimulating internal environment of the hospital. On the other hand, in North America where such interchange has traditionally been very great, the movement is in the other direction and the medical staff organization is becoming more rigorous. Proportionately more American physicians are being appointed as full-time physicians within the hospital, and the general formalities of medical staff organization are increasing.

As for the content and scope of hospital service, everywhere they are becoming wider. From its original focus on the bed care of the seriously sick, the hospital in nearly all countries has been giving proportionately more attention to outpatient services and also to professional education and medical research. This is quite aside from the widening range of diagnostic and treatment services offered to inpatients, due to the advances of medical science. In fact, many new medical procedures are so complex or delicate that they can only be carried out within hospitals where expensive equipment and qualified technical personnel can be assembled.

Generally speaking, in the economically developing countries the range of hospital services tends to be very wide, especially in rural districts. In such areas other medical resources are often lacking and the hospital must be a center for preventive health service as well as all aspects of therapy. This is more obvious in public hospitals than those under voluntary auspices.

Another important determinant of the range of hospital services anywhere is the size; generally a large hospital can offer a wider range of services than a small one. For any given size of institution, however, the diversity of internal programs will naturally tend to be greater in countries with more localized authority than in those with highly centralized hospital systems. Many interesting innovations have originated in the general hospitals of the United States of America, like organized "home care" programs or "progressive patient care" (that is, intensive, intermediate, and long-term units in the same facility)—but they have not necessarily been widely applied. (Most American hospitals, in fact, do not offer such programs.) On the other hand in the more centralized patterns a specific practice which has been found by the ministry of health to be effective is more likely to be applied across the country.

In a few countries the broad concept of the hospital as a center for all health services in an area has taken on special significance. This is the philosophy of the Chilean National Health Service and also of the Soviet and Bulgarian health systems. Administratively the hospital director in these countries is theoretically responsible for all health activities in the geographic area served by that hospital, including ambulatory and preventive services. In many developing countries, the main hospital in a rural region is made responsible also for smaller ambulatory service health centers around it. In the United States of America the concept of the hospital as a generalized "community health center" has been widely discussed, but has not yet been implemented except in a few places. In England, the concept of the "general, general hospital"—with acute, chronic, mental, and other special patients being served flexibly under one administration—has been advanced, but only rarely applied.

Considering the totality of health services there is no question that everywhere the hospital is playing a larger proportionate part. Its share of total health expenditures over the last several decades has gradually been rising, not because of price inflation which applied to out-of-hospital services as well, but because many services formerly offered outside of hospitals or not offered at all are now part of the normal hospital programs. Many health leaders are concerned about the need for greater strengthening of out-of-hospital services which are generally less expensive and more preventively oriented. Nevertheless, the widening scope of health services coming under the wing of hospitals—for either inpatients or outpatients—has an important hidden advantage: namely, the placement of services within an administrative framework, through which they may be more readily integrated. Such integration, in the long run, ought to promote greater economy and higher quality.

FINANCIAL SUPPORT OF HOSPITAL SERVICES

Regardless of the ownership, the system of external controls, or the pattern of internal administration of hospitals, their financial support throughout the world is predominantly from social sources. This applies to both hospital construction and operations, and it is becoming increasingly so. By "social sources" is meant not only various levels of government, but also social insurance and even voluntary insurance as distinguished from the private payments of sick individuals.

The source of financing of hospital construction has been discussed earlier. The cost of operation of a hospital, however, is a much larger financial question. The life of an average hospital building in recent times may be forty or fifty years or more (this is highly variable, of course, in relation to the style of construction) during all of which time the operating costs must be met. The cost of construction, however, is equivalent on the average to only about two or three years of operating costs. Not only are the operating costs vastly higher than construction costs, but they are also naturally more sensitive to the changing requirements of medical science, to economic inflation, and to all the other changes occurring in a nation from year to year.

As discussed in the historical review, hospital operating costs were originally met mainly by religious or other forms of charity and this method was satisfactory so long as the technical content of services was meager and the relative number of patients was small. But as hospitals came to serve a higher proportion of the population (in the more economically developed countries, it is common for about ten percent of the population or more to be hospitalized during an average year), and the norms of medical technology advanced steadily, more substantial and dependable sources of financing became necessary. This came to be provided initially through the mechanism of governmental revenues and then through sickness insurance (compulsory or voluntary) while private charity still continues to a small extent.

In the countries with the most localized hospital authority patterns, the financial support of hospital operations tends to be the most highly diversified. While the great bulk of support is from social sources, it is from many different social sources. In the United States of America the largest single sector in recent years has been voluntary insurance (of many different types—Blue Cross plans, commercial insurance companies, consumer cooperatives, etc.), although with the "Medicare" legislation of 1965 this may soon change to governmental social insurance revenues.[2] Another large sector is the revenue of local governments for general hospital care and of state governments for mental or tuberculosis hospital care. The federal government also contributes hospital operating costs not only for military personnel and veterans (even for disabilities not connected with military service), but also for assistance to state and local governments in meeting the hospitalization costs of indigent persons (about five percent of the United States population). Purely private payments of sick individuals now sustain about twenty percent of hospital operating costs, either for meeting certain charges not fully covered by insurance or for the full costs of patients not insured nor eligible for governmental assistance. A small balance of about four or five percent of hospital operating costs is still met by charitable donations, the income from previous charitable endowments, or the direct contribution of an occasional private company.

This is a greatly oversimplified summary of the American financial patterns which are diversified not only among different types of hospital (according to sponsorship, specialization, and size) but also within single hospitals. The very composition of a hospital's "operating costs," moreover, differs among different types of institution, in some of which the salaries of physicians are considered part of the total (as in Europe, Latin America, and most countries), while in most United States general hospitals physicians are remunerated privately by patients and their fees do not enter into the hospital budget.

In Israel, the diversity of financial sources for hospitalization costs is almost as great, although the voluntary insurance sector in this small nation is more consolidated under the wing of a single agency, the Kupat Holim of the Federation of Labor. Charity from overseas plays a larger role as does governmental revenue at the national level. Purely private payments play a very small part. The Netherlands illustrate a European country with similar diversity of financial sources, including many different voluntary insurance funds (with different religious affiliations), local governmental revenues, charity, and private payments.

In the economically weaker countries, where the great majority of the people are poor, government makes a larger relative contribution to hospital operating costs even when the authority pattern is quite localized. In Peru, charity and lottery proceeds play a large part, but about half the costs of operating the *beneficencia* hospitals (with forty-two percent of the beds) comes from central government subsidies. The social security funds, separately for manual and for white collar workers, support eighteen percent of the beds, but their expenditures per day of care are two or three times higher than in other public hospitals. The Ministry of Health hospitals, of course, are financed almost wholly from central revenues. Private payments support a small fraction of the costs of those hospitals and all of the private hospitals containing six percent of the beds. This distribution of hospital costs among charity and lotteries, central government revenues, social security funds (and sometimes private enterprises for noninsured workers), and private payments is found in many of the Latin American countries. The proportion met by social insurance tends to be rising more rapidly than that met by general revenues, although both of these are essentially governmental economic sources.

In the moderately centralized hospital patterns, the sources of support for operating costs are also highly diversified, especially in the economically weaker countries. The high proportion of private beds in the Philippines and the legal ceiling on governmental expenditures for public beds mean that private expenditures must play a very large part. The same effect operates in South Korea, where a substantial share of costs even in governmental hospitals is met by personal charges to patients. In Iran, on the other hand, the central government revenues from oil have permitted nearly full support of not only public hospital but also voluntary hospital costs. Social insurance also plays a large part in Iran, and it is growing as the worker's insurance program expands. In Chile, the bulk of hospital costs comes from central governmental revenues, the second largest share from the social security fund, and a small balance from charity and private fees.

In the economically stronger countries of the moderate authority pattern (France and Sweden), hospital costs are divided almost entirely between general governmental revenues and social insurance. Very little money is derived from voluntary insurance, charity, or private payments. Swedish hospitals are supported mainly from the revenues of local government (county councils), with a balance from social insurance and very small amounts from private fees. French hospitals are financed mainly by social insurance payments on a per diem basis, with the principal balance from local governmental revenues.

One feature of hospital financing in several countries, especially in Latin America, calls for special comment—the use of public lotteries. These are sometimes operated by governmentally chartered charitable societies and sometimes by government directly. The lottery, of course, takes advantage of the common human tendency to gamble, but unfortunately most of those who gamble—and seldom win—are poor persons who can ill afford the losses. Moreover, it dramatizes a philosophy of "getting rich without work." Most important, examination of the accounting figures of Latin American lotteries shows a huge and costly administrative infrastructure necessary to produce a relatively small donation to hospitals. In a typical program, only about thirty percent of the money raised by sale of lottery tickets ends up with the hospitals or other institutions, the rest going for prizes, commissions to ticket sellers, general administration, etc. In a few countries, like Costa Rica or Ireland, lottery income may make a substantial contribution to hospital operating expenses, but in general the share is probably less than ten percent of the total costs.

In the most highly centralized nations the financial support of hospital operations is easiest to describe because it is simplest. The USSR and other socialist countries support nearly all operating costs from the revenues of the central government (even though much of the construction cost may have come from local government or collective farm resources). The actual spending of this money is delegated through an administrative hierarchy from national to local agencies, but the ultimate origin is central. In England, with its National Health Service, about ninety percent of hospital costs are met by the Ministry of Health and about eighty-five percent of these monies come from general revenues of the central government; the balance of National Health Service monies comes from a social security fund, which is devoted mainly to providing nonmedical benefits (the old-age pensions, disability insurance, etc.) and from other lesser sources. The overall balance of British hospital costs comes from purely private payments and from a small program of voluntary health insurance ("provident funds").

In the less economically developed countries of highly centralized authority patterns (Togo and Malaysia), the vast bulk of hospital operating costs also come from the central government. In the few main cities, however, there are usually some small private hospitals financed entirely by private payments. In Malaysia, the voluntary Chinese maternity hospitals are typically operated at the expense of their patients, charitable donations, and government grants; the industrial hospitals on rubber estates and tin mines are supported by the enterprise along with government grants. In African countries like Ethiopia or Tanganyika, which also represent the highly centralized authority pattern, voluntary religious missions appear to play a larger role in hospital financing than in Togo. A careful study in Tanganyika estimated that voluntary agencies contribute about fifteen percent of the costs of organized health services, most of this being for hospital operations. In none of these countries does social insurance or voluntary health insurance play any part.

The precise method of collecting the money or preparing budgets for hospital operations tends to correspond to the patterns of financial support just reviewed. Where there is a diversity of sources, the hospital management must usually undertake accounting procedures to calculate the average cost per patient day or even the cost of specific items of service, like a laboratory test or a drug injection. These amounts are then charged to the individual patient or the responsible agency (insurance fund, governmental department, etc.) for the services provided. It is expected by the hospital that, by the end of the year, assuming a certain occupancy level, all the earnings necessary to meet its total annual budget will have been collected. In practice, hospitals under this system may earn a "profit" or suffer a "loss" depending on many circumstances. The avoidance of losses may sometimes induce admissions of patients which are medically unjustified while, on the other hand, it may induce sound efficiencies in hospital administration.

In the most centralized countries, the mechanisms of hospital financing tend to be simpler. An annual or prospective budget is prepared, estimated to meet all the costs of personnel, supplies, etc. This amount is then allocated through some sort of hierarchy to local units of government and finally to individual hospitals. The preparation of the budget is initially by the hospital management, but is subject to review, of course, at higher echelons. If a particular hospital wishes to expand its services its director must convince the higher authorites of the soundness of this idea and he may not always be successful. There are also inevitably limitations in the total national allotment for hospitals, which compel the higher authorities to make choices among competing claims for funds. Thus, there are certain inherent restrictions in this system of budgeting, but once an allocation is made to a hospital its financial support for the coming period (usually one year) is assured.

Between the two extremes the countries of moderately centralized authority patterns use systems of hospital budgeting which are, in a sense, a combination of both the above approaches. In the main, hospitals operate on a fixed annual budget which they are allocated by the principal ministerial or social security agencies that support them. In addition, however, they calculate specific costs per patient day, which certain insured persons or private patients are charged. This applies to public or voluntary nonprofit hospitals, and private proprietary hospitals are meanwhile financed entirely by individual per diem payments. The entire subject of hospital budgeting is quite complex, and this discussion is only an oversimplification of its main features.

It is evident that the financial support of hospitals, both in terms of sources and mechanisms, is intimately related to the whole system of hospital organization in a country. There is perhaps no economic factor with more influence on the quality of medical care in a country than the amplitude of financing of its hospitals. This in turn is largely dependent on the degree of social, as against purely individual, financing. Fortunately for the advancement of medical care, such social financing has steadily increased almost everywhere, both absolutely and relative to total health expenditures.

At the same time the heightened social financing of hospital services sets in motion political forces which lead to the heightened organization of hospital services. When large groups of people or even a whole national population are financing hospital operations, there is naturally more concern for efficiency, economy, and effectiveness of the services than when hospital operations are supported solely by the small percentage of persons who at any one moment happen to be sick. Therefore, the social and largely governmental financing of hospital operations—while it takes different forms in different countries—is nevertheless leading everywhere to a heightened organization of hospitals, both internally and in larger georgraphic areas, in the interests of both economy and quality.

REGIONAL RELATIONSHIPS AMONG HOSPITALS

As medical science has advanced, increasing specialization has become necessary and a great share of this has been implemented in hospitals. In many countries specialty service in medicine is associated almost exclusively with hospitals, while out-of-hospital medical services are provided only by general practitioners.

At the same time not every hospital can provide services in all the medical and surgical specialties; it is not economically feasible or ecologically sensible (in terms of the numbers and distribution of people to be served) to provide a full range of specialties—some twenty or more principal ones in medicine—in small hospitals of, let us say, under 100 beds. Associated with each of the specialties are certain technical paramedical personnel, equipment, or supplies. In addition there are related fields of dentistry, social work, physical therapy, etc. Hence, it has been necessary to develop specialization of hospitals as well as personnel.

Yet populations are unevenly settled in all countries. Hospitals naturally are established in cities, but millions of people live in rural areas. Transportation problems of varying degrees stand between the patient and the medical care he may need; they are most severe in the rural districts of economically developing countries, but are found even at the other extreme—in the great cities of the most developed countries. The goal of health service planning in most countries has been to make available to persons, wherever they may live, the scientific techniques necessary to treat their ailments, wherever these techniques may be located.

The solution to this problem offered in many countries has been the concept of "hospital regionalization." This involves the establishment of a network of hospitals in a geographic area, such that patients are treated in a facility appropriate to their medical needs—neither too simple nor too specialized. Thus, throughout the region and especially in rural areas there would be small general hospitals (perhaps of fifty beds or less), close to where the people live, which would be capable of treating the common ailments, such as injuries and other minor surgery, normal maternity cases, rehydration of infants, respiratory tract infections, etc. At the next level, and typically in a medium-sized town, would be the "intermediate" hospitals (about 100 to 300 beds), which would have a fairly wide range of medical and surgical specialties, for the more difficult cases, such as serious infections, major abdominal surgery, severe injuries, etc. At the center of the region would be a "base" hospital or regional medical center, typically in a large city; it would have perhaps 500 to 1,000 beds and sometimes be associated with a school of medicine. Here would be located the full range of specialties, including the "superspecialties" for brain or cardiac surgery, complex radiation therapy, etc. In the intermediate and regional hospitals, however, there would also be some beds reserved for the simpler conditions to treat persons with these ailments who live nearby.

This framework of hospitals, it is theorized, would function in two directions: by transportation of patients from the peripheral toward the central facilities, and by dispatch of certain consultant services and technical supervision from the central or intermediate levels outward. Moreover, if a patient is helped to recover from the critical phase of an illness or surgical operation at a central facility, he might be sent back to the more peripheral facility if it is nearer to his home, for convalescence. It must be realized that this "network" concept embodies two aspects: hospital construction and hospital operation. For regionalization to be functional the hospital facilities must first be established or be existent at particular locations; then, the services or patients must flow in the two directions as outlined.

This, in brief, is the theory of hospital regionalization, and it has caught the imagination of health leaders throughout the world. Its actual implementation, however, is fraught with many problems. It is probably fair to say that most countries are working in one way or another toward its achievement but nowhere has it yet been achieved in the idealized form just described.

In the countries at the more localized end of the range of hospital authority patterns, regionalization has been a major force in the planning of hospital construction. In the United States of America a nationally subsidized program of hospital construction, developing since 1946, has been carried out along these lines—that is, to encourage the construction only of hospitals that find a logical place in a regional network. Most hospital construction in the nation, however, is not affected by this subsidy program. On the functional side, regionalization programs with the two-way flow of patients and technical services have been achieved only at a few places where specially subsidized "demonstrations" have been launched; even in these places the range of re-

gionalized activities has been rather limited, stressing mainly a flow of educational services for physicians and hospital personnel.

Nevertheless, a certain amount of informal or unstructured regionalization appears to occur in the United States of America, simply by reason of location of the highly specialized physicians in large urban hospitals and without any deliberate administration. Moreover, within certain subsystems of American hospitals, such as the federal Veterans Administration facilities or hospitals associated with certain health insurance plans, there is some functional regionalization. New legislation launched in 1966 for "regional medical programs" to treat patients with "heart disease, cancer, or stroke" is also intended to promote this idea further. In many large urban metropolitan areas, moreover, hospitals have formed voluntary councils for several purposes, including the exercise of informal influences on new hospital construction (consistent with regionalization concepts), the bulk or cooperative purchasing of hospital supplies, the joint engagement of certain administrative consultants, etc.

In other countries of localized hospital policies but of lesser economic development, the regionalization concept has had a larger impact, both for construction and operations. In Peru it is the basis for location of all Ministry of Health hospitals and for construction grants to assist in the alteration of *beneficencia* hospitals. Within the social security hospital system, this is also the policy. The differently sponsored hospital networks, however, are not regionally integrated with each other. The same applies to Israel, where the Kupat Holim hospital network and the Ministry of Health network are each separately regionalized. Across-the-board regionalization of all hospitals in defined geographic areas, however, has been impeded by the autonomy of hospitals under different types of ownership.

In the countries of middle-range hospital authority patterns, the achievements and problems are similar to those in the Philippines—that is, regionalized relationships within the Ministry of Health institutions, but not outside them. In Iran the situation is similar, except that the growing social security program is implementing regionalization within its own network of new facilities. The strong place of voluntary agency hospitals and of university hospitals—despite their heavy governmental subsidies—has generated a great sense of pride and sovereignty in these institutions which is said to inhibit their cooperation with governmental hospitals.

In the more economically advanced middle-range countries, the strong role of local governments affects policies. Within the individual counties of

Sweden or the *départements* of France, there are cooperative relationships among hospitals. All new hospital construction, moreover, must be centrally approved, and a master plan for the entire country is encouraging the development of certain principal centers, affiliated with medical schools, which will serve as places for referral of difficult cases from several local jurisdictions. Up to the present, however, these larger regions composed of several local hospital authority areas, have no legal power and the functioning of regionalized services (professional consultations, training programs, patient referrals, etc.) is left on a voluntary basis.

The countries with the most highly centralized hospital control patterns have carried out the regionalization concept most fully for both construction and operation. In Malaysia, the staffing and equipping of all public hospitals are based on a concept of two echelons of facilities, "district hospitals" and "general hospitals." Plans call for adding a series of smaller "rural hospitals" below these and developing three large "regional medical centers" above them, to result in a four-echelon national network in all.

In the more economically developed countries of highly centralized policies, the intention of implementing full regionalization is present, but the heritage of the past causes some difficulties. These countries have all entered the twentieth century with an existing framework of hospitals which is seldom completely reasonable in relation to the current distribution of population and the people's medical needs. England has had an especially large and complex layout of old and some new hospitals, which only gradually could be modified along regionalization lines. The administration of virtually all of these facilities, however, has been placed under regional hospital boards responsible for almost all hospitals in defined areas. These boards are continuously exploring new methods of interhospital cooperation. Yet, for various historic reasons, the important university teaching hospitals in England are not directly under these boards (although they do come under the National Ministry of Health), a separation that is not found in Scotland.[3]

In the Soviet Union hospital system or that of Bulgaria and other socialist countries, the regionalization concept is the theoretical foundation for all hospitals. From rural *uchastok* to *rayon* to *oblast* levels, there are hospitals of increasing size and complexity, which come under a common framework of administration. In practice, there are no obstacles of separate ownership or autonomous administration to impede full functional regionalization, although human factors still play a part—like the pride of a local surgeon who wishes to do an operation in a small rural hospital which ought properly be referred to a higher echelon facility.

At all points on the scale of hospital authority, it is apparent that countries with less industrial development and a more rural character tend to achieve the regionalization concept more easily. Their quantitative hospital resources are less, but by the same token their backlog of existing hospital autonomy and sovereignty is also less. Therefore, when they set out to develop new hospitals in the current period they can start, so to speak, with a clean slate and can establish them both structurally and functionally along regional lines with less difficulty. The problem, of course, in these countries is more one of deficient economic resources for needed hospital construction than one of hospital organization.

This discussion has focused on general hospitals, but the regionalization concept applies, of course, to specialized facilities as well. In a regional network there may also be hospitals for mental disorder, tuberculosis, or other chronic disorders; hospitals for children; nursing homes for aged persons; leprosaria; rehabilitation centers; etc. Relationships between these and general hospitals are just as important as those among various echelons of general hospitals. Such relationships may be achieved regardless of hospital ownership and control, though it is easier when the controls are under a single public agency. The problem is simplified by the fact that, in all countries, hospitals for long-term illness are more frequently under central or at least provincial government sponsorship than are the general hospitals serving mainly the acutely ill.

There is also the whole question of relationships between hospitals and various types of facility for ambulatory health service. The regionalization concept has been applied mainly to hospital services because these are most specialized and costly, but the principle is appropriate to ambulatory services as well. A patient with a disease problem not requiring bed care can well be sent from a peripheral to a central outpatient facility for more careful examination and diagnosis; after a diagnostic conclusion is reached, he might be sent back to his local health center or physician for appropriate therapy.

The full implementation of the regionalization idea, therefore, applies to a continuum of health service starting with the person who is still in his own home and requires only ambulatory care or perhaps medical or nursing care at home. The outpatient department of the hospital at all three or four echelons in the regional network can provide such care, or it can be provided at health centers (without beds) or rural health posts; in the more industrialized countries, of course, most of such care is provided in the offices or clinics of individual doctors (whether they are paid privately or by an insurance fund or public agency). Home care of the patient likewise may be provided through the organized arrangements of a hospital or public health agency (e.g., visiting nurses) or by individual medical practitioners. Finally, regionalization may also be extended to include the personal preventive services, such as immunizations or periodic examination of children and adults.

Whether this full spectrum of ambulatory and hospital services, general and special, is systematically regionalized or not, it is found to exist to some extent in all countries. The degree of integration and coordination, however, varies in accordance with the overall governmental philosophy of countries in the same way as does the pattern of hospital authority. In the most localized countries, numerous voluntary efforts are encouraging coordination, even though hundreds or thousands of autonomous medical personnel and facilities are responsible for day-to-day medical care. A large sector of private medical practice, both outside and inside hospitals, presents the greatest challenge for coordination. In the moderately centralized countries, regional coordination is being actively achieved within hospitals, but is still weak in its linkage with the out-of-hospital ambulatory services. In the most highly centralized countries, the ambulatory services and preventive programs tend to be most closely integrated with hospitals at each of the regional echelons. It is of much interest that the separations of ambulatory and hospital services which were the historic heritage of the British National Health Service are now being tackled through new plans to develop fully integrated "health area" jurisdictions which will supervise all preventive and curative, ambulatory and hospital, services for populations of about 1,000,000 persons.

In the economically weaker countries at all points on the scale of localism to centralism, full integration of hospital, ambulatory, and preventive services is being more readily achieved than in the older industrialized countries. The tradition of private medical practice is not so strong in rural areas, and health centers can readily be established as the normal channel for ambulatory care. Such centers are commonly regarded as satellites to hospitals. Auxiliary health personnel at small rural stations usually come under the supervision of physicians at the nearest health center or hospital. In countries at all stages of economic development, moreover, the rural areas present the greatest need for and the most feasible opportunity for full regionalization of all health services.

GENERAL PHILOSOPHY AND TRENDS

This brief and somewhat oversimplified review of systems of hospital organization throughout the world reveals both similarities and differences among countries. The broad trend appears to be toward greater similarities, although the paths taken vary, on the one hand, with the stage of industrialization and urbanization of a country and, on the other hand, with its hospital policies along the scale of localized to centralized authority structures. Perhaps a few generalizations are permissible in the light of the study of a selected sample of thirteen countries.

Everywhere the hospital is becoming more important in the overall system of health services. Its importance relates not only to its mobilizing resources for treatment of seriously sick bed-patients, but mainly to its being a place where all sorts of skilled health personnel and equipment are conveniently assembled. Hence, the hospital becomes likewise a center for ambulatory health service, for preventive services, for education of health personnel, and for medical research.

Because of complex historical origins, hospitals today are owned and operated by many social entities. They have sprung from the sponsorship of religious bodies, of local and central governments, of nonsectarian voluntary societies, of social insurance funds, of industry, and of private business interests. These multiple sponsorships are found in differing mixtures among the nations, but the trend is clearly toward a greater proportion of governmental sponsorship. The level of government (local, provincial, or national) differs with the size of country and its political tradition, as does the precise public agency—as between ministries of health, social security agencies, or other entities. Even in countries where national policy has encouraged a great deal of new hospital development by voluntary bodies, the continuing financial support of such hospitals depends increasingly on governmental payments for patient care. The net effect of new construction by any type of public or private agency is to increase the total national supply of beds, all of which become eventually subject to national planning.

Ownership of a hospital depends mainly on the agency or group that originally constructed it, but increasingly the costs of hospital construction have come to be derived from governmental revenues. This is true, even for hospitals initiated by nongovernmental bodies. As medical science has advanced, costs of construction as well as operation have risen sharply, and in nearly all countries they can be met only by substantial contributions from the tax resources of government. Regardless of hospital ownership, governmental standards for the physical design of hospital buildings are being increasingly applied.

While hospitals were historically independent local entities, their operation has come to be increasingly subject to standards and controls by higher authorities. These controls may involve the appointments of key personnel as well as the policies of administration and the organization of services. Such controls operate sometimes through systems of hospital licensure or review and sometimes through the inherent existence of hospitals in a governmental hierarchy. The range of external controls is widening from concern for elementary environmental problems to surveillance over the more complex features of patient care.

Internal hospital administration is also becoming more systematized everywhere. In each institution there is a governing authority, whether this is a board of trustees or a single director. Various complex relationships are maintained between personnel concerned with purely medical matters and administrative matters, with the trend being toward a cooperative balance of responsibilities. Hospital administration, as a specific professional skill, is advancing, either in the hands of physicians or others. The range of health activities carried out in hospitals is steadily widening, in the way of complex diagnostic and treatment services for inpatients, as well as outpatient service, prevention, professional education, and research.

The financial support for hospital services is being increasingly assumed by social sources. Charity and individual payments are becoming proportionately less important, while support from governmental revenues and insurance (either compulsory or voluntary) is becoming more important. Budgeting is being executed increasingly on the basis of overall annual estimates, rather than collection of individual fees. The heightened social financing of hospital services is inducing a rising concern for economy and effectiveness in hospital operations. Rising costs, on the other hand, are leading to increasing attention for soundly organized and less costly out-of-hospital services.

As health planning for large geographic areas and whole nations is occurring, greater attention is being given to interhospital relationships in "regionalized" systems. These relationships vary from informal ties in some countries to highly formalized networks in others, but the goal is everywhere the same: to attempt to assure every patient the technical services he needs, regardless of where he may live. Regionalization involves not only relationships among different levels of general hospitals, but also between general and special hospitals and between hospitals and ambulatory care facilities. Such relationships are believed to promote both quality and economy of service.

With respect to all the above movements, a kind of equilibrium seems to be evolving between centralized standards and local hospital responsibilities. The advancement of a governmental role appears to be setting minimum quality standards on local performance, without eliminating a sense of local responsibility. Of course, there are great variations in the character of this equilibrium in different countries, but the overall trend in quality of hospital service appears to be upward.

The importance of hospitals in the total spectrum of health services is matched by their importance also in the general political arena. Hospitals are visible to the people; they are concrete centers of health recovery and life. For this reason they are of widely recognized value in political debate about all community affairs. This value can be exploited by health leaders for the overall advancement of health services. It also provides a social and psychological rationale for the continued development of the hospital from its humble origins as a hostel for the bedridden sick and destitute, toward a technical and administrative center for all health services provided in the geographic area around it.

NOTES

[1] In the 1970s, known as "certificate of need" laws, enacted by many states.

[2] By 1975, the U.S. Medicare program was financing about forty percent of general hospital costs.

[3] The reorganization of the British National Health Service in 1974 finally brought all teaching hospitals into the regionalized networks (see chapter 11).

Chapter XXIV
Social Security for Medical Care
in Developing Countries

After World War I, social insurance for medical care spread from Europe to the developing continents. In these countries, however, the percentage of persons insured has typically been small, so that "inequities" are created relative to the larger noninsured population. Ministries of health, theoretically responsible for the health of the total population (although actually concentrating most of their efforts on the poor), often look upon social security agencies as rivals, especially since the latter often have more funds to spend for their relatively small covered population than does the ministry have for its wider responsibilities.

Nevertheless, there are many socio-political reasons why the social insurance approach is justified in developing countries. In this chapter, the arguments are marshalled on why this approach is, in the long run, promotive of social and economic development as well as actually supportive of the objectives of ministries of health. This text was originally presented to a meeting of the United States-Mexico Border Public Health Association in 1971 and published as "Social Security for Medical Care: Is It Justified in Developing Countries?" in the International Journal of Health Services, *(Vol. 1, No. 4, November 1971, pp. 354-361, Greenwood Periodicals Co., publisher). It is reprinted here by permission of Baywood Publishing Company, Inc.*

The social insurance device for supporting the costs of general medical care was first introduced outside of Europe in Japan in 1922 followed by Chile in 1924. Although the idea had started in Germany in the 1880s, it was forty years before it spread to any of the developing and mainly agricultural continents. It is surely no accident that the early leadership for the Chilean program was provided by medical immigrants from Germany.[1] Soon social security programs for medical care of various groups of workers spread to nearly all other Latin American countries; the sequence of this spread is shown in table XXIV.1.[2] It may be noted in this table that nine of the Latin American programs were started before the end of World War II (1945), and ten of them after this date. Only Argentina among the twenty Latin American republics is still without a social insurance program for general medical care, although it has had, since

1934, a social insurance program limited to maternity care for women workers, and it does have wide coverage of its population for general medical services through voluntary and nongovernmental *mutualidades* and *obras sociales*.[3]

Other developing continents applied the social insurance mechanism to general medical services somewhat later. In Asia, the first move was made by India, with its Employees State Insurance Corporation (ESIC) in 1948, followed by Iran in 1949, China (Taiwan) in 1950, People's China in 1951, Burma in 1954, Indonesia in 1957, North Vietnam in 1961, Lebanon in 1963, Turkey in 1964, and West Pakistan in 1965. In North Africa, the sequence was Algeria in 1949, Libya in 1957, Tunisia in 1960, and Egypt (United Arab Republic) in 1964. Sub-Sahara or Negro Africa has applied social insurance, outside of maternity benefits for women workers, only in

Guinea (1952) and in Kenya (1946), and in the latter country, the insurance benefits are limited to hospitalization. Beyond these countries, the developing world has provided general medical care through social insurance in Cyprus and Malta, starting in 1956. This review, it should be realized, does not include social insurance for work injuries and the associated treatment (workmen's compensation in North American terminology) but refers to programs offering general medical care.

Table XXIV.1
Social security for general medical care in Latin America, by year of initiation in each country

1924 Chile	1946 Colombia
1934 Brazil	1946 Guatemala
1935 Ecuador	1947 Dominican Republic
1936 Peru	1949 Bolivia
1940 Venezuela	1949 El Salvador
1941 Costa Rica	1954 Honduras
1941 Panama	1955 Nicaragua
1942 Mexico	1958 Uruguay
1943 Paraguay	1963 Cuba
(1945-End of	1967 Haiti
World War II)	

From U.S. Social Security Administration, *Social Security Programs throughout the World, 1969*, Washington, D.C.: Government Printing Office, 1970.

In nearly all of these countries, the insurance mechanism has been able to achieve medical coverage only for a small minority of the population—usually about ten percent or less. Mexican social security programs are outstanding in reaching as much as eighteen percent of the population.[4] (The programs in Chile and Cuba have reached much higher proportions, only by shifting from social insurance to predominantly general revenue financing.) Because of this minority coverage and because social security everywhere in the developing world has been able to support a higher quality of medical care for this minority than that available to most of the national populations, serious questions of equity have arisen.

THE ISSUE OF INEQUITIES

The problem is illustrated by the findings of a study of the Pan American Health Organization on the expenditures for hospital care in social security facilities, compared with ministry of health facilities in several Latin American countries.[5] In this study it was found that the outlays in social security hospitals were two or more times higher per patient day of care than in hospitals operated by ministries of health.

The differentials with *beneficencia* hospitals would doubtless be even greater. Moreover, the ratio of hospital beds available to insured workers is also higher than that available to the general population, as was found in my own studies in the early 1960s.[6] On top of this, the ambulatory services for insured persons in polyclinics or health centers and the prescribed drugs are also usually more abundant, and of better technical quality, than those available to the great majority of Latin American people who cannot afford private medical care and must depend on public resources.

The same sort of differentials will be found in Iran or Turkey or other developing countries that have launched social security programs for medical care of relatively small segments of their populations. In these countries, as in nearly all the Latin American countries, insured persons are served in separate facilities and by separate professional staffs, with better resources than those available to the general population. In other developing countries, such as Tunisia, India, or Kenya, differential expenditures prevail, even though the social security bodies have not built separate hospitals for their beneficiaries (except for a few recently in India).

The economic explanations of these differentials are everywhere essentially the same. The socially insured workers, and often their dependents, are provided greater per capita resources for their care because the money is raised through special taxes on the most productive sectors of the economy: industry, commerce, or mining—as distinguished from the less productive sector, agriculture, to which most of the population is attached. These special taxes are called "social insurance contributions," paid by both employers and workers, but basically the money is derived from the sale of the entrepreneurial products. In both national and international markets, these products command higher prices, per hour of human labor, than most agricultural products. Whether this is due to the lesser mechanization of agriculture, the supply-and-demand dynamics of the market, or other factors is for economists to debate, but there can be no doubt of the differential consequences for medical care resources.

The effects of these differentials on medical care quantity and quality are caused not only by the disproportionately larger per capita monies available for insured persons, but also by the autonomous channels through which the money is usually spent. It was in Lima, Peru in 1940 that the first *hospital obrero* was built, exclusively for insured workers. Until then, the Latin American countries (that is, Chile, Brazil, and Ecuador) had followed the European pattern of using social insurance monies for purchasing care in existing public, governmental, and private hospitals. But in Peru and, indeed, most developing countries of the world these hospitals usually had serious deficiencies. The decision in 1940, therefore, and with increasing frequency since then, has been to build separate social security hospitals for insured persons. Through these facilities, as well as separate ambulatory care centers, the higher financial resources derived from social insurance can be dramatically converted into better quality medical resources.[7]

Thus, the question raised earlier about equity in the distribution of medical resources between insured and noninsured persons in a developing country has been posed with increasing sharpness. Why, it is asked, should industrial workers or commercial employees be a favored group, in contrast to agricultural families who usually constitute a larger proportion of the population in developing countries? (This issue is as clearly demonstrated in Mexico, with its impressive *Instituto Mexicano del Seguro Social* and related programs, focused on a minority of the population, as in any other country.)

THE RATIONALE FOR SOCIAL INSURANCE

The answer—or the defense of what may be a short-term inequity—must be sought, in my view, through examination of historical, political, and economic realities. The rationale may be formulated as follows:

1. The social insurance device—that is, imposing special taxes on workers and employers exclusively for the benefit of workers and their families—is a method of tapping a source of money for social investment in health service which would otherwise not be so spent. In the absence of social insurance taxes, these monies would simply not be allocated to health service at all or, if they were, they would be spent largely through the private sector.[8]

2. By placing these monies in an earmarked fund, separate from the national treasury, a high degree of stability is achieved. Social insurance monies are, by statute, protected from the political ups and downs of parliamentary debate. Their amplitude does, of course, vary with the level of economic activity—the amounts of wages and payrolls—but they do not require legislative appropriations each year, in competition with the demands of all the rest of government and in response to the vicissitudes of political debate. Moreover, the customary administrative structure of social security programs gives a voice to the workers (or consumers) as well as the employers in the management of the funds raised.

3. Insofar as the earnings of working people are spent for private medical service, they would be spent with less efficiency (that is, less sound service per dollar expended) than applies to their expenditure through a social security program. The latter is a *planned* use of funds, with an organizational structure of personnel and facilities which promotes rational delivery of service. Many studies, especially in Latin America, indicate that self-prescribed medications of dubious value account for an extremely high proportion of purely private expenditures for health service. Studies in Brazil, Puerto Rico, Colombia, and Chile have demonstrated this.[9] In addition, fee-for-service medical care delivery in private offices is much costlier than service through organized clinics which make optimal use of paramedical personnel.

4. By tapping an additional source of money for health or other welfare purposes, the social security device probably allocates a higher proportion of the gross national product (GNP) for such purposes than if only the general tax sources—that is, from land, income, exports, imports, excise duties—were used. I say "probably," because I have not been able to collect data which would firmly prove or disprove this point. From the World Health Organization studies by Brian Abel-Smith, it would certainly appear that nations with social security health care programs spend, through social mechanisms, a higher proportion of GNP on health than do countries without such programs.[10] For example, Iran, with a social security program, spent in 1962 about 1.4 percent of its GNP on socially organized health services, in comparison with the Philippines (without social security), which spent 0.9 percent of its GNP on such health services. Or looking at *total* health expenditures (both socially organized and private), one may compare the health outlay of 5.6 percent of GNP by Chile—with its well-developed social security program—to the outlay of 4.0 percent by Ceylon—without such a program. Admittedly, however, these are very spotty data, and we must have much more complete information before this hypothesis can be reliably proved.

5. If the above argument proves to be correct, it would probably follow that the resources available to a ministry of health for serving the general population are *not* reduced by reason of the allocation of monies to a social security program. Indeed, the resources may even be relatively increased, since part of the health care load, previously borne by a health ministry (that is, for industrial workers and so forth), is shifted to an agency supported by other monies. This point also I cannot firmly prove with statistical data, but it certainly appears true by general observation of trends in Latin America. Mexico and Venezuela, for example, where eighteen and fifteen per-

cent of the populations, respectively, are covered by social security for medical care, may be compared with Colombia and El Salvador, where about four and three percent, respectively, have such coverage.[11] Do we have any evidence to suggest a stronger ministry of health program in the latter countries than in the former? I doubt it.

Indeed, while I have not seen firm data to settle the point, I suspect that countries with a strong social insurance program for health services probably also have a stronger ministry of health program than do countries with weak or with no social insurance programs. The reason for this hypothesis is political, rather than economic. Thus, I suspect—on the basis of conversations with public health leaders in many countries—that the existence of a strong and impressive health program for insured workers *heightens* the bargaining power of the minister of health in the total arena of national government. This minister can then effectively point to the modern hospitals of the social security agency and say, "Why do we not have similar facilities for rural people?" In other words, the competitive influence of a strong social insurance program establishes high medical care standards which other branches of government soon try to emulate.

6. Quite aside from the above arguments, one can appreciate that the construction of health facilities or the support of health personnel out of social insurance funds adds to the nation's total medical resources, leaving aside for the moment the question of equity. This can be observed in Iran and India, as well as in the Latin American countries, where the total national supplies of hospital beds have clearly been expanded as a result of social security capital investments. It can also be inferred from the very high proportion of doctors in Latin America who are engaged by social security institutions, thus enlarging their annual incomes. There is little doubt in my mind that the steadily improved ratios of medical manpower to population in nearly all Latin American countries from 1940 to the present are directly related to the increasing potential for their remuneration, after training, by the expanding social security programs in those countries.

7. There remains, then, the question of equity, or more accurately, the distribution of health care resources in relation to the needs of diverse population groups. Why, in a word, should city workers get more service than poor peasants or *campesinos*? One answer to this may be on a purely pragmatic political level: the city workers carry more political weight because they are generally better educated and are more likely to vote in elections; also, they are often in labor unions which achieve a louder collective voice.

A second answer is on the level of health administration and logistics. By reason of better urban than rural transportation, as well as higher urban than rural levels of education, the health service demands and expectations of city workers are greater than those of rural people. I am not suggesting that this is sound or reasonable, but it is a reality that has been found in all countries, including the United States, where extensive documentation of the point has been issued in the U.S. National Health Survey.[12] Thus, even for the same income level or social class, city families utilize higher rates of medical care than rural families. It would seem justified, therefore, to provide relatively greater medical resources in cities, in response to the heavier demands of urban people.

A third answer to the equity question is on the axis of national development, and this is probably the most decisive. In large degree, the economic development of a country depends upon industrialization. Even the improvement of agriculture depends largely on the production of farm machinery, transport, fertilizer, and other items requiring industrial processes. Thus, it is reasonable for a developing country to give priority in health resource allocation to its industrial workers. A skilled industrial worker represents a social investment; that is, the attainment of the skill ordinarily requires long training and experience. Thus, preservation of the worker's health is especially important for maintenance of industrial productivity. In rural areas of developing countries, there is typically much unemployment and underemployment, so that farm labor is in surplus supply and less scarce than manpower in industry. These remarks should not be interpreted as callous indifference to the health needs of rural people; quite the contrary, the long-term welfare of rural people—as has been shown in Europe and North America, in Japan and the Soviet Union—depends directly on industrial development and on reduction in the whole rural proportion of national populations.

COORDINATION OF THE HEALTH SERVICES

Having offered these seven arguments for social insurance programs in developing countries, despite the initial inequities they seem to cause, it does not follow that these programs should evolve in complete independence of the efforts of ministries of health or other organized health activities. Many of the problems faced by ministries of health in Latin America and elsewhere have been caused, not by the existence of social security programs, but by their independence and separatism, with respect to salary levels, location of health facilities, and other matters.[13] It is not sound social policy for one public agency to pay a higher salary to doctors or nurses than another, thereby immediately attracting the better qualified manpower. It is hardly good policy for a social security agency to construct a special hospital or health center in a town, across the street from a similar facility operated by the ministry of health, without any professional or administrative connection between the two.

In other words, coordination in both construction and operational policies, between social security and ministerial bodies, makes sense regardless of any priorities in the receipt of services that may be accorded to certain insured workers.[14] The same sort of coordination, of course, is called for between or among multiple social security bodies, covering different classes of workers—manual or commercial, private or governmental, blue collar or white collar—such as are found in Mexico, Peru, or Brazil. Fortunately, this need for coordination has been increasingly appreciated in recent years, as reflected in important conferences that have been convened in the Americas, as well as at the global international level.[15, 16]

If, then, social insurance is a reasonable stage in the national development of health services—provided that coordination with health ministry activities is achieved—can one offer a criterion on *when* it is sound to launch such a program in a developing country? The answer to this question must be partly political and partly economic. I would not venture a guideline on the political dimension, but on the economic dimension one might suggest the following criteria: (1) There should be a large enough number of regularly employed workers to yield a population base adequate to spread health care risks on an actuarially stable basis; this could be as few as 25,000, although a larger number would, of course, be better. (2) The average earnings of these workers should be high enough to render them either ineligible for or not desirous of using public services, so that—in the absence of social insurance—they would tend to make use of the private medical market with all it extravagances and inefficiencies. This level would, of course, have to be determined empirically in each country.

Finally, one may ask whether it is always historically necessary for a developing country to go through the stage of social insurance for supporting medical care in the course of its economic development. One can point to countries such as Chile or Cuba which, today, make very little use of the social insurance device and yet—mainly through general revenues—provide a very extensive entitlement to

medical care for their entire populations. One can point to currently industrialized countries such as Great Britain or Soviet Russia—which in past decades were, of course, once "underdeveloped"—that now have "national health services" for everyone supported almost entirely through general revenues.[17]

In reply, it may be noted that all four of these illustrative countries, in the course of their development, went through a stage of social insurance for selected population groups. Even in modern People's China, with its highly collectivistic ideology, health services for urban workers—in contrast to those for rural people—are financed along social insurance lines, although all contributions come from management payrolls rather than wage deductions.[18] In the United States today, we also see a great debate on national health insurance for the whole population—following six years of such insurance limited to the aged.[19] In the Soviet Union, it was some twenty years after its 1917 Revolution before the financing of medical services for the industrial population was shifted from social insurance largely to general revenues.[20] In New Zealand, which started a national health insurance program in 1938, it was only a few years ago that the shift was made to general revenue support.[21]

Thus, it seems to me that in countries of all types—industrialized and developing, capitalist and socialist—the social insurance mechanism is virtually an inevitable stage in the political and economic process of attaining effective distribution of personal health services to a total population. In the course of this evolution there may well be temporary inequities, favoring certain social groups as compared with others, but this is in the very nature of social progress. It is realistically not a great price to pay for the advantages of stability, planning, the achievement of a higher priority for health, and all the other advantages of the social insurance approach discussed earlier.

The waves of social change do not move forward evenly on all fronts. This is true within countries, no less than it is between countries. Improvements in health service come along many different paths, even if a country has policies of careful and systematic planning. One of the most important of these paths, in the experience of nations throughout the world, is the use of the social security mechanism for supporting medical care.[22]

NOTES

[1] B. Viel, *La Medicina Socializada y su Aplicación en Gran Bretaña, Union Sovietica y Chile.* Santiago: Universidad de Chile, 1964.

[2] U.S. Social Security Administration, *Social Security Programs throughout the World 1969*. Washington, D.C.: Government Printing Office, 1970.

[3] La Comision de Consultores Internacionales designada por el Director de la Oficina Sanitaria Panamericana, *Estudio de los Servicios de Salud Publica de la Argentina*. Washington, D.C.: Oficina Sanitaria Panamericana, 1957.

[4] Instituto Mexicano del Seguro Social, *La Seguridad Social en Mexico (Doctrina, Servicios, Legislacion, Information Estadistica)*. Mexico: 1964.

[5] A. L. Bravo and A. P. Ruderman, *Costs and Utilization of Ministry and Social Security Medical Care Facilities in Latin America*. Washington, D.C.: Pan American Health Organization, 1966.

[6] See chapter 7.

[7] M. I. Roemer, *The Organization of Medical Care under Social Security*. Geneva: International Labour Office, 1969.

[8] G. F. Rohrlich, "Social Security and Economic Development: The Evaluation of Program Needs at Successive Stages of Development." In E. M. Kassalow (ed.), *The Role of Social Security in Economic Development*. Washington, D.C.: U.S. Social Security Administration, 1968.

[9] Republica de Chile, Ministerio de Salud Publica, *Recursos Humanos de Salud en Chile: Un Modelo de Analisis*. Santiago: 1970, pp. 67-70.

[10] B. Abel-Smith, *An International Study of Health Expenditures and Its Relevance for Health Planning*. Geneva: World Health Organization, 1967.

[11] A. L. Bravo, "La Medicina de la Seguridad Social y los Programas Nacionales de Salud." *Revista Seguridad Social*, No. 56, March-April 1969.

[12] U.S. National Health Survey, *Selected Health Characteristics by Area: Geographic Regions and Urban-Rural Residence (United States 1957-1959)*. Washington, D.C.: Public Health Service, March 1961.

[13] Pan American Health Organization, *Administration of Medical Care Services*, Scientific Publication No. 129. Washington, D.C.: P.A.H.O., June 1966.

[14] See chapter 28.

[15] Pan American Health Organization, *Coordination of Medical Care* (Final Report of a Study Group on the Coordination of Medical Care Services of Ministries of Health, Social Security Institutes, and Universities). Washington, D.C.: P.A.H.O., 1970.

[16] Joint ILO/WHO Committee on Personal Health Care and Social Security, *Report of the Meeting 10-16 November 1970*. Geneva: 1971.

[17] J. Fry, *Medicine in Three Societies: A Comparison of Medical Care in the USSR, USA and UK*. New York: American Elsevier Publishing Company, Inc., 1970.

[18] F. T. Fox, "Medical Care in Communist China Today." *American Journal of Public Health*, Vol. 50, June 1960, pp. 28-35.

[19] H. M. Somers and A. R. Somers, *Medicare and the Hospitals: Issues and Prospects*. Washington, D.C.: Brookings Institution, 1967.

[20] H. E. Sigerist, *Medicine and Health in the Soviet Union*. New York: Citadel Press, 1947, p. 111.

[21] G. M. Emery, "New Zealand Medical Care." *Medical Care* (London), Vol. 4, July-September 1966, pp. 159-170.

[22] Research done after this article was published demonstrated the validity of the fifth hypothesis offered—namely, that in Latin America, countries with stronger social security programs tend to be associated also with stronger, rather than weaker, ministries of health. Both types of "strength" were quantified in several ways. An article presenting these data is published, with the coauthorship of N. Maeda, as "Does Social Security Support for Medical Care Weaken Public Health Programs?" *International Journal of Health Services*, Vol. 6, No. 1, 1976.

Chapter XXV
Social Insurance as Leverage for Changing Health Care Systems

In the social debates about national health insurance, both in the United States and elsewhere, it is often pointed out that the problems of improving medical care distribution involve more than money. The pattern of delivery or method of organization of health services is equally or more important.

In this chapter, the experience of several nations is explored from the viewpoint of social insurance serving as a step leading to the improved organization of health care systems. While the course of events, of course, differs in various political settings, there is much historical evidence to suggest that mandatory health insurance leads to modification in patterns of delivering medical care. This paper was presented to the New York Academy of Medicine in 1971 and published as "Social Insurance as Leverage for Changing Health Care Systems: International Experience" in the Bulletin of the New York Academy of Medicine, *Second Series, Vol. 48, January 1972, pp. 93-107). It is reprinted here by permission.*

Most if not all of the issues on the financing and organization of the health services in the United States today have been or are being faced also in other countries. While comparisons of health care solutions in different nations, which differ in their social, political, and economic settings, have hazards too obvious to recite, one may still gain perspective for wise decisions in the United States by cautious observation of foreign experience.

In these remarks I shall focus on one issue, which has become especially salient in the present American scene: the feasibility of social insurance providing leverage for modifying patterns of delivering health service. What has been the experience of other countries, where social insurance has been developed, with respect to modification of medical care patterns which had prevailed before the insurance program? In exploring this question, I shall try to examine countries at various points on the political spectrum and at different stages of economic development.

SOCIAL INSURANCE AS A BUTTRESS FOR THE STATUS QUO

In Western Europe, where the social insurance movement had its start, the initial purposes were essentially limited to providing economic protection of workers against the cost of certain risks, including sickness. The pioneer German law of 1883 simply required workers to belong to a local sickness fund which would (1) compensate them for loss of earnings due to illness, and (2) pay for the costs of medical care.[1] The laws that followed later in Austria, the Scandinavian countries, Belgium, France, Great Britain, and elsewhere were fashioned basically on the same model—that of compelling enrollment of workers in local societies which would pay for doctor's services, drugs, and hospital care obtained in the open market. Hospitalization had previously been supported mainly from general tax funds, and this continued after social insurance, the latter paying only the partial charges levied on a patient above the indigency level.[2]

The existing nineteenth century patterns for the delivery of medical care were taken for granted in Western Europe. Indeed, it has been pointed out by many that the social insurance schemes largely fortified the patterns of private individual medical practice in these countries, along with commercial pharmacies, private dental practice, and local autonomous hospitals. Massive poverty in many European cities and the strength of socialist movements threatened to lead to more radical forms of "state medicine." Far from being a revolutionary approach, social insurance was generally put across by conservative political parties as a palliative social reform; Bismarck's original proposal, in fact, was opposed by the Social Democrats (i.e., socialists) of the day on the ground that—limited as it was initially to low income workers—it was "beggar's insurance" designed to compel the poor to look out for themselves. It was also attacked as merely treating the ills of the working class, without getting at the basic causes of their misery. Later, of course, as social insurance broadened its coverage of people and its scope of benefits, the left-wing parties supported it. With such origins, in any case, the European programs of health insurance could hardly be expected to launch any wholesale changes of the system of furnishing medical care.

Yet it is an oversimplification to suggest that social insurance had no effects at all on the patterns of serving patients. After not many years of operation, the sickness insurance societies in Europe came to recognize the value of preventive medicine, and undertook to promote it in various ways. As long ago as 1928, Franz Goldmann and Alfred Grotjahn compiled a review of these efforts entitled *Benefits of the German Sickness Insurance System from the Point of View of Social Hygiene*.[3] In this book we learn of the provision of x-ray examinations by special clinics for early detection of tuberculosis, general periodic health examinations in factories, health education through literature, exhibits, and health visitors sent to homes, and of special subsidies from the insurance funds to local public health authorities for the strengthening of maternal and child health or venereal disease control services. To encourage services for the promotion of health, a number of German insurance societies paid cash "nursing benefits" to the mothers of newborn infants only on presentation of a certificate showing that the baby was receiving regular check-ups at a child welfare station. Similar preventive services were promoted by the French social security system after its extension to include medical benefits in 1928; support was and is still given to tuberculosis control, maternal and child health services, and a general corps of *assistantes*

sociales, who help French families cope with health problems in various ways.[4]

While these preventive activities involved only a small percentage of health insurance expenditures, they did constitute a modest modification of conventional patterns of private medical care. The point is that these efforts to influence the procurement of health services, rather than merely paying doctor's bills, were being made before World War I, long before any significant voice was being raised in America or in Europe to change the system of health care. In those days the office of the private family doctor, the compounded prescription, the home call, specialized consultation, service at the general hospital outpatient clinic or inpatient ward were the mainstays of medical care; the problem was to ease the payment for these services. The social insurance programs addressed themselves to this problem with much success.

Here and there, nevertheless, the European health insurance funds took steps to modify patterns of curative services also. A few of the German sickness funds provided medical care to their members through full-time salaried doctors working in organized dispensaries. In some of the larger cities, moreover, special diagnostic institutes were established, providing laboratory equipment not available in the private doctor's office. Such an institute was operated in Berlin, for example, by the Association of Berlin Sickness Funds in 1925; on its staff were five salaried doctors along with twelve technical personnel. Special centers were also established for physical therapy and for orthopedic gymnastics; in Dresden the funds established a clinic devoted to the treatment of varicose veins. In connection with large factories, the insurance societies sometimes established clinics for rehabilitative treatments. University polyclinics also came to be used for insured persons through special contracts with the funds, thus providing ambulatory specialist services in organized frameworks which had otherwise been restricted to the poor.

The deficiencies of private solo practice did not pass unrecognized by some medical leaders in the social insurance movement. Drs. Goldmann and Grotjahn wrote in 1928:

> It is not the fault of the practitioners who work single-handed that they cannot achieve all that might be desirable from the standpoint of social hygiene, either in the matter of curative treatment of individual cases or of prevention. . . . The idea has therefore been put forward that the basis for such a reorganisation of the medical service might be found in institutes in which a group of doctors can cooperate in the treatment of individual cases and in social welfare work alike. . . . The possibility of examining,

of establishing a diagnosis and of advising a great number of patients with as little waste of time as possible, and few overhead costs, through an association of efficient general practitioners and specialists under an able head, assisted by a trained staff and the best diagnostic and therapeutic equipment, offers patients, doctors, and fund administrations such great advantages over the present system of isolated sickness fund doctors, that it is unthinkable that this systematising of services . . . should not end by becoming general, despite all opposition.

The opposition, as we know, largely prevailed in Western Europe, but even within the context of private medical practice the social insurance movement had the important influence of increasing the general utilization of health services. This, in turn, provided an economic foundation for expanding the supply of doctors. In the decade from 1889 to 1898, for example, the German population increased twelve percent while the number of physicians rose by fifty-six percent; this was a much greater expansion than characterized the medical profession in Great Britain and the United States, which lacked social insurance, over the same decade. The great improvement in hospital equipment and staffing after the turn of the twentieth century, moreover, required financial support which the social insurance programs helped to provide. We have seen the same dynamics at work in America, where the voluntary hospitalization insurance movement undoubtedly facilitated the great expansion of hospitals, both quantitatively and qualitatively, over the last thirty or forty years.

SOCIAL INSURANCE OUTSIDE OF EUROPE

In the countries outside Western Europe, social insurance has usually had a different background, and its impacts on medical care have accordingly been different. The first non-European application of social insurance to general medical care occurred in two countries much influenced by Germany in their general cultural and industrial development: Japan in 1922 and Chile in 1924.[5] In Latin America the idea spread to every other sovereign country except Argentina over the next forty years. In 1938 New Zealand launched its national health insurance program; Australia enacted a law in the same year, but it was not implemented until ten years later. After World War II the idea spread to India (1948), Iran (1949), Indonesia (1957), and several other countries of Asia and North Africa. Canada enacted its national insurance program for hospitalization in 1957 and for physician's care in 1966.

In the substantially industrialized countries

among these—Japan, Australia, and Canada—conditions were somewhat similar to those in Europe, with a prior existence of many voluntary or nongovernmental health insurance plans and a strong sector of private medical practice. In these countries, the health insurance programs applied the "indirect pattern" of purchasing services, on a fee basis, from independent doctors and hospitals. In the numerous developing countries, however, conditions were different. Local health insurance societies, with administrative experience and vested job interests, were rare. The great majority of doctors had to struggle hard to make a good living in the private market, and were only too glad to accept salaried employment in organized programs. To provide an adequate quality of medical care for insured persons, therefore, direct action could be taken at the national level in the way of mobilizing medical resources and services. This meant, in effect, a substantial alteration of the health care delivery patterns that had previously prevailed for persons who had now become insured.

In Chile, after 1924, this meant the construction of a network of health centers and polyclinics for both primary and specialized medical care of insured persons.[6] Urban industrial workers, who were the first beneficiaries, had previously obtained ambulatory medical care at the crowded and understaffed clinics of charity hospitals or from private doctors, if they could afford them. Well-equipped ambulatory care facilities, staffed by doctors paid a salary for their time—rather than being called upon to serve the poor free, in a condescending spirit of noblesse oblige—meant a considerable change. Hospitalization for insured persons in Chile was arranged in existing hospitals, but special amenities and semi-private rooms were provided instead of care in the large traditional charity wards. In 1940 the Peruvian social security program broke away from dependence on existing hospitals by constructing the Hospital Obrero de Lima—the first hospital devoted exclusively to care of insured persons in Latin America. Since then, this pattern of separate hospitals, as well as separate health centers, for insured persons has spread throughout Latin America. The same pattern has been adopted in most of the social insurance programs of other developing countries, such as Iran or Turkey.

The insured populations of these developing countries, it must be realized, constitute only a small proportion of the total—typically less than ten percent. Since the financial resources of social security programs are usually greater than those of ministries of health in proportion to the number of persons served, the quality of medical care offered is correspondingly higher than that available to the great majority of people.[7]

Numerous questions have been raised about the inequities of these patterns with respect to the noninsured portions of the population; the justifications, in terms of the special requirements for national economic development, have been explored by international committees of the United Nations.[8] Whatever position one may take on the ethical and economic issues involved, there can be no question that these social insurance programs in developing countries have, indeed, modified the prevailing patterns of medical care for important segments of the national populations. Moreover, there is indirect evidence that the relatively high medical care standards, applied to the favored minority of insured persons in these countries, have had an influence in upgrading the standards of care offered to the rest of the people.

SOCIAL INSURANCE AS A PROLOGUE TO NATIONAL HEALTH SERVICES

Beyond the original Western European health insurance programs and the more innovative patterns in developing countries, there is a third route through which social insurance has influenced health care delivery systems. This has been by serving as a prologue, by paving the way to massive modifications of the whole national system of medical care. Such extensive changes, of course, depend very much on larger political events, but the health care developments launched tend to be built upon the prior accomplishments of the insurance programs.

The most spectacular of such changes in health care systems have occurred in countries undergoing socialist revolutions. I do not suggest that social security itself paves the way to socialism—as shrilly argued by early antagonists to health insurance, even voluntarily sponsored, in this country—for the effect has probably been exactly the opposite: to help preserve capitalism by correcting its worst ills. When the first socialist revolution occurred in 1917 in czarist Russia, however, the plans for the new medical care system did not ignore but were rather built upon the statutory health insurance schemes which had been operating in the main cities since 1912. Under the Soviet government the social insurance program, which had previously covered about one-fifth of the wage-earners, was expanded to cover 100 percent of them. The basic mechanism of financing medical care through social insurance funds, derived from the earnings of each industrial enterprise, was continued.[9] Initially medical care was obtained from private doctors or local hospitals, paid for by the insurance agencies, until the socialized framework of health facilities with salaried staffs could be established. Since agricultural people, the vast majority of the population of the Union of Soviet Socialist Republics, were seldom wage-earners, and since special district doctors and feldshers had previously served them (albeit inadequately) under the czarist zemstvo medicine program, the peasants and other country dwellers were not included under the social insurance program; a separate rural health service was organized for them. It was not until 1937, about twenty years after the Revolution, that this dichotomy between urban and rural medical care financing and organization was dissolved in the Soviet Union, and the whole system was integrated under general revenue financing.

Similar evolutionary processes have characterized medical care developments in the other Eastern European countries undergoing socialist revolutions after World War II. In each case the social insurance mechanisms, with payment for each unit of service rendered by individual practitioners, were continued until a structured state medical service could be developed. In Poland, for example, up to the present day, the entitlement to medical care of wage-earners, coming within social security financing, is much greater than that of peasants or small shopkeepers. These self-employed persons may use the organized state system of health centers and hospitals, but they must pay for these services (reportedly at about fifty percent of their true cost).[10] Alternatively, noninsured persons may still obtain ambulatory care from private doctors and dentists. Cuba is another socialist country which, since its 1959 Revolution, has retained much of the framework of former local mutual aid societies for furnishing care to certain groups of urban workers.[11]

Less radical but still profound changes in medical care organization have occurred in a few other countries that had several decades of experience with social insurance. In Great Britain a program of national health insurance for manual workers was enacted in 1911. The benefits were limited to care by general practitioners and prescribed drugs; other services, such as hospitalization and specialist care, were financed through voluntary insurance, governmental revenue, charity support, or private payment. When the National Health Service covering the total population was put into effect in 1948 the thirty-seven years of health insurance experience were not ignored.[12] Care by general practitioners previously remunerated through capitation panels continued in the same way, and duties of the former "friendly societies" and local "insurance committees" were assigned to the new executive councils. Other branches of the tripartite National Health Service—the regional hospital boards and the local health authorities—did not emerge from the social insurance framework, but did come from other prior programs in the British health scene. It is only now, in 1971, that we are seeing serious moves to integrate the three sectors of the British health care system under a new network of "unitary authorities."[13]

Can there be any doubt that the experience of British health insurance from 1911 to the outbreak of World War II paved the way for the current National Health Service? The limited social insurance program worked but, as the Beveridge Report pointed out, it did not do enough. The lessons of the experience were that, if needs were to be met, both the coverage of people and the scope of services had to be extended, with substantial changes in the management of hospitals. By the same token the experience of the National Health Service over the last twenty-three years is exposing the deficiencies of its least organized sector: the general practitioner service. In the last few years the clustering of general practitioners in small group practices has been increasing rapidly, along with more frequent location of such medical groups in government-owned health centers.[14] These trends constitute further important changes in British health care delivery.

Chile is another country where experience with social insurance for medical care of a limited minority of the population paved the way for a much more extensive program. In 1952, after twenty-eight years of experience with social insurance for manual workers, Chile enacted its National Health Service (NHS) serving about seventy percent of the population; coverage was extended to all low income people, in agriculture as well as urban industry, and to all children in families of any income level. The great majority of hospitals were taken over by the Ministry of Health, and all health centers or polyclinics, under previously diverse auspices, were integrated with the hospitals into regional networks. Each region or health zone (thirteen in all) is administered by a medical officer responsible for the total health service: ambulatory, hospital, and preventive. In 1969 the coverage of the Chilean NHS was broadened to include white collar employees, previously covered under a separate insurance program, although permitting them to have free choice of a private doctor if the individual is willing to pay half of the private fees. It will be interesting to observe the further evolution of the Chilean system under its new left-wing coalition government, headed by a physician and former health minister.

New Zealand and Sweden illustrate other coun-

tries with national health insurance, where after several years substantive changes in delivery patterns are taking place. In New Zealand, for example, legislative amendments in 1970 have authorized hospital boards, which administer several hospitals in a region, to establish and maintain health centers for ambulatory care as well.[15] The intent is clearly to encourage and facilitate movement of general practitioners from their private "rooms" to organized facilities, where they can work in close alliance with the local public health staff of visiting nurses, social workers, health educators, technicians, etc. After thirty years of the national insurance scheme, the New Zealand practitioners themselves are very much in favor of this idea.[16]

In Sweden one can identify several steps of significance in the evolutionary process. After a century of purely voluntary health insurance societies, national legislation brought the local funds under governmental surveillance in 1931. Enrollment remained voluntary, however, until 1955, when the total population became protected and the medical benefits were increased and made nationally uniform.[17] Then, in 1970, the previously autonomous local hospitals, mostly under county government control, were brought under the general influence, if not actual supervision, of regional hospital authorities—seven of these covering the nation.[18] At the same time hospital-based physicians, who account for most of Sweden's specialists, have been made strictly full-time, instead of being allowed to have private practices on the side; ambulatory cases are seen by specialists in the hospital outpatient departments. These developments clearly mark rationalized changes in the Swedish health care system.[19]

THE BASIC CHANGES IN
HEALTH CARE PATTERNS

Having reviewed, although superficially, the modifications of health care patterns occurring under social insurance programs in a number of countries, it may be helpful to analyze these developments according to their technical nature, rather than their mode of evolution. In my view health system innovations, for the attainment of which social insurance may provide leverage, come down to four major types: (1) disease prevention, (2) medical teamwork, (3) regionalization, and (4) general quality controls.

With respect to the promotion of preventive services we have noted the activities of local sickness funds in Germany of more than fifty years ago. Other present examples may be cited. In Great Britain special fees are now paid to general practitioners, over and above their capitation receipts, to encourage them to give immunizations and prenatal examinations. In Belgium the local insurance carriers organize screening programs for chronic disease at places of work, physical examinations of schoolchildren in some districts, and cancer-detection cytological tests for women. In Tunisia the medical care financed by social insurance is administered through the Ministry of Health rather than by a separate social security agency, and preventive services—such as trachoma control—are rendered to insured persons at health centers, along with curative services.[20] An especially interesting program of this sort has been operating in Chile since 1938 under its preventive medicine law, as it was called. This required annual examination of all insured workers for early detection of tuberculosis, syphilis, and heart disease; cancer was added later to the statutory list. After a while the burden of performing these examinations became greater than could be borne by the resources of the Chilean health insurance system as a whole, and the tests became applied only to selected groups of white collar employees, mainly in governmental jobs.[21]

In regard to the promotion of medical teamwork the influence of social insurance in establishing health centers staffed by teams of physicians and allied personnel has been observed. This is the prevailing pattern in Latin America, the Mediterranean region, and developing countries generally. It should be realized that if there were no social insurance in those countries skilled workers with relatively stable incomes would tend to become patients in the purely private medical sector. One can observe this vividly in South Korea or Malaysia where, lacking social insurance, moderate income urban workers and their families get their ambulatory care predominantly through privately practicing doctors on a fee basis.[22] Thus the "direct pattern" of organized ambulatory care facilities for insured persons, used in many developing countries—not to mention the socialist societies—constitutes a promotion of teamwork medicine that does not otherwise seem to come about for this social class.

Even in Western European countries, where individual medical practice outside the hospital has been so firmly established, the teaming up of doctors in private group clinics or in community health centers has been growing in recent years. We have already noted the trends in Great Britain; the Ministry of Health there has actually encouraged group practice for some years through low-interest loans to doctors for the construction or remodeling of clinic facilities. Also in France, Germany, the Scandinavian countries, Japan, and Australia, there has been a small but definite tendency for group practice to grow in a variety of forms.[23] The social insurance programs may not be directly responsible for the founding of these group clinics but they obviously provide indirect financial support and, insofar as group practice yields internal economies of the medical care production process, the payment of standard insurance fees can provide incentives to organization of medical groups by yielding higher net incomes for the doctors. In France local health centers, for both curative and preventive services, have recently been promoted by the social security authorities, and a National Association of Health Center Doctors has backed up this movement.[24]

Regionalization, as a basic strategy for changing health care delivery, is evident under many of the social insurance programs. It is relevant that the first clear elaboration of the concept came from a British committee, of which Lord Dawson of Penn was chairman, which issued its report in 1920, only nine years after the national health insurance program had been started.[25] This called for organization of all personal health services, both curative and preventive, through regional networks of health centers and hospitals. Although the concept was not implemented until 1948 under the National Health Service—and then only partially—the Dawson Report had an influence on health care organization in many British colonies overseas. The recent British "green papers" on reorganization of the health services are extending the idea. In Sweden we have noted other forms of implementing regionalization under a social insurance framework, and somewhat similar policies are being pursued by regional authorities of the national Ministry of Health in France. Where social insurance has evolved into general revenue financing, as in Chile and New Zealand, not to mention all the socialist countries, the concept of regionalization has been most actively implemented.

Finally, the influence of social insurance on general promotion of the quality of medical care should be appreciated. When care is provided through organized frameworks, professional surveillance over quality is built into day-to-day work. In the Mexican social security program, for example, there are systematic medical audits of the work of individual doctors. In the Polish system, there is a hierarchy of technical supervision from national to district to local levels; there are also periodic inspections by consultants from the specialist associations. Postgraduate education of doctors is encouraged in Poland, although it is not required regularly, as under the health system of the Soviet Union.

When medical care is provided through private

practitioners and local hospitals, the quality controls are most tenuous, but many measures have been applied. In Great Britian, for example, a maximum number of persons is allowed on a general practitioner's panel in the interest of protecting quality. In the German program there are statistical analyses to identify doctors whose patterns of practice deviate markedly from the average; these give a signal for discussions with the practitioner by a medical consultant or "control doctor" from the insurance administration. In several countries exceptional patterns of prescribing drugs are also followed up. Persistent deviance by a doctor that cannot be justified may lead to his exclusion from the social insurance program. In Belgium certain modalities that might be subject to abuse, such as physical therapy, are subject to prior authorization. The quality of in-hospital services is protected in all the Western European health insurance programs, as well as in Canada, by governmental inspection of the facilities to make certain that they meet technical standards. While such monitoring of private medical care is always somewhat awkward, and while much of it is focused on cost controls, the existence of the surveillance undoubtedly influences quality through enhancement of the self-discipline of all participating providers.[26]

CONCLUSION

This review of foreign experience, it is hoped, may have demonstrated that social insurance programs have exercised many influences on the patterns of medical care delivery, over and above their role in financing. The degree of this influence is obviously dependent on the general political and economic realities of the country. It is greater where the political ideology is more collectivized and where the economic level is somewhat lower. Where individualism and affluence are greater, the leverage of social insurance to modify medical care patterns tends to be less.

It does not require great imagination to see the parallels between various current legislative proposals for health insurance in the United States and the experiences in various other countries. The proposals which would encourage but not require enrollment of people in voluntary insurance plans, with subsidies for low income persons, are mindful of the present law in Australia.[27] Proposals which would mandate membership of wage-earners and certain others in some existing or new local health insurance plan, also subsidizing the poor, are similar to the design of the original German legislation, as

well as the Belgian. Much obviously depends on the precise governmental standards imposed on these local plans and the rigor with which any standards are enforced. Proposals which would cover the entire national population by law, with support through social insurance and general revenues, are more like the programs in New Zealand or Sweden. On the other hand, the systems in these countries for specialized care and hospital organization, both internally and regionally, would not be instituted by any present American proposal. Moreover, the provision of strong personal incentives to private providers, as well as consumers, to join in new forms of "health maintenance organization"—which figure prominently in several American bills—are not found in any of the foreign programs.[28]

This use of the profit motive, so to speak, to encourage local modifications of the health care delivery system seems to be a uniquely American idea. In it there are great attractions but there are also hazards if strong safeguards are not established against the deterioration of quality in the interest of maximizing earnings. It remains to be seen how these ideas, if legislatively implemented, will work out. In all nations, however, the difficulties emerging under a social insurance program tend to generate their own reform. No better example could be found than the current discussion of national health insurance for the whole population of the United States, growing out of the experience of the Medicare law for the aged and the difficulties in our system that its operations have exposed for everyone to see.[29] In the same vein we may be confident that any program of social insurance for general medical care enacted in this country would probably, before long, induce many changes in our delivery patterns, as has happened in other countries throughout the world.

NOTES

[1] H. E. Sigerist, "From Bismarck to Beveridge: Developments and Trends in Social Security Legislation." *Bulletin of the History of Medicine*, Vol. 8, 1943, pp. 365-388.

[2] I. S. Falk, *Security Against Sickness: A Study of Health Insurance.* Garden City, New York: Doubleday, Doran, 1936.

[3] F. Goldmann and A. Grotjahn, *Benefits of the German Sickness Insurance System from the Point of View of Social Hygiene.* Geneva: International Labour Office, 1928.

[4] P. Laroque, "Social Security and Social Services." *Bulletin of the International Social Security Association.* October-November 1952, pp. 317-352.

[5] U.S. Social Security Administration, *Social Security Programs throughout the World 1969.* Washington, D.C.: Government Printing Office, 1970.

[6] See chapter 7.

[7] See chapter 24.

[8] Joint ILO/WHO Committees on Personal Health Care and Social Security, *Report of the Meeting 10-16 November 1970*. Geneva: 1971.

[9] H. E. Sigerist, *Socialized Medicine in the Soviet Union*. New York: W. W. Norton and Company, 1937, pp. 85-92.

[10] E. R. Weinerman, *Social Medicine in Eastern Europe*. Cambridge, Massachusetts: Harvard University Press, 1969, pp. 117-155. In 1973, however, Poland extended its public medical care system to cover the entire population.

[11] W. P. Butler, "Cuba's Revolutionary Medicine." *Ramparts*, May 1969. Also, R. John *et al.*, "Public Health Care in Cuba.: *Social Policy*, January-February 1971, pp. 41-46.

[12] A. Lindsey, *Socialized Medicine in England and Wales: The National Health Service 1948-1961*. Chapel Hill: University of North Carolina Press, 1962.

[13] Department of Health and Social Security (United Kingdom), *The Future Structure of the National Health Service* (Green Paper II). London: 1970. Also, see chapter 11.

[14] M. Curwen and B. Brookes, "Health Centres: Facts and Figures." *Lancet*, No. 7627, November 1, 1969, pp. 945-948.

[15] Government of New Zealand, *Hospital Amendment*, 1970, No. 12. Wellington: Government Printing Office, 1970.

[16] See chapter 13.

[17] C. G. Uhr, *Sweden's Social Security System*. Washington, D.C.: Social Security Administration, Research Report No. 14, 1966.

[18] A. Engle, "Areawide Hospital Planning in Sweden." *World Hospitals*, Vol. 4, 1968, p. 214.

[19] A. R. Somers, "The Rationalization of Health Services: A Universal Priority." *Inquiry*, Vol. 8, 1971, pp. 48-60.

[20] M. I. Roemer, *The Organization of Medical Care Under Social Security: A Study Based on the Experience of Eight Countries*. Geneva: International Labour Office, 1969, pp. 121-128.

[21] B. Viel, *La Medicina Socializada y su Aplicación en Gran Bretaña, Union Sovietica y Chile*. Santiago: Universidad de Chile, 1964.

[22] M. I. Roemer and O. Manning, *Assignment Report on Strengthening of Health Services and Training of Health Personnel (Malaysia)*. Manila: World Health Organization, February 1969.

[23] First International Congress on Group Medicine, *New Horizons in Health Care: Proceedings*. Winnipeg: Wallingford Press, 1970.

[24] "Evolution des Centres de Santé et Organisation Sociale de la Medecine (III Congres National des Médecins de Centres de Santé—Soins et Prevention)." Supplement to *Centre de Santé*, April 1964.

[25] Ministry of Health, Consultative Council on Medical and Allied Services, *Interim Report on the Future of Medical and Allied Services*. London: His Majesty's Stationery Office, 1920.

[26] Roemer, *Medical Care Under Social Security*, pp. 181-197.

[27] J. M. Last, "Medical Care in Australia." *Practitioner* (London), Vol. 197, 1966, pp. 177-184.

[28] P. M. Ellwood, "Health Maintenance Organizations: Concept and Strategy." *Hospitals*, Vol. 45, 1971, pp. 53-56.

[29] "Our Ailing Medical System." Series of articles in *Fortune*, January 1970.

Part Five

General Interpretations

Chapter XXVI
A Classification of Medical Care Systems in Relation to Public Health Organization

If one takes a very broad view of national systems of medical care throughout the world, it is possible to classify them into categories. The predominant mechanism of economic support for services plays a large part in the administrative pattern by which those services are delivered, so that this mechanism-ranging from individualistic to collectivistic–may serve as a useful basis for classification. On this basis, four major types of medical care system may be identified in the world; each of these types bears a different relationship to the administration of community preventive services by "health departments" or public health agencies.

Because the relationship between public health agencies and medical care programs has long been a contentious issue in the United States, a brief review of the world scene in this regard was presented at the annual meeting of the American Public Health Association in 1958. Since then, of course, organizational changes have occurred in all countries: social insurance has extended in the United States, Canada, and elsewhere; the Cuban Revolution has brought a completely socialized health care system to one Latin American country; governmental services have been greatly expanded in Africa and Asia; and so on. Yet the concept of a range of medical care systems, depending on the predominant (not the only) mechanism of economic support, is probably still valid. This chapter was originally published as "Health Departments and Medical Care–A World Scanning" in the American Journal of Public Health (Vol. 50, February 1960, pp. 154-160) and is reprinted here by permission.[1]

Every public health worker knows how difficult it is to define the meaning and scope of functions of a health department in the United States—so different are activities among the states, counties, and cities. On a world scale, the problem of definition is obviously greater. For the sake of simplicity, and to provide a convenient basis for comparing administrative patterns in different countries, we may use "health department" to mean that agency of government which, among other things, is responsible for most organized preventive health services in a nation, province, or community. In addition, this agency may supervise or provide various segments of medical care for the population. This brief review describes the predominant forms of relationship between public health and medical care administration in different nations.

AMERICAN BACKGROUND

The issues that have confronted us in the United States as to the best pattern for administration of medical care are by no means unique, nor are they of recent vintage here. Current-day readers are doubtless familiar with the official statement of the American Public Health Association in 1944, advocating administration of any program of medical care for the general population by health departments. The basic argument was that administrative integration of preventive and curative services is desirable, and this could be better achieved under a unified health department rather than dual agency administration.[2]

Less well known, perhaps, is the fact that America's public health leaders advocated the closest possible connection between medical care and public health administration long before this. In 1916, the

Conference of State and Territorial Health Authorities, meeting in Washington, D.C., adopted a report on "Health Insurance." This report advocated general medical care insurance for all employed persons earning less than a specified annual income. It favored the establishment of state funds from employee and employer contributions, but it criticized European health insurance programs because they did not provide for "correlating the system with existing health agencies." In contrast, this report recommended that in America:

> There must be close connection of the administration of any health insurance system with the health agencies of the country and with the medical profession. It is believed that this can be done in three ways: (1) by providing efficient staffs of medical officers in Federal and State health departments to carry into effect the regulations issued by the central governing boards or commissions; (2) by providing a fair and sufficient incentive for the active cooperation of the medical profession; and (3) by providing for a close cooperation of the health insurance system with State, municipal, and local health departments and boards.[3]

Especially familiar to contemporary ears is the ring of a later paragraph which states:

> Health officials should realize now the necessity for correlating the administration of the medical benefits of any proposed health insurance system with existing health agencies. If health departments are at present inefficient, they should be strengthened and made adequate to meet all demands.

Despite these views, going back over forty years, health insurance programs developing in the United States have had little if any administrative connection with health departments. Even programs of medical care for the needy, workmen's compensation, medical care for veterans, the operation of hospitals for mental disorders, or other significant programs of medical care are generally not under health department jurisdiction. One may see a small trend toward increasing health department concern for medical care in the last fifteen or twenty years, but the predominant pattern today remains one of divided rather than unified responsibilities for preventive and curative health service administration.[4]

WORLD PERSPECTIVE

A scanning of the administrative schemes in other countries may help to provide a better understanding of the pattern now found in the United States. For, if we take the world as our social laboratory, we can observe a range of differing patterns of health service organization, and the relationships of the health department to medical care can be defined more or less by the place of a country in this theoretical framework.

The health service programs of different countries can be characterized as falling into four principal types: (1) free enterprise, (2) social insurance, (3) public assistance, (4) universal service. Of course, no such classification can be made too rigid, for social phenomena are far too complex. In every country there are some elements of all four of these patterns of health service organization. In each country, however, one of the four predominates, while the others play a subordinate role.[5]

In the United States, the free enterprise pattern predominates, with the population receiving most of its health service under privately financed arrangements. We know how rapidly this is changing, with the great extension of voluntary insurance and public medical care programs, but as of 1958 these movements have not yet affected the lion's share of medical care costs or services. On the whole, Canada and Australia are likewise in the free enterprise group, although they are moving very rapidly toward the social insurance pattern. All three countries, it may be noted, are federations of states or provinces, comparatively wealthy, highly industrialized, relatively young, and pioneering in character.[6]

In these countries, the health department tends to concentrate heavily or exclusively on the administration of preventive services. Health insurance administration is mainly under voluntary societies, having little if any official connection with the health department. Even in Canada, where national hospital insurance legislation has recently taken effect, the provincial administration is predominantly under agencies other than the public health authority. The general hospitals are largely under the control of local voluntary groups. Health centers are interpreted mainly as buildings to house a health department, rather than places for ambulatory health care of the population. Programs of medical care for special diseases and selected population groups are usually administered by agencies separate from the health department, although there are important exceptions in some of the provinces and states. School health services are often under boards of education, rural health programs under agricultural agencies, industrial injury services under other auspices. Licensure of physicians and other health personnel is usually in the hands of semiautonomous professional bodies.

In western continental Europe, the social insurance pattern of health service organization predominates. In France, Germany, the Benelux countries, Italy, and Scandinavia, most of the population receive the major part of their medical and hospital services through social insurance systems. In general, benefits are related to specific contributions. Of course, there are great differences among these systems in the methods of raising funds, population coverage, health benefits, ways of paying doctors, and in patterns of administration. On the whole, however, physicians remain in private medical practice for ambulatory care and receive payments of fees directly or indirectly from the insurance funds. Hospitals, on the other hand, are predominantly governmental, under local or provincial authorities. Most medical practice in the hospitals is by salaried specialists, employed directly by the hospital administration. This general pattern is found also in Japan and Israel, countries highly influenced by European developments. (Israel is exceptional, however, with its salaried insurance doctors in health centers.) In Sweden and Norway, health insurance coverage has recently been extended to the entire population. Under these schemes the patient is indemnified for most, though not all, medical charges and certain benefits (e.g., drugs and dental care) are restricted.

Under the social insurance pattern, the health department has little connection with the administration of the health insurance funds. These are typically under hundreds of semi-independent organizations, developed on geographic, occupational, or religious lines. They are usually supervised by ministries of labor or social welfare, which also control old-age pensions and other aspects of social security. At the national level there may be an advisory service from the health ministry or department, but at the local level the health officer is seldom involved. It is noteworthy, perhaps, that many of the social insurance institutions have undertaken their own preventive service programs—even without health department ties—a trend reported as early as 1928 by Franz Goldmann and Alfred Grotjahn.[7] On the other hand, in Scandinavia, one sees salaried district health officers, responsible for public health administration, engaged also in the provision of medical care to the rural population.

Hospitals, in general, come under much greater public health supervision in the social insurance than in the free enterprise countries. The health ministry, typically, has a major division for supervision of hospitals, the authority of which goes far beyond such measures as are embodied in the Hill-Burton construction program or the hospital licensure laws of the United States. Health officers at the provincial or district level are often responsible for supervising the operation of all public hospitals in their territory, including standards of personnel and operation as well as construction. Medical and other types of professional licensure are also usually a health ministry function. The care of tuberculosis and mental disorders in special institutions is ordinarily assigned to branches of the national health department, although the local health officer may not be involved. Health departments commonly have duties in legal or forensic medicine, especially in Central Europe. Medical inspection of factories, on the other hand, by reason of European political history is usually a function of separate officers of departments of labor.

There has been rapid movement since World War II, especially in the northern European countries, from a social insurance toward a universal service pattern of health care. Increasing shares of hospital service are financed from general revenues, rather than insurance funds; and even the insurance funds for ambulatory medical care receive increasingly larger subventions from general revenues, as coverage is extended to the entire population.

The third, or public assistance pattern of health service, is found principally in the great stretches of Asia, Africa, and most of Latin America, areas characterized as the economically underdeveloped parts of the world. Here the great majority of the population cannot afford to finance needed medical services either through insurance or private payments. They depend for the most part on services provided free by the government and financed from general revenues. Most of these services are given by salaried personnel working in hospitals, dispensaries, or health centers. Because of the prevailing shortage of doctors, extensive use is made of auxiliary personnel. In the large cities, private physicians and private hospitals are available for the relatively small upper and middle classes. A means test is theoretically applied to determine eligibility for public services, but since the vast majority of people are poor, eligibility is taken for granted in everyday life.

While the level of medical services in countries with the public assistance pattern is seriously impaired by the sheer poverty of these nations and their great shortages of personnel and facilities, the administrative pattern vests wide authority in the health department. Typically, the national health ministry is responsible for most curative as well as preventive services. Provincial and district health departments are usually responsible for all health services in their territory; they administer, rather than supervise, the hospitals and in health centers they provide ambulatory day-to-day medical care. The task for many of these health departments—in contrast to the American scene—is to give sufficient attention to the preventive services, so heavy are their responsibilities for medical care. To cope with special problems like malaria or tuberculosis control, the central government often organizes campaigns, in which the local health officer may be only indirectly involved. Since local government is usually weak, strong central control is the general rule.

In Latin America, largely under European influence, the health insurance idea has recently been spreading for certain groups of workers in industry, mining, or government. As in Europe, administration of these programs is, typically, by social security institutes, quite separate from the health ministries. Unlike Europe, however, and consistent with the overall service patterns of the public assistance countries, physicians attend insurance beneficiaries, not in a private office, fee-for-service setting, but rather in organized clinics usually on part-time or full-time salaries. Most of the Latin American populations are predominantly agricultural and, with the exception of Chile, are not covered by these insurance programs. In Chile, an estimated seventy percent of the population is entitled to some form of prepaid medical care, and it is significant that a recent reorganization of the Chilean health system places practically all responsibilities under the health ministry and a network of zone health departments.[8]

Finally, there is the universal service pattern of health organization found in the Soviet Union and other socialist countries, Great Britain, and New Zealand. In these countries, virtually complete medical care has been made a public benefit for all persons. Contrasted with the public assistance countries, there is no restriction of care to the poor, and the supply of personnel and facilities equals or exceeds that in the free enterprise or social insurance countries. In contrast to the latter, benefits are not related to contributions or payments. Almost all hospitals are owned and operated by the central government. Almost all personnel are under contractual arrangements with the government and paid through funds derived mainly from general revenues.

In the Soviet scheme, the health ministry has authority over all preventive and curative health services, supervising a hierarchy of administration at three other levels: the republic, the district, and the local area. The local health officer is responsible for all services in his area, including the management of hospitals and health centers. All personnel are on full-time salary. Hospitals are organized in functional regions, with referral of complex cases from peripheral to central facilities, as in the military hospitals of the United States. Unlike all three other country patterns, the manufacture of drugs and appliances is carried out directly by the national

health ministry. Even the education of physicians, nurses, and auxiliary personnel has, since 1930, been a function of the health ministry through special institutes separate from the universities. Other institutes also conduct all medical research.[9]

In Great Britain and New Zealand, while the impact of the national health services is as great or greater than in the Soviet Union, the assignment of authority to the health department is not so sweeping. At the national level, the authority for all public health as well as medical care—ambulatory and hospital—is, indeed, vested in the Ministry of Health. Social insurance for cash benefits is supervised by a ministry of labor or social welfare, but medical services have been separated from the other benefits and assigned with public health to the national health agency. Peripherally in Britain, however, concessions have been made to various interest groups. Hospitals and specialty services are administered by regional boards and ambulatory care, including the services of general practitioners, dentists, and drugs, by local executive councils—both of these bodies being responsible to the national Ministry of Health. Traditional preventive health services are provided by local health departments, along with certain auxiliary curative functions, such as the services of visiting nurses, home helpers, and ambulances. It is significant that one of the most pressing problems of the British National Health Service is the need for coordination of all these activities at the local level, for which the logical resource would be the local health department.

COMMENT

The ultimate test for the effective administration of health services is how it functions at the local community level, where the services reach the people. Even in the United States, with its free enterprise pattern, a great deal of coordination has occurred at the national level, through the Hoover Commission studies; the formation of a national Department of Health, Education, and Welfare; and in the voluntary field with a National Health Council, a national Blue Cross Association, and others. At the state level, interdepartmental committees on health services are becoming common. But at the local level, health authority generally remains highly dispersed with scores of agencies typically involved—155 playing a role in one rural county studied in 1948.[10]

In a number of countries, consciousness of the need for improving local administration has been shown by launching demonstrations of fully integrated public health and medical care programs in selected localities. Space permits only mention of the names of some of these bold experiments: for example, the programs at Nancy, France; at Beth Mazmil, Israel; at Pholela, South Africa; at Swift Current in Saskatchewan, Canada; at Bayamon, Puerto Rico; at Quezaltepeque, El Salvador; and in the Sindhibis Valley, Egypt. Perhaps in every country there is some special effort at integration of all health services in one or more local areas. The approaches are different, of course, but the goal is always the same: to develop a comprehensive health program, involving both preventive and curative service, ambulatory and institutional care, with governmental and voluntary sources of financing, under a unified administration.

One word about the role of the general hospital, which many see as "the health center of the community." If the hospital is to be the center of preventive service, education, and research, as well as patient care on all levels, what becomes of the integrating role of the health department? There is no doubt of the strong position occupied by the general hospital everywhere in the professional lives of doctors and the emotional lives of people. Where the hospital is a public facility, as in most countries of the world, there is no reason why it cannot serve as the key physical instrumentality of a unified community health agency, along with health centers and other peripheral facilities. In the United States, however, where most local general hospitals are voluntary organizations, it is difficult to envisage their serving as coordinating administrative agencies. Hospitals have an enormous community task in almost every aspect of health service and medical science, but the job of supervising the whole community's health—with all its legal and organizational complexities—must be vested in a public body. While health departments in America seldom exercise such wide authority, they obviously offer the nucleus for such a future role.

The skeptic may ask, what is the point of all this? Why does it matter whether there are multiple agencies for multiple services, except to satisfy the compulsive demands of students of administration who like to see tidy organization charts? I would answer that there are sound human and social reasons for promoting unified health administration in general, and health department participation in medical care programs in particular.

The first reason is that such arrangements are most likely to have a preventive approach incorporated into day-to-day medical care administration—a point which can be well documented on this continent in the experience of Saskatchewan. Second, unified administration is most likely to be balanced, giving appropriate attention to different health needs in proportion to their quantitative importance, rather than in response to the strengths and weaknesses of various special interests. Third, unified administration can permit engagement of the highest calibre administrative skill at lowest overall cost, by combining funds from many sources but avoiding duplication of work. Fourth, it can strengthen the competitive position of health services in the arena of government and in the larger arena of overall national goods and services which must be financed. Finally, and most important, unified administration allows individuals to be served as whole persons—rather than as representatives of different diseases, age levels, social status, or other categories by which health service is divided—so that continuous, sensitive, technically proficient, and comprehensive health care can be rendered. The person rather than the agency becomes the focus.

On a world level, one cannot help but see a trend in all countries toward more and more socially organized and financed health service. In a way, this is a trend from the free enterprise toward the universal service pattern. This is not an advocacy but an observation. If this observation is valid, it means that the need for health service coordination at the local level will become more and more manifest, both to the technical specialists and to the public at large. What we see in America today as the local health department, with its specified list of functions, may become the true community health administration agency of the future.

NOTES
[1] Paper presented before the Medical Care Section of the American Public Health Association at the Eighty-Sixth Annual Meeting in Saint Louis, Missouri, October 28, 1958.

[2] American Public Health Association, "Medical Care in a National Health Program (An Official Statement)." *American Journal of Public Health*, Vol. 34, December 1944, pp. 1,252-1,256.

[3] "Health Insurance: Report of Standing Committee Adopted by the Conference of State and Territorial Health Authorities with the United States Public Health Service, Washington, D.C., May 13, 1916." *Public Health Reports*, July 21, 1916, pp. 1,919-1,925.

[4] J. W. Mountin, "Participation by State and Local Health Departments in Current Medical Care Programs." *American Journal of Public Health*, Vol. 36, December 1946, p. 1,387.

[5] M. I. Roemer, *Medical Care in Relation to Public Health*. Geneva: World Health Organization, unpublished document, December 7, 1956.

[6] Since 1958, in all three of these countries, socially insured medical care has been greatly extended, and in Canada since 1966 it has become the predominant source of health service financing.

⁷ F. Goldmann and A. Grotjahn, *Benefits of the German Sickness Insurance System from the Point of View of Social Hygiene*. Geneva: International Labour Office, 1928.

⁸ After its 1959 Revolution, Cuba also united all its health services under the Ministry of Health.

⁹ World Health Organization, "First Report on the World Health Situation." Geneva: WHO (All-P-B-6), May 1958, chapter VIII, pp. 372-377.

¹⁰ M. I. Roemer and E. A. Wilson, "Organized Health Services in a County of the United States." Washington, D.C.: Public Health Service Publication No. 197, 1952.

Chapter XXVII
Health Consumerism in Global Perspective

With extension of democratic concepts everywhere, the general population is demanding more and more of a direct voice in the management of all social affairs. In no field has this been more evident, especially in the United States, than in the health services. A new social movement of "health consumerism" has taken shape, and especially prominent in it have been demands from ethnic minority groups.

Yet, if we examine the role of consumers historically and globally, we find that in many aspects of health service organization the people served have long played a decisive role. The birth of hospitals, of health insurance, of countless agencies to tackle specific diseases has come from the initiative of consumer or citizen groups, rather than from doctors or other providers of health service. A brief overview of this consumer role was presented to a Canadian audience in 1969 and published as "Sponsorship of Health Care Programs: The Role of Consumers in World Perspective" in the proceedings of the Conference on Costs and Organization of Medical Care *(J.Z. Garson and J.D. Bury, editors, Saskatoon, Saskatchewan (Canada): Saskatoon Community Health Foundation, 1970, pp. 12-19); it is reprinted here by permission.*

This chapter will explore trends in the diverse forms of sponsorship of health services on the world scene. The principal forms of sponsorship are usually defined as (1) governmental, (2) consumer, (3) providers of service, and (4) commercial. To discuss all these forms of health program sponsorship properly would be a big order, but I will try by focusing especially on the role of consumers. That form of sponsorship has, we all know, special interest for North America. It is also recognized as being of the greatest importance in the health services of countries throughout the world today.

MULTIPLICITY OF SPONSORSHIPS
OF HEALTH PROGRAMS

In almost all countries of the world there is a mixture of sponsorships of health care programs. By "sponsorship" I refer to the social character of the people or organizations who exercise control or power over the operations of a program. Usually this constitutes the same body as that which initiated the program, but this is not always so. For example, in Mexico the majority of general hospitals were started years ago by the Catholic Church, but later, after the 1910 Revolution in that country, these facilities were taken over and controlled by the central and state governments.

Aside from historical changes, the concept of sponsorship is complicated further by the fact that many health programs or facilities are sponsored by one body, but heavily influenced by others. The Blue Cross plans for hospital insurance in the United States, for example, were initially and still are sponsored by the hospitals themselves, but in due course they have become heavily influenced by governmental agencies (such as state insurance commissioners), by medical societies, labor unions, and other forces. The voluntary general hospitals themselves in the United States—while they are sponsored by various local religious or other nonprofit associations—have become heavily influenced by such national professional bodies as the Joint Commission on Accreditation of Hospitals or the American Medical Association Council on Internships and Residencies, as well as by the state hospital licensure authorities in virtually every state.

The sources of power, in back of the various types of sponsorship of health care programs, are several. They may be best conceived, I think, in relation to the medical care process itself. Fundamentally this process involves a healer or provider, on the one hand, and a patient on the other. Once a large number of persons become involved in the process, and money flows through some collectivized channel, then there arise administrative tasks which require a middleman between the two basic parties. Thus, the organized medical care process, involving numbers of patients and numbers of providers, can be represented by a triangle in which one corner represents the provider, a second corner the middleman, and the third corner the patient.

The sponsorship, then, of a health care program may be assumed by any one of the three parties involved in this basic medical care process. Furthermore, it may be by an agent or a secondary offshoot of any one of these three parties. For example, the patients or consumers in the medical care process may theoretically be represented by their employers—as we see in certain industrial medical service programs. Or they may be represented by a labor union, as in other programs of health service. Or the patients may be represented by a combination of union and management jointly, as in the health care programs of various labor-management trust funds.

Theoretically, moreover, all three basic parties in the medical care process may sponsor a program through a designated common agent—in the form of an elected government. This governmental sponsorship may be at different jurisdictional levels— local, state, or federal.

Thus, the various sponsorships of health care programs, in summary, may be considered as being of four types: (1) the providers of health service, (2) middlemen or commercial entities, (3) consumers (or their agents), and (4) government at different levels.

In many countries certain sectors of health service are controlled predominantly by one or another type of sponsor. For example, services for the protection of health through environmental controls are predominantly sponsored by government. The services of bedside nurses in the patient's home are predominantly sponsored by associations of consumers— voluntary visiting nurse associations. Or the sponsorship of private ambulatory care facilities, bringing together different types of medical and surgical specialists—that is group practice clinics—is usually

(though not always) by the providers of service themselves.

On the other hand, certain forms of health care program typically have a wide multiplicity of sponsorships. Insurance plans for provision of general personal medical care are an important example. In the United States this pluralism is seen strikingly. The providers of health service, for example, sponsor the Blue Cross and Blue Shield plans, with which the reader is familiar. There are also a few insurance plans utilizing group practice clinics (like the Ross-Loos program in Los Angeles—started incidentally by Canadian prairie doctors) which are sponsored also by physicians. Secondly, the middlemen in the process sponsor literally hundreds of different health insurance plans through the commercial insurance mechanism. It is interesting to note that this sponsorship of health insurance plans—that is by private insurance companies—while coming into the field relatively late, about 1940, has now acquired the largest enrollment of any type of health insurance sponsorship in the nation. Thirdly, consumers sponsor many health insurance plans in the United States. Most of these are small, and their aggregate enrollment is only about five percent of the total insured population. Finally, governmental authorities sponsor the new health insurance program for the aged, known nowadays as Medicare, not to mention the older programs of health insurance for industrial injuries or workmen's compensation in each of the states.

This mixture of many sponsorships of health insurance programs or indeed other types of health service, is especially prominent in North America, where there has been great freedom of experimentation and local initiative. On other continents, a proportionately larger role tends to be assumed by agencies of government at all levels. On all continents, moreover, there has been a decided trend over the decades toward greater governmental responsibility for health services, in order to extend the coverage and benefits of various programs and to achieve long-term stability. This is seen strikingly here in Canada where, after many years of hospitalization insurance sponsored by various voluntary entities, there evolved in 1957 one major national governmental program of social insurance for hospital care, operated jointly with the ten provincial governments.

In spite of this rising worldwide importance of governmental sponsorship, the role of consumer action has always been and continues to be important in the development of health care programs. We can now examine this role in a little more detail.

CONSUMER RESPONSIBILITY HISTORICALLY

On a world scale, the technical organization of health services has been heavily influenced by the establishment of hospitals, and the initiative for this came mainly from consumers. This was often expressed through religious organizations, leading to the church-supported hospitals of Europe, Latin America, and elsewhere. Many types of voluntary nonsectarian association in England, North America, and elsewhere have also established hospitals. Sometimes these institutions were later taken over by government, but boards of citizens usually still remain in positions of authority. Perhaps these boards have not been sufficiently representative of rank and file consumers, but the concept of a hospital board of directors is classically intended to represent the general community in sponsorship of hospitals. Physicians, in fact, are explicitly barred from hospital board membership in most of North America.

Specific diseases or the health needs of specific populations, have been the focus of many types of voluntary health society. In nineteenth century Germany and France, tuberculosis associations were organized to help the victims of this disease. There have been societies for the care and treatment of crippled children throughout Europe, and also in Moslem countries, for several centuries. Everywhere in the world the Red Cross is found, as a voluntary agency devoted to giving service in emergencies or public disasters. It is interesting to note that in most Latin American countries the Red Cross societies remain voluntary bodies, although they are typically financed by governmental grants up to ninety percent of their budget. A whole variety of special societies for meeting the health needs of children, women, or old people have long been operating in Europe and elsewhere.

The historical role of consumers in sponsorship of health insurance plans has been especially strong. Going back to the Middle Ages, craftsmen's guilds developed systems to finance both medical care and cash benefits, in replacement of lost earnings, for their sick or disabled members. In Germany, these evolved into the "Kranken Kassen" or sickness chests; in England they became the "friendly societies," playing a strong role among the factory workers of the industrialized cities. In other countries, including the United States, the development of health protection plans was through so-called "mutual benefit societies." In Yugoslavia and Poland farmers, as consumers, formed health cooperatives in the early twentieth century, to help provide medical care in the rural areas.

From these various forms of consumer-sponsored health insurance plan there evolved the movement for social security. It was in Germany in 1883 that the first social insurance law was enacted under the conservative Chancellor Otto Bismarck. It is worth noting that this initial law did not set up a national insurance program for medical care, but rather required that working people, of certain low income levels, be obligated to become members of some existing sickness chest. Various regulations were enacted to assure minimum levels of benefit and maximum premium rates among these sickness chests, but their sponsorship remained voluntary and local. Similar legislation was eventually enacted by all the other countries of Europe and then of other continents. Today about sixty nations throughout the world have programs of social insurance providing for medical care. The scope of population coverage and medical benefits is quite diverse, but the trend has been toward extension of both. The administration of social insurance or social security programs usually incorporates a significant role for consumer groups. Typically the top policy board of a program is tripartite, including workers, employers, and government. Workers, of course, are equivalent to consumers, and they are usually represented through the channel of labor unions. This pattern is seen not only in Europe but also in Latin America, Japan, India, New Zealand, and elsewhere.

In recent years, however, the consumer's role in health care programs has changed its form. As medical care costs have escalated everywhere, the money-raising side of health care programs has come to be increasingly assumed by government. This is done either through the device of general revenues or the various social insurance schemes just mentioned. This trend is observable in all countries, both the industrialized and the developing. It is especially prominent in the developing countries, where the mass of people cannot afford medical care or even small social insurance contributions.

The main role of consumers, therefore, has shifted from that of fund raising to two other functions: (1) an advisory role in the policy-making councils of government, and (2) the direct organization of personal health service programs, the financing of which is assumed by government.

Regarding the advisory role of consumers, one may look to the composition of the various regional hospital boards or local executive councils in the British National Health Service. Indeed, the consumer's role may be somewhat more than advisory in these bodies since, along with others, he participates in actual policy decisions, at least on the local level.

In the health system of the Soviet Union, centralized and government-sponsored as it is, there is at every level a host of committees for surveillance over program operations; consumers have a strong voice in the operation of these committees. In the United States, almost every new health program enacted by Congress in the last twenty-five years has had its "national advisory council," on which consumer or citizen representatives sit. The hospital construction (Hill-Burton) program, for example, has its National Advisory Hospital Council, as does the national program for mental health services, for comprehensive planning, for training of health manpower, for control of cancer or other diseases, etc. These advisory committees operate at state and local levels as well.

Regarding the role of consumers in the direct organization of personal health service programs, there is more to be said, which may also be of greater interest to the reader.

CONSUMER ROLES IN HEALTH SERVICE ORGANIZATION TODAY

The direct initiative of consumers in organizing health service programs is seen strikingly in the hospital field. On the voluntary hospital boards of North America it has been the consumer voice that was mainly responsible for the important innovations in recent years. I would include among these the launching of organized home care programs, started by the board of the Montefiore Hospital in New York City twenty-five years ago. The trend toward expansion of organized outpatient clinic and emergency services in many hospitals can be credited to the leadership of hospital boards of directors. Typically the expansion of these ambulatory services has been opposed by medical staffs, for fear of competition with their private practices, but socially conscious boards have developed such programs in response to public demands.

The development of tightened patterns of medical staff organization itself can be largely attributed, in my opinion, to the leadership and stimulation of hospital boards. In the United States increased organization, to achieve more disciplined medical work in hospitals, has typically been opposed by doctors, but the pressure of hospital boards to upgrade the quality of patient care has prevailed. The Joint Commission on Accreditation of Hospitals has, of course, played an important part, but it is interesting to note that in its early years the "hospital standardization movement," as it was initially called, was opposed by most private physicians.[1] A final type of innovation, important in modern hospitals, is the concept of "progressive patient care." This concept of hospital design organizes services not according to medical specialties, but rather according to patient needs for intensive, intermediate, or long-term care. While the progressive patient care idea has been induced by a search for economies, which are indeed felt most keenly by consumers, the effects are to improve the quality and particularly the sensitivity of patient care. These and other innovations have been brought about mainly by alert hospital boards.

Outside of hospitals, the consumer voice is heard loud and clear in the development of improved patterns for organized ambulatory health services. In my opinion, nothing is more important for the improvement of overall health services in a nation than a sound system for providing comprehensive personal health service to the ambulatory patient. From this primary service there follow referrals to the hospitals, the dispensing of medications taken at home, the pursuit of rehabilitation efforts, and all the other modalities of medical care.

Organized ambulatory health care programs take many forms. They may take the shape of large polyclinics attached to hospitals, seen in all countries. They are embodied in health centers, sponsored by the ministry of health or sometimes by social security agencies in Latin America, India, Africa, the Soviet Union, and nearly all the developing countries. Recently I saw an impressive network of such health centers in Malaysia, where a special Rural Health Services Scheme has been under development for fifteen years. It is of significance, in the light of other tragic events observable in Southeast Asia today, that these rural health centers were built in response to the revolutionary guerilla movement that arose in the former British Malay Federation just after the Second World War.[2]

Another type of organized ambulatory health service is seen in the "neighborhood health centers," developed to serve the people in certain pockets of poverty in the United States under the sponsorship of the national Office of Economic Opportunity (O.E.O.). These health centers, like those of Malaysia, were also constructed in response to a crisis situation—namely, the riots occurring in the ghettos of many of our large cities. There are now about forty of these neighborhood health centers in operation, and they demonstrate the feasibility of providing comprehensive multispecialty service to poor people, close to where they live. There is also an important emphasis in these facilities on the key role of the primary physician. I understand that in Montreal and Halifax, under the sponsorship of medical schools, similar neighborhood health centers are now being developed. In these Canadian cities, as in several American cities, medical students are playing a key role in launching and staffing the health centers. National policies of the United States O.E.O. mandate a strong voice for consumers—representatives of the poor people—in the administrative structure of these health programs.

Another form of organized ambulatory service is the prepaid group practice clinic. In the United States there are some 250 to 300 of these, associated usually with health insurance plans sponsored by labor-management or consumer groups. The best known are the Health Insurance Plan of Greater New York and the Kaiser-Permanente Health Plan of the West Coast, but there are many smaller group health associations, with their associated clinics, in Washington D.C., in Minneapolis, Minnesota, in Detroit, Michigan, in Cleveland, Ohio, in St. Louis, Missouri, in Elk City, Oklahoma, and elsewhere. At Sault Sainte Marie, Ontario, there is an important new prepaid health program with a group practice clinic, sponsored by the Canadian steel workers union. All of these programs are, of course, the result of initiative—often against great opposition—of consumer groups. The Group Health Association of America has played an important role in stimulating and supporting this movement.

Private group practices should also be mentioned, although they are not sponsored by consumers. There are now about 4,300 such private clinics, with 28,000 doctors associated in them, throughout the United States. While the vast majority of these group practice clinics are operating on a purely private basis, without any consumer control, I believe that their steady growth over the years can be partially attributed to consumer support. Group practice clinics often face bitter opposition from private medical societies, and they can survive only with the steadfast support of their patients.

Finally, among various types of organized ambulatory service, we can identify the community health clinics of Saskatchewan. These are almost a unique development on the world scene, in having consumer sponsorship of teams of doctors, without a prepayment basis. The financial support comes from governmental revenues, while the clinics themselves are sponsored by consumer groups. I understand that there are now five such community clinics in operation—in Saskatoon, Regina, Prince Albert, Lloydminster, and Wynyard. This program again illustrates the trend, noted earlier, toward governmental financing of health service patterns which have been organized and sponsored by consumer groups. These clinics are certainly a remarkable and positive response by consumers to the opportunities for

socio-medical innovation, presented by the enactment of the Saskatchewan Medical Care Law in 1962.

THE SIGNIFICANCE OF CONSUMER SPONSORSHIP

What is the real significance, however, of consumer sponsorship of these organized centers for ambulatory health service? One can speculate on many possible meanings, but an empirical study was made in 1963, the results of which we may consider. An investigation was made of twelve prepaid group practice organizations in five states of the United States—six of them sponsored by physicians and the other six by consumer groups.[3] After detailed research, it was found that the two sets of prepaid clinics actually had greater similarities than differences in their policies of basic coverage, benefits, costs, quality controls, etc. I think that this suggests that the pattern or concept of prepaid group practice has several inherent features and consequences, regardless of the sponsorship.

There were, nevertheless, certain important differences between the plans sponsored by consumers as against doctors. The consumer-sponsored plans were found to have:

• More liberal enrollment policies—being less restrictive of membership by persons considered "bad risks"

• Greater sensitivity in handling complaints of patients

• Wider provision of supplementary benefits such as dental care, psychiatric services, or prescribed drugs

More important perhaps, it should be noted that in the current dynamics of health services in North America, it is the initiative or demands of consumers that usually stimulate the establishment of prepaid group practice systems. If one examines the history of prepaid group practices—even those ostensibly sponsored by providers rather than consumers—one nearly always finds a consumer group, often an industrial population, involved in the initiation of the program. The Ross-Loos Clinic Plan in Los Angeles, California, is doctor-sponsored, but it was a population of public utility workers that was responsible for its origin, and the whole Blue Cross movement, while hospital-sponsored, got its start from the initiative of schoolteachers in Dallas, Texas.

I am stressing this concept of prepaid comprehensive ambulatory health service because it has great importance in the overall dynamics of medical care today. The comprehensive clinic, in which payments are made by capitation rather than the archaic fee-for-service system, leads to many beneficial consequences. It makes possible the care of the total patient and his family, with all the technology that medicine can offer. It promotes primary economies in the delivery of medical service, through the advantages of a larger scale "production" process. It also yields important secondary economies, in fostering lower rates of utilization of hospitals, the prescription of generic name drugs which are less costly, the maximum effective use of nurses and social workers, and other sound approaches to medical service. There is abundant evidence of these secondary economies, as well as the primary economies, in the operation of prepaid comprehensive health clinics.[4] Furthermore, such clinics facilitate a preventive orientation, which is seldom feasible in the practice of a solo doctor. Finally the multidisciplinary staff of a group practice clinic makes possible continuity of care, with follow-up of the patient by social workers, nurses, rehabilitation counselors, etc., if necessary. At the same time, the primary doctor or family physician can play his proper role as the practitioner most steadfastly concerned about the care of the patient, with backup by specialists and others as necessary.

The prominent issue today, then, is the *organization* of health services. Financing of health care, through various social measures, is on the way to solution. It is not fully solved, but the progress is clear. This is certainly obvious in Canada, with the 1966 national Medicare Law a major milestone. Saskatchewan and British Columbia have participated in this new national program since its onset, and I understand that this very week Manitoba and Nova Scotia joined in. It seems likely that most of the other six Canadian provinces will participate in the national Medicare insurance program before long.

The bigger challenge now, however, is to achieve sound patterns of teamwork in the delivery of personal health services. We must move forward from the ancient model of solo practice toward a pattern that is responsive to the requirements of the world we live in. Thirty years ago, Henry Sigerist—who in 1944 was the first Health Services Planning Commissioner in the province of Saskatchewan— described individual medical practice as a historical hangover, a social anachronism that no longer matched the technical developments of science or the human needs of patients.[5] This is far more true today than when Doctor Sigerist pointed it out.

It is up to consumer bodies, such as the sponsors of this conference, to demand and work for more rational and sensible patterns of health care organization, as well as economic support.

FUTURE ISSUES IN CONSUMER PARTICIPATION

This brief review of the past roles of consumers in health care programs, and some of the features of their current role, may provide some basis for looking ahead and perhaps offering some suggestions.

In my view, the consumer will continue to play a salient and enlarging role in the planning and operation of health care systems. This will be not only through direct sponsorship of new patterns of personal health service, as discussed above, but also through his exercising a voice in the councils of government at all levels. In public medical service programs, the voice of consumers will become steadily stronger, in step with the general enlargement of democratic principles in our society. The consumer will contribute to the advancement of health services, I believe, in relation to both goals and methods.

As for the formulation of *goals* for improved health service, I believe that we may look to consumers for achievement of the following objectives:

1. Universal coverage of the population with a health care system which provides prompt access both financially and geographically.

2. A truly comprehensive scope of services for both physical and mental illness and involving all the personnel and facilities on which modern science depends.

3. Methods of technical organization of health services which will promote economy, since it is the consumer who must pay the costs.

4. Patterns of health service organization which promote the highest quality of service, since it is the consumer's life and well-being that are at stake.

Among the many *methods* or approaches to health service organization, the consumer voice will call for other things. I think that these will include:

1. Patterns of health service which show full sensitivity to the needs of patients. This means large enough numbers of personnel of all types, so that they have the time to be kind and considerate.

2. Coordination of the many classes of personnel—specialist, paramedical, etc.—so that the patient is treated as a whole. This obviously means health care teams with a pivotal place for the personal family doctor. (The new provision of specialty status for "family medicine" in the United States is a step toward assuring the well-trained general physician his proper role.)

3. Provision of services that are physically close to people. This means neighborhood health centers of various sorts, with ties to hospitals and larger medi-

cal centers as necessary. It means regionalization of health services over large geographic areas, so that any person may receive the services he needs with promptness and efficiency, no matter where he lives.

4. Full social financing of health care. Hence, there is no real place for payments by the patient at the time of sickness, as is required with the use of deterrent fees. It is often overlooked that the great bulk of medical care costs arise from services which are decided upon by the doctor rather than the patient—that is, all ambulatory services beyond the initial office visit, all hospital services, laboratory and x-ray procedures, prescribed drugs, and nearly all the rest. To impose a utilization fee for these services is to shift to the patient a part of the cost of decisions which are made by the doctor.

This question of utilization fees is a complex matter. Despite the imposition of such fees in Saskatchewan in April 1968, world experience suggests that this "cost sharing" (as it is called in Europe) has no enduring effect on utilization rates, unless the amounts charged are so high as to discourage the procurement of needed care among low income people. If a utilization fee is low enough to avoid this serious difficulty, then it will not have any effect on utilization rates; it may indeed even increase utilization rates, by giving patients the feeling that since they are paying for services, they are entitled to use them on the slightest provocation. The application of cost sharing mechanisms, however, does have a second effect that cannot be denied. It reduces the extent of social financing of health services (through taxes or social insurance), replacing it partially with individual financing by those who are sick. Such a policy gives the false impression that the costs of a system are being held in check, merely because the social insurance premiums or tax rates—which are easily visible—are reduced. The total costs, counting the individual outlays, may actually be rising more than ever.[6]

Consumer groups, in order to play these constructive roles—involving both goals and methods of health service organization—need to educate themselves. I do not personally believe that every patient, by reason of being a good citizen, automatically knows how to solve technical problems in health care organization or any other complicated field. He needs advice from technical experts. He needs education and perspective.

The consumer, however, can formulate goals and even methods, as suggested above, getting advice on strategies and tactics from the professional experts in the health field—professional persons whom he can

trust. The combination of the educated consumer and the professional friend is the winning team. To forge such teams would seem to be the value of a conference like this one. It is the purpose, I gather, of the Saskatoon Community Health Foundation.

We are also seeing such partnerships of consumers and health professionals taking many forms today in my country. There is a new "Committee of 100" for promotion of national health insurance, which has been recently sparked by Walter Reuther, a distinguished labor leader. In California, there is a new Council on Health Plan Alternatives, representing the seven largest labor unions in this large state. This organization is building upon the strength of several million labor families to achieve improved health insurance plans. It is seeking to strike a better bargain with the various health insurance carriers, to promote greater surveillance over the quality of care received by patients, to speak for the consumer in various planning agencies of government, and to develop new and alternative programs of organized health service on its own. The American Public Health Association—the professional society of public health workers in the United States—held a conference last week to launch a new nationwide plan for broadened partnership with involved citizens, as a basis for achieving greater social action toward health objectives. There are citizen groups devoted to an endless variety of specific health issues: fluoridation of the water supply to reduce dental disease, improved mental health services, extension of family planning and reform of antiquated abortion laws, restriction of cigarette advertising to reduce the hazard of lung cancer and other diseases. In local communities, there are innumerable local committees tackling problems of drug addiction, air pollution, achievement of a better hospital, development of a livelier public health agency, getting a square deal for racial minorities, and other small and large issues in the health arena.

Such consumer actions, as we have seen, have been expressed throughout history and in all countries. Today, the voice of the consumer is perhaps stronger than ever, because he is more educated, because the potentialities of science are greater, and because man's expectations are higher, as they should be. With clarity of purpose, the initiative and dedication of consumers—of all the people—are certainly our strongest hope for achieving in Canada and elsewhere a system of health services which will apply our knowledge effectively and sensitively for the welfare of everyone.

NOTES

[1] Loyal Davis, *Fellowship of Surgeons.* Springfield, Illinois: Charles C. Thomas, 1960.

[2] Milton I. Roemer, *Strengthening of Health Services and Training of Health Personnel in Malaysia: General Overview and Analysis.* World Health Organization, Regional Office for the Western Pacific (Assignment Report), February 3, 1969.

[3] Jerome L. Schwartz, "Consumer Sponsorship and Physician Sponsorship of Prepaid Group Practice Health Plans: Some Similarities and Differences." *American Journal of Public Health,* Vol.55, January 1965, pp. 94-102.

[4] Milton I. Roemer and Donald M. DuBois, "Medical Costs in Relation to the Organization of Ambulatory Care." *New England Journal of Medicine,* Vol. 280, May 1, 1969, pp. 988-994.

[5] Henry E. Sigerist, "Medical Care for All the People." *Canadian Journal of Public Health,* Vol. 35, July 1944, pp. 253-267.

[6] Milton I. Roemer, *The Organization of Medical Care Under Social Security.* Geneva: International Labor Office, 1969, "Cost Sharing," pp. 204-207.

Chapter XXVIII
A Coordinated Health Service
and National Priorities

The health service systems of most countries are characterized by a multiplicity of agencies to serve particular population groups or to tackle certain diseases. The major exceptions are the Soviet Union and other socialist nations, but elsewhere priorities are determined by selective allocation of resources among different and often competing agencies. This very multiplicity of programs, however, causes waste which reduces the effectiveness of the whole system.

Priorities for certain persons or diseases, nevertheless, are rational in the face of scarce resources. The question arises, therefore, whether priorities may be applied within a unified health service system–that is, without the wastage of fragmented authority patterns. This question was explored at a medical conference in Venezuela in 1965, and this chapter was published as "A Coordinated Health Service and the Problem of Priorities" in the Israel Journal of Medical Science *(Vol. 1, July 1965, pp. 643-647); it is reprinted here by permission.*[1]

The American sociologist, C. Wright Mills, spoke of the importance of a "sociological imagination" in understanding the problems faced by individuals in a community or a nation. Without such imagination, one does not see beyond the pains or troubles in a patient to the larger social environment responsible for them. Without this understanding, there can be no effective leadership, no intelligent planning to make a better world for people.

THE NEED FOR PLANNING

A woman dies of breast cancer, which, if detected early, might have been cured. A child dies of malnutrition. A young man develops far-advanced tuberculosis before it is discovered. A patient dies of postoperative hemorrhage because there is no blood bank from which to give a transfusion. But these tragedies cannot be blamed on the individuals immediately involved—the unfortunate patient or the individual doctor or even the local hospital. Their causes must be sought in the whole national (or even international) system of health services. They must

be sought in the whole national production and allocation of resources for preventive and curative medicine which led to the failure to diagnose a breast cancer when the lump was small or the lack of a blood bank in the hospital at the proper time and place. If avoidable death and preventable disease and suffering did not occur, we would have no need for the national planning of health services. But the persistence of unnecessary tragedy makes planning urgent.

Everywhere in the world, East and West, there is a movement toward greater planning of health and welfare services (not to mention industry, agriculture, and other sectors of life). In countries of all stages of economic development, the demand is for greater coordination, greater integration of health services. The reason everywhere is basically the same: to achieve more effective use of limited resources in relation to the needs of people. If existent resources were wisely used, better health services could be provided—even before the total national resources are increased.

In nearly all countries progress has been made

against the ravages of certain diseases, like malaria, or the liabilites of certain persons, like pregnant women, through specialized programs. Intensive efforts have been applied to protect favored groups, like military personnel or railroad workers or white collar employees. Enormous energies of citizens, often in small voluntary groups, have been mobilized to carry out campaigns against specific diseases, like cancer, blindness, or poliomyelitis. All these specialized efforts have made contributions to the total welfare, but sometimes the price has been high. There is in Latin America (and elsewhere) often destructive competition for scarce personnel, sometimes bitter clashes between agencies.

MOVEMENT TOWARD COORDINATION

After many decades, we see a crazy quilt of organized health programs, with numerous duplications and serious gaps. The net allocation of resources in personnel and facilities may bear only a very crude relation to an objective assessment of the relative needs of people at different times and places. The advocacy of coordination of health services, therefore, is based on such considerations as the following:

1. Each doctor or other health worker should be used to the full. Hence, if one physician is partially idle, while another one is overworked, it is wasteful of resources. If one clinic is half empty, while another is overcrowded, the total welfare of patients is reduced.

2. Skilled administrative leadership is rare. It should not be squandered by requiring several different health administrators for different programs in one locality, when one qualified person could do the job.

3. Travel and transportation are costly; if patients or health personnel must travel to point A for one service and to point B for another service, or a man must attend clinic C if he is employed and clinic D if he is unemployed, there is vast wastage of time and money. Health services for all conditions and all persons should be at locations as near as possible to where people live or work.

4. Recruitment and training of health personnel and purchase of medical equipment and supplies are laborious tasks. Great effort can be spared by doing these tasks on a unified rather than fragmented basis. There are also basic economies from the purchase of commodities in large, rather than small quantities.

5. Expensive resources in laboratories, x-ray departments, or surgical operating rooms should be used to the full. Duplication of new equipment and technical staff, while some existing units are stand-

ing idle, is extravagant. This is especially true of infrequently used items like cobalt bombs or artificial kidneys, but it is also true of ordinary laboratory technicians or microscopes.

6. Sound technical standards can be more readily applied throughout a system if there is a free flow of information. The results of scientific research can be promptly put into practice if there are clear lines of communication, rather than sovereignty and anarchy amidst many different professional units. Likewise, patients can be more easily referred from one part of a system to another, rather than across administrative barriers.

OBSTACLES TO COORDINATION

For these and other reasons, after decades of independent growth of diverse health care programs, integration is being advocated everywhere. But what are the obstacles? Why is there so much more discussion than action?

The fact is that separate and independent programs of health care serve various reasonable purposes. There are large political reasons for favoring military personnel with abundant and high quality medical care. There are good economic reasons for protecting the health of industrial workers under social security programs. There are sound epidemiological reasons for conducting a special campaign against yaws or schistosomiasis. There are reasons of humanity as well as future investment for focusing attention on infant and maternal health. In other words, these specialized programs do not lack justification. Each can be defended as meeting a special need. Each has made progress by reason of the energies and motivation inspiring it. Nevertheless, the very multiplicity of these programs creates wastes, either hidden or open, and it means that resources are not being used optimally.

The question, therefore, is whether a nation can successfully meet the special needs recognized in certain population groups or certain disease hazards, while at the same time achieving the advantages of an integrated health service system? Put in another way, is it possible to apply priorities for certain diseases or certain persons within the bounds of a unified system. In the past, priorities have been achieved through competition; can they be achieved within an arena of cooperation?

PRIORITIES WITHIN A COORDINATED SYSTEM

After study of the health service systems in a number of nations of differing economic and political settings, I think the answer is "yes." Within a nationally unified health service system, it would not only be possible, but also necessary and wise, to incorporate priorities for certain disease problems and certain populations.

In most nations of the world, medical emergencies make a high claim on available resources; the patient with serious trauma, with hemorrhage, with heart attack, demands immediate attention. Likewise, an infectious disease demands prompt identification, isolation, and treatment, so that it will not spread to others. Any disorder that can be readily prevented through environmental controls (like clean water) or immunization obviously warrants action.

Moreover, the health of industrial workers is of enormous importance everywhere, but especially if an agricultural nation is to develop the vast advantages of industrialization. The health of schoolchildren and of teachers is extremely important if there is to be mass education and enlightenment. The military forces must be healthy to protect the state, and governmental employees must be able-bodied to carry out their functions that are essential to the welfare of everyone.

But all these priority actions can be carried out within a unified medical system. It is not necessary to have a separate campaign under the ministry of health to tackle diphtheria, a traumatology or emergency service under the municipal governments, a separate social security program of medical care for industrial workers, an elaborate military medical department, an independent health service within the school system, to achieve these several ends. This separatism of the past has been a product sometimes of political rivalry, sometimes of selfish interests, sometimes of impatience with the weaknesses of an old program which has provoked the establishment of a new one. But seldom has separatism been a response to strictly technical requirements. While it has produced short-run benefits for certain persons it has worked to diminish the long-run benefits of everyone.

APPLICATION OF PRIORITIES

Within a unified system of health service organization, it is quite feasible to apply priorities. The task essentially is to allocate resources deliberately for the tackling of certain disease problems or the service of certain population groups. This can be done by three basic approaches: (1) policy decisions on certain diseases or accidents, (2) geographic location of manpower and facilities, (3) identification of certain persons and time allotments. I shall try to explain these approaches.

Let us picture the simplest and most efficient system of health service organization. There would be a coordinated network of health centers distributed so that they are close to where people live. Each center has the physicians, nurses, technicians, the equipment, the drugs, and the supplies needed for the treatment of all common ailments as well as for prevention. The general physician would be the leader of the team, backed up by a surgeon, a pediatrician, a midwife, and perhaps others. If hospitalization is required, the patient is sent to the nearest appropriate hospital—closer if it is a relatively simple condition, farther perhaps if it is a more complex condition requiring elaborate diagnosis and treatment. This regionalization of facilities is matched by deployment of personnel with various levels of technical skill. Physicians and others would be paid salaries appropriate to their training, skills, and levels of responsibility. Quality of performance would be maintained by a system of supervision, careful records, medical review, and rewards for excellence. The many technical skills required for effective prevention and good patient care of the sick would be blended into a teamwork operation.

Now, how would people have access to this system? Under a pure philosophy of "free economic enterprise," the answer would be simply: through the price tag. What each person could pay for, he would get, and "the market" would regulate the entire flow of services. Fortunately, no modern nation is this callous (or foolish) in its philosophy, and various patterns of social financing have been devised to replace the pocketbook or the peso with a better means of access to medical resources at given times and places. In an ideal system, however, the problem of financial tickets to service would be eliminated completely. There is no question that all nations are moving in this direction.

Qualifications or entitlements to this ideal system of medical services, however, would still be necessary—since nowhere in the world are the resources adequate to meet all the needs. As mentioned above, the first qualification might be the nature of the disease. Thus, a critical emergency case would always be seen first, regardless of the person affected. Likewise for a communicable disease. By the same logic, immunizations would have a high priority in order to prevent contagion—and, indeed, at low cost.

The second basis for applying priorities would be through geographic location of resources. Since industrial populations have great importance for the general socioeconomic development of a nation, health personnel and facilities would be more abundant at places close to where they live. Some services might be located right at the place of work. The same could apply at schools or military installations or governmental offices. But this would not mean the exclusion of nonschool or nonmilitary or nongovernmental or nonindustrial persons from access to these resources, if they came. Simple location of resources, however, could have the effect of favoring the designated groups.

The third basis of priority would be through personal identifications and time allotments. If more medical attention is to be given to industrial workers or governmental employees, then there is a task simply of allotting the hours of the days for their care. The high priority groups would be allowed a higher proportional share of the medical hours in each day. The lower priority groups would be entitled to less time, since their contribution to the total community welfare has been deemed to be less. They should not—as is now often the case—be permitted to "buy" with money a disproportionately greater share of the available resources.

EVALUATION AND PROSPECTS

At first glance, this system of priorities may seem harsh, but it is less so than the current system of hidden priorities based upon wealth and tradition. It is less harsh than a system of medical care which includes a large private sector, where anyone with money may claim an extremely high share of scarce skills, at the expense of perhaps hundreds of others of great social usefulness. But one may argue that purely medical or biological need, and not social usefulness, should be the ideal criterion of priorities. Certainly this should be the ultimate goal, but it cannot be achieved overnight. In the meantime, even such an egalitarian philosophy would not be so compromised by a pattern of social priorities as might at first appear.

The fact is that—for better or for worse—the demands for medical care tend to rise when education increases. Along with education usually goes greater skill, responsibility, and social usefulness. The more skilled industrial workers and the more responsible public officials tend to voluntarily seek medical services more readily than others. Therefore, the natural demand for health service would, to a large extent, be congruent with priority allocations, rather than clashing with them.

The goal of any health service system, of course, must be to so increase the total resources—the general supply of personnel and facilities—that no pain-ful priority decisions would be necessary. One would even like to see a surplus above basic needs, so that a substantial private sector might possibly operate for those who wished to purchase "luxury" service, without thereby reducing the minimal essential services for anyone else. No country has yet reached that utopian level. We must, in the meanwhile, work steadily to increase the net resources and apply priorities on the way.

It is not that we lack a priority approach in our health service systems now. We have distinct priorities, but they are based on competitive economic and political power. To some extent they are rational, as I suggested above, but the relationships to an objective assessment of the health needs in overall national development are, at best, crude. Moreover, the very mode of operation of these priorities—through separate, competitive health programs full of duplications, gaps, and wastages—is an extravagance in all countries, and especially in underdeveloped countries which can ill afford the loss.

Aside from the question of intelligent priorities, there is one more reason for an integrated health service system. It is the need for an effective doctor-patient relationship. Much of the fragmentation of modern health service has been not only between different persons in the same community or family, but even between different ailments or organs in the same person. An integrated health service system, as sketched above, would provide a personal physician backed up by a team of specialists and paramedical personnel, for each citizen. These services would be as close as possible to his home. He would come to be known in the local health center as an individual. The medical team would likewise come to know the environment and the people it served. The very economies of this pattern would permit a more rapid expansion of aggregate resources, so as to hasten the day when human need, rather than the nature of the disease or the person, would be the only basis of priority.

This approach to social medicine, in any nation, may demand a bit of sociological imagination, but I believe we must use it if we are to move ahead effectively.

NOTES

[1] Paper presented at the First Medico-Social Congress of the Venezuelan Medical Federation, in Caracas, Venzuela, August 20, 1965.

Chapter XXIX
Regulation in Different Types of Health Care System

As health care systems have become more complex, involving more people and greater expenditures of funds, regulation through various social processes has become increasingly necessary to assure that investments of effort and resources are kept "on track" toward their intended objectives.

In connection with an educational project of the Association of American Medical Colleges, a review was made of worldwide approaches to the regulation of health care. To simplify the analysis, the health care systems of the world were categorized into five types: (1) free enterprise (typified by the United States), (2) welfare state (exemplified in Western Europe), (3) developing countries of two levels: severely underdeveloped, such as in Africa, and (4) transitional, such as in Latin America, and (5) socialist. All five of these types of system exercise regulation over the health services, although in several different ways. This chapter was written in 1976 and has not been previously published.

A definition of "regulation" is not easy, since almost any social action may exert an influence, direct or indirect, on the behavior of people. This chapter, however, employs the concept in a relatively modest or restricted sense. First, we will examine the regulatory influences, both governmental and voluntary, on the preparation of health manpower and their legal authorization to serve the population in various types of country. Next we will consider the regulation of other types of health care resource, particularly health facilities and drugs. Third, we will review briefly the different ways that the continuing performance of personnel is monitored under various health care systems.

REGULATION OF HEALTH PERSONNEL

To assure or attempt to achieve a certain quality of services in a health care system, there are numerous methods of regulation of the qualifications of health personnel. The policies vary among the types of country and for different categories of health profession or occupation.

Free Enterprise Systems

In the free enterprise setting, governmental licensure of physicians and many (though not all) other forms of personnel is the basic approach to regulation of health manpower. Licensure of the health professions is highly diversified among the American federation of fifty state jurisdictions. In California, as many as twenty-one different health service disciplines are subject to licensure under a State Department of Consumer Affairs. There are eleven health fields that are licensed in some form in all fifty states, although the type of state agency varies. The smallest number of different health occupations subject to licensure is in Iowa and four other states, where twelve fields are licensed.

The American policy on licensure of physicians reflects the consequences of a free enterprise ideology with respect to educational institutions. Since universities and medical schools were (until the 1910-1920 period) essentially free from governmental or any other regulation, the state authorities could not "trust" the quality of graduates. As a result, special state medical examinations were required for licensure—a practice that is relatively uncommon around the world. The first such state law was enacted in Texas in 1873, followed soon by all the other states. In most states, the members of the medical examining board are chosen by the governor from nominations submitted by the private state medical association; only in recent years have non-physician members been appointed to these boards, as a hedge against their promotion of the commercial self-interest of doctors.

Gradually reciprocity grew among the states, in recognition of each other's licensees; today this permits mobility of doctors among about seventy-five percent of the states. In 1915 a nongovernmental National Board of Medical Examiners was formed; this voluntary body offers a relatively rigorous three-part examination (basic sciences, clinical fields, and practical), which has come to be accepted by all but a few states. In 1966, about three-fourths of the nation's medical schools required their students to take the first two parts of this examination. The fifty state examining boards have also cooperated recently in establishing a uniform examination prepared by the Federation of Licensure Examining Boards (FLEX) to achieve technical uniformity; this examination has been especially useful in licensure of foreign medical graduates, whose numbers have greatly increased since the immigration law changes of 1948. (In addition to the examination, state boards may require internships and other credentials.) There is also a nongovernmental Examining Council for Foreign Medical Graduates (ECFMG) which offers a test both overseas and in the United States as a screening procedure for foreign graduates who intend to seek postgraduate training or restricted employment (e.g., in a mental hospital) in an American state.

The specialties in medicine have been subject only to nongovernmental regulation in the free enterprise American setting. Under the pressure of competition from nonphysician optometrists, the first American specialty board was established in 1915 for the field of ophthalmology. Gradually additional specialty boards, stipulating criteria for training as well as formal examinations, were founded and became affiliated eventually with the American Medical Association. Today there are about twenty principal boards for certifying specialty competence, and an additional fifteen subspecialty (e.g., cardiology as a subdivision of internal medicine) disciplines. It is noteworthy that, while nationwide in operation and impact, this regulatory program is not governmental; yet specialty-board certification is recognized for participation and payment purposes by many governmental programs (e.g., the state crippled children's services) and by most hospitals for staff appointments. Yet there is no law requiring specialty board certification as a condition for engaging in various types of medical practice—for example, surgery or radiology. Hospitals may establish their own rules for physician appointment or definition of professional "privileges," but these are not statutory.

The most recent "specialty" in the American medical scene is "family practice," designed to increase the training and status of generalists. This is also the only specialty field now requiring periodic recertification; a family practice specialist must keep taking a certain amount of continuing education, to reestablish his specialty status each five years. For maintenance of overall medical licensure, the state of New Mexico has also mandated a minimum amount of continuing education each five years since about 1970, and a number of other states are now following suit. Only in this way, it is argued, can the population be assured that a doctor is keeping informed on new advances in medical science.

Most other health science disciplines in the United States have followed the model of medicine in their state licensure requirements, but there are a number of noteworthy variations. Dentistry, for example, has a statutory rather than purely voluntary basis for specialty status in several states. Registration of trained nurses requires a formal examination in every state, but a national federation has established one uniform set of questions. As a result, reciprocity in recognition of R.N. qualifications is universal among the fifty states. Examinations in pharmacy are also required in all states, and in twelve jurisdictions relicensure is periodically required on the basis of a minimum record of continuing education.

Some health professions are not required to have government licensure at all in certain states; this applies, for example, to laboratory technology. In those states mandating licensure, the candidate must usually pass an examination, in addition to having credentials from an approved school. In the other states, the laboratory technologist or technician may simply offer to prospective employers a voluntary credential: certification by the American Society of Clinical Pathologists. This is based on attendance at a school approved by the Society and passage of its examination. Certain new health disciplines, such as inhalation therapy, are licensed in only a few states; likewise for clinical psychologists. Hospital administration is a field defined as subject to state licensure only in one state, Minnesota. On the other hand, "nursing home administrator" is the first field which, by national law, requires state licensure (meeting minimal requirements) under certain conditions. This was due to serious deficiencies detected in the administration of nursing homes serving patients under the federal Medicare program, and the national requirement was imposed as a corrective action. Nursing homes are reimbursed for Medicare patients, only if they are headed by licensed administrators.

While the state licensure of health professions in the United States is highly variable, several voluntary professional societies have attempted to fill some regulatory gaps. Nonofficial approval of various types of auxiliary personnel, such as pharmacy or laboratory assistants, is being offered by the corresponding national societies (pharmacists or laboratory technologists), based on examinations or proof of satisfactory training. Probably more important is the role of these societies in the approval or "accreditation" of educational programs. Since neither state nor federal governments have taken initiative in approving professional training programs, this is being done by the private societies. The roles of the American Medical Association and the Association of American Medical Colleges in approving medical schools have been noted previously. The same sort of approval has been carried out by the American Pharmaceutical Association with respect to schools of pharmacy, the National League for Nursing regarding schools of professional (i.e., offering R.N. awards) nursing, and so on. There is, furthermore, a National Commission on Accrediting, another voluntary body, which helps to establish general criteria for reviewing educational programs in all fields. Finally in the federal U.S. Office of Education there is a unit, recently formed, to approve of the accrediting associations; only at this point has government come to enter the picture.

Welfare State Systems

The diversity of patterns of regulating health manpower in the many welfare states is too great to permit anything but a few examples. In general (with several notable exceptions), one finds that in these countries greater control is exercised by national governments over the educational programs; as a result, the establishment of qualifications for engaging in various forms of health service is usually much simpler than in America. Proof of graduation from a governmentally approved training program usually grants the legal right to engage in the profession more or less automatically.

In Sweden or Norway, for example, all the medical schools must be approved by the national Ministry of Education or its equivalent. Then a medical graduate need only present his credentials to the health authorities in the national Ministry of Social Affairs (Norway) for registration. The same general sequence in these countries applies to nurses, except that the maintenance of registration records has been delegated by the government to the voluntary nurses association. In France and West Germany, the basic governmental controls apply also to the educational institutions. No further examination is required of medical graduates. In Germany, the new graduate must then have two years of hospital training, after which registration with a provincial (not national) health authority becomes a *pro forma* matter. In France, the new medical graduate simply registers, on the basis of his academic credentials, with the local government (prefect) in the area where he settles; for ethical and professional surveillance, he must also register with the national *Ordre des Médecins* (Order of Physicians). Similar policies are followed in Belgium and Holland.

Great Britain differs slightly from most welfare states in requiring its medical schools and their examinations to be approved by the General Medical Council—a prestigious voluntary body—even though all the educational institutions are also approved and supervised by the Ministry of Education. Canada even requires passage of a national examination, given by the Medical Council of Canada. It is claimed that this "second examination" does not reflect distrust of the schools, but rather is intended to help them maintain their standards. In Great Britain, there are still further examination hurdles, which are, however, voluntary: these are for fellowship in the Royal College of Physicians or the Royal College of Surgeons. The latter are more rigorous and specialized examinations; their passage entitles the doctor to add FRCP or FRCS after his name, as a mark of additional status and competence.

Japan illustrates the influence of politics on regulatory processes. Before World War II, it followed the German model of more or less automatic registration of medical and other health science graduates, after schooling—relying on supervision of the schools by the national educational authorities. Then during the postwar occupation by United States armed forces, the American pattern of a second examination was imposed. Some years later, great resistance to this came from the students, and the prewar policies were reinstated. Generally speaking, the procedures for licensure or registration of nurses, pharmacists, and other health personnel follow the model of physicians in each country. There may be slight modifications in certain fields— as in Norway, where, although there is no second examination of nursing graduates by the government, the final examination administered by each nursing school consists of a nationally uniform set of questions.

Verification of specialty status in medicine varies among the welfare states, although it is primarily left up to professional bodies. In France, there are two classes of specialist: (1) those who are exclusively devoted to a specialty or *médecins specialists* and (2) those engaging in a specialty but also continuing with some general practice or *médecins compétents*. Both types are so registered with the Ministry of National Education, after completing appropriate training and passing examinations given by the several specialty societies. They are also so registered in each *département* or province. In Norway, the national medical association simply maintains a committee, which regulates specialty training requirements and gives credentials. In Belguim, there are no examinations, but an especially rigorous sequence of training is required in every field, and it must be approved in advance by the national medical association; if the medical candidate passes through all the stages successfully he is awarded specialty credentials by the medical association. In Belgium and, indeed, in most welfare state countries, specialty status must be registered with a governmental authority, if the doctor is then to be entitled to payments from the health insurance program at specialist (higher) rates.

Less Developed and Socialist Countries

In both the transitional and the underdeveloped countries, the role of government is generally stronger and of the professional bodies weaker than in the welfare states. Within the Ministry of Health in Colombia (South America), for example, there is a Council of Professional Practice which registers all physicians and other health personnel who have had prescribed training. No examination is required, but the candidate must simply show his credentials from a school recognized by the Ministry of Education; physicians must also, however, show proof of a one-year internship in a hospital plus a second year of service in a public health post or a rural facility of some type. Many Latin American countries require the latter form of service as an approach to solving the worldwide problem of rural doctor shortages.

Beyond these *pro forma* registrations, physicians, dentists, and others engaged in individual practice must usually join a professional society (*Colegio Medico de Chile* for example) for purposes of ethical controls over their behavior. These societies may also engage in bargaining with government agencies on rates of payment for services, or they may establish parallel nongovernmental bodies for such purposes.

In the deeply underdeveloped countries, regulation of personnel tends to follow patterns laid down earlier by colonial authorities. Professional societies tend to be quite weak and virtually all responsibilities are vested in ministries of health. Registration with the ministry follows automatically from completion of prescribed courses of training. Nurses and allied health personnel are registered in substantially the same way as physicians.

The socialist countries likewise require no examinations by a government authority beyond completion of specified educational programs. The Ministry of Health of Poland, for example, simply registers all nurses, physicians, and others when their training is completed. Even the educational institutions for the health disciplines are usually controlled by the national health, rather than education, authorities, so that there is no need for interchange between two ministries (education and health). Physicians, as noted earlier, may be required to serve for two or three years in a rural area as a condition for registration. Ethical and behavioral matters are also supervised by the health ministry. There are nonofficial professional societies, but their functions are essentially in the field of postgraduate or continuing education. Since the overall health care systems in the socialist countries are in structured frameworks, the hazards of malfeasance by an isolated practitioner are generally much less. Regulation, one might say, is built into the course of day-to-day work.

REGULATION OF OTHER HEALTH CARE RESOURCES

Beyond health manpower, all countries exercise some supervision over the structure of health care facilities, the production and distribution of drugs or medical supplies, and certain other inputs of the health care system.

Facility Approval

As the importance of hospitals in total health service has increased, standards for their construction and operation have increasingly come to be imposed by governmental authorities. The application of these controls varies with the overall political ideology of countries.

In free enterprise America, there were very few public standards for hospital construction until the federal law to subsidize state projects in 1947; as a condition for hospital construction grants, each state was required to enact a hospital licensure law. Under these laws all hospitals are periodically inspected with respect to physical standards, laboratory facilities, kitchen sanitation, fire safety, radiological protection, and related matters. Enforcement of these laws is rather weak, however, since the staffing of the state inspectional authorities (usually the state department of health) is generally meager. Moreover, most of the state laws stress standards on the hospital's physical features, and demand little in the way of standards for functioning of the staff. Compensating for the latter, in a sense, there was established in 1950 in the United States a nongovernmental body: the Joint Commission on Accreditation of Hospitals (JCAH), representing several professional associations. Accreditation by the JCAH is entirely voluntary, but it emphasizes the performance of the medical staff, the diligence of patient care, and various functional aspects of the hospital. This approval has become a generally more prestigious badge of merit than the official licensure by a state government.

Until about 1960, any hospital in the United States could be built or enlarged, so long as it met state licensure requirements. As bed-population ratios increased, along with expansion of voluntary insurance for hospitalization, it became apparent that under fee-for-service medical practice almost any new beds constructed would soon become occupied by patients. In response, one state (New York) enacted a law in 1961, requiring that any construction providing new hospital beds had not only to meet the licensure standards but also to satisfy the state government that there was a "social need" for these additional beds. Such "certificate of need" laws were soon passed by twenty-five or thirty other states. In 1974, a national law was enacted (the National Health Planning and Resource Development Act), requiring that every state must have such legislation controlling the supply of hospital beds as well as their quality standards

Hospital construction in the welfare states has generally been more subject to governmental controls, although the levels of public authority differ. Voluntary accreditation bodies play no role. In British and French systems, standards for both construction and operation are promulgated by the ministries of health at the national level, although they are monitored by regional or provincial authorities. In Great Britain, where virtually all hospitals are now actually owned and controlled by the central government, exercise of this authority is not difficult; in France, where government sponsors about seventy percent of the beds, the implementation of standards, while theoretically universal, is not so perfect for the nongovernmental thirty percent. The authority in Sweden is lodged in local units of government for ninety-five percent of the beds, but national government standards for both construction and operation of hospitals are typically followed on a voluntary basis.

Regarding the supply or bed-population ratios of hospitals in Western Europe, the constraints becoming necessary in the free enterprise setting have not arisen. With salaried hospital doctors or, at least, selectively small hospital medical staffs, the problem of "overhospitalization" (with its serious cost burdens) has evidently not been felt. As a result, any local community or, in some countries, any voluntary group has been free to build hospitals, so long as they met technical standards. The high cost of construction to meet such standards is an inherent constraint.

In Canada and Japan, on the other hand, where "open staff" hospitals and fee remuneration of doctors for inpatient care prevail, the situation is different. Canada, after its federal-provincial hospital insurance program was enacted in 1957, soon recognized that almost any beds constructed would quickly become filled with patients, for whose care the entire population had to pay under the insurance system. Therefore, the provincial governments now exercise control over all new hospital construction or enlargement, requiring that there be proven a definite need for any additional beds. In fact, some provinces—faced with spiralling hospitalization costs—have even ordered the closure of certain small hospitals to limit the bed availability; enforcement is implemented through the insurance program. In Japan, similar action has been taken recently at the national level.

In both types of developing country, the need for hospital beds has been so great and the economic resources to build them so limited that controls over either quality standards or bed supply have been very limited. Many of the national ministries of health maintain technical offices to prepare architectural plans for hospitals and health centers of various sizes, along with rosters of appropriate equipment. These offices are concerned with any facilities constructed by the ministry itself (or by a ministry of public works at the request of the health authorities), and they offer advice, if requested, to private or charitable bodies building hospitals. In Latin America and several Middle Eastern countries, some social security agencies have similar architectural design offices. But disciplinary controls are rarely exercised if a nonofficial body establishes a private hospital that does not meet central government standards. The concept would seem to be that almost any sort of hospital, in countries desperately short of beds, is better than none.

Hospital construction in the socialist countries, being entirely governmental, presents no special problems of surveillance. Depending on the degree of centralized authority, hospitals are simply built according to the plans of the national or local government bodies. In the highly centralized model of the Soviet Union, the national Ministry of Health plans all construction or must approve projects originating at a local level (such as a collective form), since the operating costs are eventually to be met from the national health budget. In the more localized model of China or Yugoslavia, the provincial or republic authorities make their own hospital or health center construction decisions, but they may obtain advice on technical standards, if they wish, from the central health ministries.

Drug Control

The manufacture and distribution of pharmaceutical products is probably more dependent on the overall operations of a country's economic system than any other aspect of the health services. Thus, in an essentially capitalist economy, even when the delivery of all health care has largely come under the control of government, as in the British National Health Service, the production and sale of drugs remain mainly a responsibility of private commerce.

The free enterprise ideology in American health services is especially well illustrated in the provision and distribution of drugs. Their manufacture is by private corporations, they are widely advertised to both physicians and the general population, their sale is by private pharmacists (either small merchants or corporate chains of drugstores), and their consumption depends overwhelmingly on private (noninsured) payments. The harm to patients resulting from exercise of the profit motive in this field has generated a series of federal legislative responses from 1906 to 1962, which have imposed increasing controls on pharmaceutical production and distribution.

Because of the actual or potential harm done by toxic substances, sold as remedies or publicized by false claims in labeling or advertising, or because of the sale of substances of unproven safety or efficacy, the federal Congress and many state legislatures have enacted increasingly restrictive legislation. As a result, today the United States paradoxically has more rigorous controls over drug marketing than many other countries, where the general health care system is more disciplined. In reaction to a succession of tragedies, in which patients have been poisoned or killed by innocently purchased drugs, American law now requires the manufacturer to offer rigorous proof (presented to a federal government agency) of a new product's safety as well as efficacy before it may be distributed. There is also careful surveillance of advertising claims.

Nevertheless, the freedom of hundreds of manufacturers to produce and sell their products, usually under patented brandnames, results in a bewildering array of tens of thousands of drugs. Excellent university hospitals have found that a "formulary" or list of a few hundred preparations is adequate to deal with almost all human ailments. Yet, the free market for both production and distribution results in the sale of numerous compounds with identical chemical composition, under different names and with widely varying prices. Moreover, there may be scores of medications with very similar pharmacological action, even though their chemical composition may differ slightly or substantially. To cope with the confusion caused by this plethora of drug products, many organized health care programs have issued defined lists of drugs—often under the "generic" chemical name (typically less expensive), rather than the brand name—which will be financed; other products may be used only at the patient's personal expense.

The social insurance programs, which usually cover prescribed drugs in the welfare states, have led to many more controls over the distribution of pharmaceutical products. In countries where few drugs are domestically manufactured, such as Norway, the legal controls over production may be relatively limited. Even in West Germany, where many drugs are manufactured, the tests mandated for drug safety have not been very strict, so that it was possible for a company to market "Thalidomide" for years, before its tragic deformative effects on the babies of pregnant women taking the drug were detected.

The marketing of drugs in the Western European countries, on the other hand, is subject to many constraints. Ministries of health, usually with the advice of expert committees of medical practitioners and pharmacologists, often issue a list of compounds which may be legally imported or sold—with periodic updating. Thus, Norway authorizes the sale of only 2,000 drugs within its borders—far fewer than the number in the United States or, in fact, West Germany. In Great Britain, the number of marketable drugs is greater, but there is a "recommended list" of products covered under the National Health Service; drugs not on this list and prescribed by the doctor must be paid for by the patient personally, unless the doctor can specifically justify their use in a particular case. The Belgian social insurance program requires some cost sharing by the patient for all prescriptions, but it is a lower percentage of the price if the drug is on the officially approved list.

Pharmacies come under greater control in several welfare state systems than in America. In Norway, pharmacies are inspected by the central government periodically to assure their compliance with defined standards. Also there are controls over the establishment of new pharmacies. In certain areas—especially the large cities—where pharmacies are abundant, new ones will not be permitted; hence a pharmacist may be employed only in an existing pharmacy at such locations or else he must go to an underserved area if he wishes to open a new pharmacy shop. In Belgium, there is an unusual law placing responsibility on the dispensing pharmacist for ill effects from any prescription—even though the doctor's written orders have been accurately followed. As a result, to protect both their members and the general population, the Belgian Association of Pharmacists has long operated its own elaborate drug-testing program, over and above the controls imposed on manufacturers (within Belgium) by the Ministry of Health.

In the developing countries, drug controls are relatively weak. The vast majority of modern drugs are imported; even if the packaging or the preparation, for example, of capsules is done in the country, the required chemical compounds come from outside sources. Once a company has been authorized to open a pharmaceutical plant, there is little if any government surveillance over its operation. Likewise, most drugs are readily dispensed by a pharmacy, or even a general food shop, with or without a prescription. There may be limitations on the sale of certain narcotics, but even these are seldom enforced. With respect to the remedies sold or administered by traditional healers in the developing countries, there are virtually no attempts at government controls. In organized programs, such as the health centers of a ministry of health or the polyclinics of a social security program, the drugs dispensed usually come from central depots and are therefore more carefully controlled.

The socialist countries control both drug production and distribution along lines parallel with the rest of their health care systems. In the Soviet Union, the number of drugs available is much smaller than in Western Europe, since only one or two compounds are produced for each pharmacological purpose. Controls are simply built into the planning of pharmaceutical production by the Ministry of Health. In People's China, the manufacture of "Western" drugs, such as antibiotics or contraceptive steroids, is planned and carried out by the Ministry of Health; the herbal drugs of traditional Chinese medicine, however, are freely produced in every local area.

REGULATION OF HEALTH CARE PERFORMANCE

After the licensure of personnel, the approval of health facilities, or the control of drug production

and distribution, there are many further forms of regulation feasible to assure effective performance within a health care system. These are sometimes built into the delivery patterns, such as the discipline implicit in the "closed staff" salaried doctor model of hospital organization in Europe, compared with the "open staff" model with numerous private visiting doctors in America. The same applies to the health center model, compared to private office practice, for delivering ambulatory medical care. Here, however, we may examine other less direct regulatory influences: those exercised by payment agencies, professional societies, or judicial systems.

In the United States, the laissez-faire economic approach to most medical care has led to a long-term escalation of prices; the rate of inflation has been especially rapid over the last thirty years. Largely in response to this—although concerns about the quality of health care also play a part—various payment agencies have come to apply increasing controls. Thus, with fee-for-service payments being used in most government programs of medical care for the poor (such as Medicaid), many states require "prior authorization" by a government medical consultant before elective surgical procedures are paid for. Such regulations, of course, influence both the costs and the quality of the service. Other government programs, such as those for rehabilitation of disabled workers, may stipulate that only board-certified specialists may participate and be paid. Voluntary health insurance programs may also review payment claims with a special eye for abuses, such as excessive numbers of injections, diagnostic tests, or surgical procedures of dubious value, like tonsillectomies. On the other hand, many voluntary insurance organizations have been criticized for being relatively loose in their surveillance, including their exercise of the "fiscal intermediary" role under the governmental Medicare program for services to the aged.

Within the Medicare program, in which costs have risen very rapidly, the federal government has been impelled to introduce more and more regulatory constraints. The rules for determining "usual and customary" fees have become increasingly restrictive and legal actions have been taken against doctors suspected of submitting fraudulent fee claims. In 1973, amendments to the federal law required establishment of professional standards review organizations (PSROs), to exercise peer review over all Medicare and Medicaid payment claims for services in hospitals. The United States is to be covered by some 200 PSROs, whose surveillance should hopefully lead to greater self-discipline in the American medical profession.

Professional societies of physicians, dentists, nurses, or others are theoretically expected to promote ethical behavior among their members. In America, nevertheless, it has been very rare for such societies to discipline any of their members, except for the most egregious behavior, such as that associated with drug addiction, alcoholism, or frankly illegal actions. Professional societies, however, have been effective in preventing advertising by their members or other blatantly commercialized practices. On the other hand, they have often put greater energies behind political opposition to various legislative proposals, that might extend health service to the population, but allegedly constrain the "freedom" of the private practitioner.

A third indirect channel of regulation is the right of the patient to take legal action against his doctor (or other health care provider) for injuries suffered due to negligence. In the United States, such lawsuits for malpractice have become increasingly frequent in recent years. The reasons are numerous; they probably reflect the relatively lax medical staff discipline in many American hospitals, the increasing sophistication of patients, the aggressiveness of lawyers, the high costs of medical care (often not covered by insurance or in other ways), the tendency of insurance companies (covering the doctor) to "settle" claims of even dubious merit rather than run the risk of court litigation, the jury system even for noncriminal tort actions, and so on. In any event, the rate and amounts of malpractice awards or out-of-court financial settlements have risen so much that the personal liability insurance, which nearly all American physicians carry, has become extremely costly; premiums amount to many thousands of dollars a year, being especially high for surgeons and anesthesiologists. This "malpractice crisis" has led to intense protests (including strikes) by doctors and to many legislative reforms of the tort law in this field. At the same time, the patient's right to initiate these lawsuits has exerted an influence in heightening self-discipline within the medical care system, especially in hospitals.

Regulation of medical performance through the social insurance programs of the welfare state countries is somewhat more rigorous. The British general practitioner pattern with its capitation payment, for example, uses a simple approach: to protect quality, the government sets a maximum number of persons allowable on any G.P. list. In the more prevalent fee-for-service payment pattern, regulation is always more complicated. The German sickness funds conduct computerized reviews of each doctor's practice habits, as measured by such criteria as the number of drug prescriptions per case, number of office visits and of laboratory tests per case, rates of certain surgical procedures, etc. These measurements are compared with those of other doctors in the same specialty, and highly deviant individuals are readily identified. Such identification is regarded only as a screening step, to be followed up by detailed examination of the individual doctor's work. If this reveals unjustified services, the doctor may be penalized by payment of only a fraction of his claims; in seriously irregular instances, the doctor may be ruled out of participation in the social insurance program entirely.

In Canada, several of the provinces apply similar techniques for identifying doctors whose practice customs suggest abuse. Procedures are especially diligent in the province of Quebec, where the medical care insurance program transmits to the medical licensing body the names of doctors with deviant "statistical profiles." The licensing body then calls on the doctor for an explanation, and if not satisfactory its "penalty" may be to require him to undertake a certain course of postgraduate study or to have a second consultant in all subsequent cases of certain diagnoses. These regulatory procedures, in general, probably exert more influence on the quality and costs of medical care by their mere existence than by the relatively few cases of irresponsible medical performance that they uncover.

Not that every welfare state's health insurance system is equally rigorous in its regulatory practices. Belgium and Japan are examples of countries where the private medical profession is extremely powerful politically. Doctors have successfully resisted almost any efforts of the insurance program to discipline deviant behavior. In these countries, the social insurance program is regarded essentially as a payment mechanism that cannot challenge the decisions or performance of any licensed physician.

Professional societies in most of the welfare state countries generally fall into two types: (1) the association concerned with scientific advancement, including continuing education and (2) the body concerned with negotiations on economic matters with governmental or social insurance organizations; the latter group also monitors the ethical behavior of its members. In addition, there are also various societies in the medical specialties, including general practice. In nursing, pharmacy, and other health professions, these two distinct roles are sometimes played by committees or divisions of one national association. With the prevailing separation of general medical practitioners from hospitals in the welfare states, societies of GPs tend to have a great deal of vitality, and are staunchly dedicated to advancement of the status of their members. As a result, they are particularly conscientious in promoting diligent performance.

For many reasons, the relative weights of which are not clear, legal actions for malpractice against doctors or hospitals or other providers are quite rare in the welfare states. Most prominent among the causes is probably the national health insurance legislation, under which any medical costs due to malfeasance are covered, along with other health care costs. The more disciplined medical staff organization within hospitals (compared with that in America) also probably reduces poor performance. The legal systems concerning torts generally differ: contingency fees for lawyers are either prohibited or considered unethical; jury trials are not used in civil (noncriminal) actions. Private insurance companies are not so commonly used for carrying malpractice liability insurance; instead, the medical associations often operate "protective associations" to which all their members contribute premiums. Then, whenever the doctor's behavior has been considered reasonable, he is vigorously defended, rather than offering financial "settlement" to avoid litigation. Finally, the effective personal relationships, that tend to develop between patients and their general practitioners (who, it will be recalled, are proportionately much more numerous than in America), mean that patients seldom get angry with their doctors and the whole medical establishment. (In America, patient anger is the initial provocation of many lawsuits.) As a result, malpractice insurance premiums paid by doctors in Great Britain, Canada, Norway, or Australia average only about $100 a year—a trivial fraction of the rates in America.

In the developing countries, the organized health care programs usually pay doctors by salary, rather than by fees or capitation, so that the scheme of remuneration, as such, is not relied upon for regulation of performance. Rather, it is the organizational dynamics within the delivery system—supervision, consultation, meritorious promotion, and so on—that influences the behavior of health care providers. So far as purely private professional practice is concerned, regulation is virtually nonexistent, after professional licensure or registration.

Similarly, the professional societies do little if anything to discipline practitioners in the developing countries. Their roles are to educate their members on scientific advances, and to negotiate with government and social insurance bodies on economic questions. In a sense, the diligence of medical and other societies in protecting patients against any malfeasance of providers varies with the sophistication of the general population about scientific mat-

ters; this tends to be quite weak in the developing countries.

For the same reason, legal redress for patient grievances is seldom sought in the developing countries. Rare is the patient in Africa who would challenge the effects of a doctor's acts, or the lawyer who would represent him. Grievance procedures may sometimes operate in the social security medical care systems of the transitional countries, although these generally concern problems of accessibility (e.g., a long waiting time before seeing the doctor) rather than medical performance. A rather highly educated and sophisticated population is required to generate recourse to the courts for adjudicating the claims of patients about injuries resulting from improper medical care.

In the socialist countries also, it is the structure of the whole delivery system that principally regulates the quality of medical care. The salaries paid to personnel and the responsibilities assigned to them embody rewards for competence, experience, and responsibility; correspondingly, poor performance, in the opinion of the organizational leadership, may result in failure to advance or even demotion. (In a way, the mechanism resembles that used in American universities, where the advancement of professors depends upon the judgment of their colleagues and academic supervisors.) Thus, the scheme for payment of health personnel does, in fact, exercise an influence on performance by giving incentives, through salary levels, to diligent work. The judgment of merit, however, depends on professional peers, rather than on popularity with patients.

Professional associations play only a very limited role in the socialist countries, outside of the sphere of continuing education. Ethical constraints are exercised within the governmental health system itself; since there is little if any private practice, however, the objective of opposing commercialized abuses, which generate most "ethical codes" in other societies, is not relevant. There are labor unions of health workers, including physicians, but their role is primarily to mediate grievances of personnel, to represent their members in salary negotiations, to conduct welfare programs (such as operating rest homes and vacation resorts), and so on.

Medical specialty societies in Poland, and probably in other socialist countries as well, play a semi-official role in monitoring performance in their respective fields. Committees from each specialty body make periodic visits to all hospitals and polyclinics for monitoring the quality of the work in their particular fields. They give ratings on the quality of performance of individuals, which influence their rates of promotion. If they find substandard performance, they may recommend transfer of certain personnel to another location, where the individual's work will be more closely supervised. In addition, these committees may be summoned to consult on problems at a particular facility, where the local medical director needs advice. An effort is made to include on these specialty committees doctors from both academic (or theoretical) and practical backgrounds of experience.

Judicial redress through the courts plays little part in the regulation of health care performance in socialist settings. A patient with cause for dissatisfaction, or with an injury considered attributable to poor medical work, would bring his complaint to the attention of the supervisor of the program involved. If there are complaints from several persons, they might appeal to the political party machinery, which is intended to oversee the operations of all social programs. Courts of law, however, are confined largely to adjudication of criminal acts or alleged crimes. Even such matters as transfers of property, wills, business contracts, etc., which occupy so much of the time of private lawyers in capitalist societies, are handled in socialist societies by governmental bureaus.

Thus, in all types of country and in a variety of ways—governmental and voluntary—regulation over the health services has grown. While official licensure of health personnel has been the fundamental approach, various forms of approval or control have been increasingly applied to other kinds of health resource, such as facilities and drugs. Regulation of the day-to-day performance of health services has been extended through diverse methods of surveillance or teamwork patterns for organizing health care delivery. As the financing of health care by the whole population becomes more collectivized, pressures mount for greater regulation to control both the costs and quality of services.

Chapter XXX
Future Prospects in American Health Service

In this final chapter, the view is shifted back to the American scene, where some predictions are ventured about the future, based on the trends of the last twenty or thirty years. In many ways, American trends in health service organization recapitulate European, coming about fifty years later and in somewhat different form. Observations in the older industrialized countries of Europe, therefore, give further clues on probable future developments in the United States.

The following text was presented as an address to the California Association for Health and Welfare in March 1967.[1] It was entitled "Combining Science and Humanism in the Health Services of Tomorrow" and has not been previously published.

Today we are looking twenty years ahead in the health services. Perhaps the best way to judge where we are going is to look backward and plot out the direction in which we have been moving. Unfortunately, the historians have not yet succeeded in computerizing the past on electronic machines, so we must still rely on that humble and mass-produced computer—the human brain—to study the trends and make some estimates about the future shape of things.

THE PAST THIRTY YEARS

It is relatively easy to review the span of a generation, and so my thoughts go back to thirty years ago when, as a medical student, I was stimulated to study the social problems in medicine. We were in the depths of the Depression, Fascism was growing in Europe, and everyone was worried about what lay ahead. The Social Security Act, setting up old-age pensions, unemployment insurance, and more generous public assistance for the poor, had just been enacted. The President of the General Motors Corporation had warned that this law would mark the end of the "American way of life," but the greater threat seemed to come from the persistent poverty, squalor, and sickness in the land.

One of the positive responses to the glaring needs for health care in 1937 was the initiative taken by hospitals to set up voluntary nonprofit insurance plans—a movement which a few years before had been popularized with the symbol of a blue cross. At a meeting of medical students in Chicago I was speaking of the vast problems of unattended sickness revealed in the recent National Health Survey of 1935-1936. "Hospitalization at three cents a day," as Blue Cross insurance was then epitomized, was one of the answers, I said, even though at the time it had reached only a tiny proportion (about four percent) of the American population. A distinguished surgeon on the platform thought otherwise. A leader in the American Medical Association, he spoke of the dangers of socialized medicine represented by this idea. Hospital insurance would lead to doctor's care insurance and then an inevitable decline in the quality of American medicine. Both physician and patient would lose their freedom, as bureaucratic third parties would intervene in the sacred relationship between the two. The patient's loss of individual responsibility for his hospital bills would lead to a more general deterioration of moral fiber. Moreover, this—like other socialistic ideas—could not succeed because it went contrary to the rules of human nature.

The economic pressures of half-empty hospitals, however, and precarious family incomes led to the continued and robust growth of Blue Cross. With the soundness of the idea demonstrated, commercial insurance carriers entered the field, and we all know what has happened. By the end of 1965, over 156,000,000 Americans were protected by some form of hospitalization insurance; this was eighty-one percent of the U.S. civilian population at the time, and did not include an additional eight or nine million old persons (previously uninsured) who were brought under the health insurance umbrella by the Medicare Law that took effect six months later.

There are plenty of weak spots, of course, in this success story of hospital insurance. For most people, benefits are still not comprehensive in the hospital sector, let alone the other basic sectors of physician's care, drugs, and dental service. Millions of low income and rural people are still totally unprotected. But the Blue Cross story has importance as just one example of a multitude of trends in the application of social principles to the health services, in spite of enormous opposition. It could be repeated with respect to the entire public health movement, the advancement of medical education and research, the surveillance of drug production and distribution, the medical care of the needy, the organization of private group practice clinics, and many other social mechanisms by which the health sciences have been adjusted to changing technology and human needs.

SOCIAL PROGRESS

Looking back over the past thirty years and more, we can detect great progress in reducing the gaps between medical science and its application. There is not time, of course, to review all the achievements, but I think we may get some appreciation of their nature and of the large residual problems to be solved, if we consider the trends under three broad categories.

The hospital insurance movement is a stream within the first broad channel of social adjustment; namely the provision of better economic support for health services. A second broad channel is the production of increased resources for delivery of health services—resources in personnel, facilities, and knowledge. A third broad channel is the improved organization of complex techniques, so that they may be applied with maximum quality, efficiency, and effectiveness. In most specific health programs there is, indeed, a certain blending of elements from all three of these channels, but I think we may see the issues and prospects that lie ahead more clearly if we consider each of them in turn.

Economic Support

In the development of expanded economic sup-

port for health services in America, the social progress has been enormous. In 1930, the vast bulk of medical expenses had to be paid privately by individuals when illness struck. All the support of government from tax sources, at all levels, contributed fourteen percent to the nation's health expenditures; this included the whole public health establishment, the military and veterans medical services, welfare medicine, and so on. Charity contributed about five percent, most of which went to support the construction of hospitals. Private industry, including all the health insurance plans that then existed, covered two percent of the total national costs. Thus, seventy-nine percent of health service costs had to be met from the pockets of individuals at the time of sickness.

Today the picture is very different. In 1965, of the $38,500,000,000 spent for all health purposes, twenty-six percent was derived from governmental revenues. The share borne by voluntary insurance had spiraled to twenty-four percent. Charity had declined slightly as a proportion to about four percent, and industry—for management-financed in-plant health services—to about one percent. Thus counting all forms of social financing, fifty-five percent of national expenditures for health purposes in 1965 were met through collective action, leaving forty-five percent to be borne out-of-pocket by individuals. With the implementation of Medicare in July 1966, the socially supported sector has now very likely risen to about sixty percent, leaving the purely private individual sector at forty percent. It is a very different picture from the nearly eighty percent private burden of 1930.

It must also be realized that, while we are speaking here of percentages of total health expenditures, the overall segment of such expenditures in the United States gross national product (GNP) has also risen. In 1930, barely four percent of GNP was spent for health purposes, and today it is six percent of a greatly enlarged GNP. Thus, the health services are absorbing a fifty percent larger share of a larger economic pie, and a much greater proportion of that slice of pie is derived through social devices—mainly taxation and insurance. There is much reason to believe, moreover, that the expansion of the relative claim of health objectives on the nation's total economic resources—which is so important if needs are to be met—is largely due to the very force of an increased role of social, as against individual, financing.

This increasing amplitude and social character of the economic support for health purposes has yielded a steadily rising volume of medical services for the American population. The rate of contacts between

physicians and patients and the rate of admissions to hospitals have about doubled in the last thirty years, to take only two elementary measures. To accommodate this greater effective demand for health care, we have had to develop more personnel and facilities. The economic support, therefore, has had important spillover effects on the second channel we have conceptualized: the production of basic resources.

Resource Production

Thus, to meet the rising demand for medical care the nation has trained a greatly expanded corps of health personnel. The supply of total health manpower has risen steadily in relation to the growth of population, in spite of the virtual constancy of the ratios of two key types: physicians and dentists. In other words, a greatly increased rate of consumption of health services has been made possible by the educational output of an enlarged ratio of nurses, technicians, clerks, therapists, aides, and other paramedical personnel who have, so to speak, extended the productivity of a relatively constant ratio of doctors. These personnel have been both trained and supported by the enlarged economic investment in the health sector.

Likewise, the resources in physical facilities and equipment have been greatly enlarged. Through greater social financing, hospital beds have increased as a ratio to population about thirty-three percent between 1930 and 1960. The federal government, through the Hill-Burton Act, has contributed increasingly to the construction of both public and voluntary local hospitals. Equally important, the intensity of hospital bed use has been heightened. The reduction in average length of general hospital stay from about fifteen to seven days over this period means that each bed is occupied by twice as many patients in the course of a year. Automated equipment enables many more services—for example, blood sugar tests or dispensing of drugs—to be provided by a given number of health personnel in a unit of time.

Resources in the form of scientific knowledge have also expanded enormously—some would say, as a geometric series. Social expenditures for research, largely from governmental revenues, have produced an endless flow of new knowledge. Both theoretical principles and applied techniques have come from the scientific and clinical laboratories of this nation and other nations at a rate more rapid than they could be put into practice.

Technical Organization

It is in the third channel of medico-social trends, however, that our progress has been least impressive. The organization of complex scientific techniques, in relation to the inherent demands of the technology, has moved at a very slow pace. For, in the patterns of *how* our health resources are organized, traditions and vested interests run deep. It is mainly in this sphere that the great challenges of the next twenty years, in my view, are presented. It is in this channel that I would like to probe a little more deeply, and call for your imaginative explorations.

Let me not leave the impression that problems in the first two channels of economic support and resource production are all happily solved. Far from it. The gaps in financial support for needed health services are still tremendous. Despite all our social financing, the poor still get a lesser quantity and quality of health services than the affluent, in the face of a heavier burden of sickness and death. Even in sectors like the health care of the aged, where the economic progress has recently taken a long jump, the inadequacies remain serious. Likewise, the production of basic resources is far from satisfactory, especially in the sphere of health manpower. The Presidential Advisory Commission on Health Manpower, the reorganization of the U.S. Public Health Service to establish a major Bureau of Health Manpower, the formation of a new State Health Manpower Council in California, are only a few of the signs of widely recognized deficiencies in this sector.

But much more serious than the problems in these two channels are those involved in the technical organization of the health services. With certain exceptions (which I will try to examine in a moment), the vast increases in the nation's economic allocations to health service and production of medical resources have been made within a pattern of technical organization which stems largely from the nineteenth century. In fact, there is much reason to believe that the very large rise in medical costs has been partly a wasteful consequence of our failure to do much about the systematic organization of the available health resources. It is as though we set out to improve our national transportation system by a vast increase in the production and operational financing of horses and buggies.

The crucial fact is that most of the expanded economic support for health service has been applied to a framework of medical and dental practice in isolated individual offices and a patch quilt of hospitals, drug stores, and laboratories which are characterized by extravagance, inefficiency, and frustration for the patient and provider alike. Half the nation's general hospitals (and a higher proportion in California) are of under 100 beds—a size much too

small to render optimal scientific services soundly and economically. Eighty-five percent of clinical physicians and ninety-five percent of dentists hold forth as solo practitioners despite the enormous development of specialization demanding professional teamwork. Thousands of small, independent drug stores dispense a bewildering array of drugs at very high prices, inflated by the cost of a fantastic volume of competitive advertising, robust manufacturing profits, and an elaborate network of middlemen between producer and consumer. Dental treatment absorbs the scarce and expensive time of highly trained professionals, doing tedious tasks that could be readily assigned to technicians under supervision. Preventive medicine is widely preached but seldom practiced, while geriatric rehabilitation is a fiction in the thousands of small proprietary nursing homes that accommodate the vast majority of chronically ill and aged patients whose numbers are increasing daily.

Though this is a grim capsule sketch, it could be easily documented with reams of facts and figures. While American medical science at its best is capable of wonders in reducing disability and saving lives, these wonders are applied far less than they could be. Our age-adjusted mortality rates are higher than those of many other countries of lesser wealth and, at that, spending lower proportions of their GNP on health care. The difference lies in the way we spend our health dollars. Our social machinery has simply not caught up with our scientific capacity.

Fortunately, there are exceptions to this picture of organizational anachronisms. In contrast to the great bulk of physicians in solo medical practice, there is a fifteen percent sector engaged in organized teams or group practices. Against the thousands of small, isolated, substandard hospitals, there stand the magnificent medical centers making proper use of the full range of scientific techniques. Regionalized networks of health facilities are slowly being promoted through a number of voluntary social experiments; new legislation on cooperative interhospital arrangements for tackling heart disease, cancer, and stroke is fostering this idea further. The worst abuses of drug profiteering are being combatted through new federal laws, through more systematic use of formularies, and through various drug distribution plans. Prevention is being extended through slow strengthening of the public health agencies, the fluoridation of some public water systems, the use of more multiphasic screening programs for early detection of chronic disease, and so on. Improved rehabilitation programs are being launched in hospitals, and many small nursing homes are developing professional ties with them.

Some of the most imaginative and promising innovations in the channel of health service organization are being applied in categorical programs, addressed to special disease problems or special population groups. To help cope with mental illness, for example, we are seeing the slow development of comprehensive mental health centers, where education, research, prevention, and treatment—both ambulatory and institutional—are offered for persons in the neighborhood. The huge mausoleumlike mental hospital off in the hinterland is being replaced by an active psychiatric service in the community general hospital. Alcoholism control is gaining increasing, if inadequate, public support. For the very poor in the central city slums, with aid from the federal Office of Economic Opportunity, neighborhood health centers are here and there being launched. Unlike the traditional public health clinic, they will offer comprehensive health service, both preventive and therapeutic. We all await the opening of such a center in Watts.[2] If a man happens to be a veteran with a military service-connected disability, and if he happens to live near a Veterans Administration facility, he is accessible to first-class comprehensive medical care; he is served by a system like that which General Eisenhower or President Johnson uses when sickness strikes.

But the pity is that these reasonable organizational patterns of health care are confined essentially to meeting small sectors of human need, defined either by the type of person affected or his type of illness. For the great bulk of people and of morbidity, we must depend largely on the wasteful and haphazard patterns sketched earlier. And it is more than economic waste that we tolerate.

The basic professional self-controls over quality of health service that are taught to every medical student and are regarded as mandatory in a university teaching hospital are only meagerly applied in the typical community hospital; they are hardly at all applied in thousands of private medical or dental or optometric offices throughout the nation.

INNOVATIONS IN THE FUTURE

Yet the organizational innovations that have developed for small sectors of health care give us some clues about what the future may hold. We can envisage, in perhaps a generation or two from now, a pattern of activity in which the technical and logistic provision of service will match the social level that has been achieved in the purely economic sector. This pattern would evolve from various organizational forms which we see embryonically now.

In each neighborhood, there would be a com-

prehensive health center staffed by a team of general physicians, specialists, nurses, technicians, and aides. Everyone—not just the veteran or the pauper or the crippled child—would be served by a "primary physician," as the Millis Report of the American Medical Association has recently defined him. Specialists would be called on for help as necessary. The mentally disturbed would be treated as well as the physically disabled. Dental care would also be provided, with reasonable use of dental technicians for the many simpler mechanical tasks. Laboratory and x-ray procedures would be done in the center, and drugs dispensed by the staff pharmacist. Preventive health examinations and screening tests for hidden disease would be done routinely with the aid of modern equipment and auxiliary staff. Personnel for health education and environmental surveillance would also be based at the health center.

Hospitalization, when necessary, would be provided at a good general facility of perhaps 300 to 500 bed capacity, where the full range of technical modalities could be offered. Institutional care of the mentally ill or the chronic sick would be given in special wings of the hospital or in affiliated units nearby. Several of the neighborhood health centers would be satellites to each such hospital, and their professional staffs would receive periodic continuing education in the hospital. Depending on the density and ecology of the population, the hospital would be professionally and administratively tied to other institutions in a regional network; at its hub would be a great medical center, where basic education of the health professions and medical research would be actively pursued.

The quality of health service would be subject to continual surveillance, not just in the hospitals but throughout the system. Major surgery or other serious procedures would, of course, only be done by qualified specialists. Cultists would have no place, nor would patent, self-prescribed medications. Physicians or public health nurses would make home calls, as necessary, but no time would be wasted in a doctor's travel to five or six separate hospitals—as the current lack of system compels him to do. The patient would be treated as a whole person, monitored by a unified medical record (which would move with him to a new health center if he changed his home). Whether he was a veteran or an injured worker or a welfare recipient or a parochial schoolchild, whether his illness was infectious or mental or traumatic or neoplastic—he would be treated by the unified system, starting in a nearby neighborhood health center and branching to other resources as necessary.

The economic support for all this would be de-rived from the social devices of insurance and public revenues that we have seen evolving over the last thirty years or more. The underlying resources of personnel, equipment, facilities, and knowledge would be produced likewise by social planning and investment—both governmental and voluntary—as they are now at an increasing tempo. The personnel would be rewarded for their labor according to equitable principles of skill, seniority, and responsibility, and their contributions would also be recognized by appropriate social status. But the receipt of services by an individual would not depend on the amount or source of the money paid, nor on the diagnostic category of his disease nor his social pedigree. It would be a right of his being an American and of living where he did.

SCIENCE AND HUMANISM

To some this picture may seem utterly utopian and unrealistic. To others it may seem far too highly planned and regimented. What would happen to the personal relationship between doctor and patient in such a setting? What would happen to the larger principle of individual freedom?

The answer, I believe, is that these relationships and freedoms would be enhanced. Paradoxical as it may seem to some, the greatest assaults on personal freedom in our current health care system have come, not from too much organization but from too little. Our troubles have come from the commercialization of the medical marketplace and the categorization of people and disease to save money. The crowded public clinic has been accepted for the poor because it was a cheaper arrangement. The deficiencies in quality that we tolerate spring from our hesitancy to impose standards that require organization.

Impersonality and loss of freedom are not attributes of organization; they are liabilities of inequitably allocated resources and inhibited or deficient organization. The most individualistic private medical office may yield a service that is both unscientific and insensitive—a fact tragically demonstrated by several hundred private medical records that I recently reviewed. A large and complex clinic, on the other hand, may be both scientific and humane—if it is adequately staffed and organized—as anyone can testify who has been treated at Mayo's or other first-class medical centers.

There is no question that division of labor and organization of the resultant specialized skills are necessary to achieve scientific excellence. There is also no question that organization of health services can achieve economies, as several comprehensive prepaid group practice medical care plans have demonstrated. But it is no less true, though often denied, that the personal and human needs of people can be best served by organization. Adequate quantities of manpower, facilities, and knowledge are required to meet those needs, but sound organization of these resources is equally essential.

As a nation we clearly have the economic potential. Much of it may be diverted for nonproductive purposes because of the world of international conflict in which we live. Even in the limited sphere of health services, much of it may be wasted simply because of the inhibitions of tradition and the timidity of our movements in the channel of organization. But the very increasing social visibility of the six percent of our GNP going to health purposes—sixty percent of it through social paths—is heightening the pressure toward patterns of organization that will optimize both economy and quality.[3] And the steady expansion of the hospital's outpatient role, of regional planning, of group medical practice, of mental health clinics, of rehabilitation centers, and many other forms of coordinated service constitute an evolution before our eyes.

We may be optimistic, I believe, that our society will behave with increasing rationality about a human need so pressing and intimate as preservation of health and life. The trend toward systematic planning of the health services is seen with amazing uniformity in virtually every nation of the world. We see it here in California in a hundred ways. Whether or not the picture I have painted is accurate, there can be little doubt that the direction of health service trends in the next twenty years is toward greater organization in the technical channel, as it has occurred (though not yet completely) in the economic support channel over the last thirty years. The precise lines of the future may well differ from any shape we can sketch today, but I am confident that we will move toward a health service system that combines both science and humanism in meeting social needs.

NOTES

[1] 56th Annual Meeting, Los Angeles, California, March 13, 1967.

[2] The Watts Multi-Purpose Health Center, financed by the U.S. Office of Economic Opportunity, was opened in south central Los Angeles in 1968.

[3] By 1975, the proportion of GNP spent for health purposes in the U.S. had come to exceed eight percent.

Selected Bibliography

MULTINATIONAL AND COMPARATIVE STUDIES OF HEALTH SERVICES

1. Abel-Smith, B., *Paying for Health Services: Study of the Costs and Sources of Finance in Six Countries*, Geneva: World Health Organization, Public Health Paper No. 17, 1963.

2. Abel-Smith, B., *An International Study of Health Expenditures, and its Relevance for Health Planning*, Geneva: World Health Organization, Public Health Paper No. 32, 1967.

3. "Asilomar Conference on International Studies of Medical Care" (6 papers), *Medical Care*, Vol. 9, No. 3, May-June 1971.

4. Andersen, Ronald B., B. Smedby, and O.W. Anderson, *Medical Care Use in Sweden and the United States* (A Comparative Analysis of Systems and Behavior), Chicago: Center for Health Administration, Research Series No. 27, 1970.

5. Anderson, Odin W., *Health Care: Can There Be Equity: - United States, Sweden, and England*, New York: John Wiley & Sons, 1972.

6. Babson, John, *Health Care Delivery Systems: A Multinational Survey*, London: Pitman Medical Publishing Company, Ltd., 1972.

7. Bridgman, Robert F. and M.I. Roemer, *Hospital Legislation and Hospital Systems*, Geneva: World Health Organization, Public Health Paper No. 50, 1973.

8. Brockington, F., *World Health* (second edition), London: J. & A. Churchill, Ltd., 1967.

9. Bryant, John, *Health and the Developing World*, Ithaca, New York: Cornell University Press, 1969.

10. Charron, Kenneth C., *Health Services, Health Insurance, and Their Inter-Relationships: A Study of Selected Countries*, Ottawa: Department of National Health and Welfare, 1963.

11. "Comparative Health Systems" (12 papers), *Inquiry*, Supplement to Vol. XII, No. 2, June 1975.

12. Evang, Karl, *Health Service, Society, and Medicine*, London: Oxford University Press, 1960.

13. Evang, Karl, D.S. Murray, and W.J. Lear, *Medical Care and Family Security: Norway, England, USA*, Englewood Cliffs, New Jersey: Prentice-Hall, 1963.

14. Falk, I.S., *Security Against Sickness: A Study of Health Insurance*, New York: Doubleday, Doran and Co., 1936.

15. Farman, C.H., *Health and Maternity Insurance Throughout the World 1954*, Washington: Social Security Administration, Department of HEW, February 1954.

16. Fendall, N.R.E., *Auxiliaries in Health Care: Programs in Developing Countries*, Baltimore: John Hopkins Press, 1972.

17. First International Congress of Group Medicine, *New Horizons in Health Care*, Winnipeg (Canada): Canadian Association of Medical Clinics, 1970.

18. Fry, John, *Medicine in Three Societies* (A Comparison of Medical Care in the USSR, USA, and U.K.), New York: American Elsevier Co., 1970.

19. Fry, John and W.A.J. Farndale, editors, *International Medical Care: A Comparison and Evaluation of Medical Care Services Throughout the World*, Oxford (England): Medical & Technical Publishing Co., 1972.

20. Fulcher, Derick, *Medical Care Systems: Public and Private Health Coverage in Selected Industrialized Countries*, Geneva: International Labour Office, 1974.

21. Gish, Oscar, *Doctor Migration and World Health: The Impact of the International Demand for Doctors on Health Services in Developing Countries*, London: G. Bell & Sons, 1971.

22. Glaser, William, *Paying the Doctor: Systems of Remuneration and Their Effects*, Baltimore: John Hopkins Press, 1970.

23. Glaser, William, *Social Settings and Medical Organization: A Cross-National Study of the Hospital*, New York: Atherton Press, 1970.

24. Hogarth, James, *The Payment of the Physician: Some European Comparisons*, New York: Macmillan, 1963.

25. *International Journal of Health Services*, all issues February 1971 to date.

26. International Labour Office, *International Survey of Social Security: Comparative Analysis and Summary of National Laws*, Geneva: 1950.

27. International Labour Office, *The Cost of Medical Care*, Geneva: 1959.

28. International Labour Office, *The Cost of Social Security*, Geneva: 1949-1971.

29. International Social Security Association, *Relations Between Social Security Institutions and Members of the Medical Profession*, Geneva: 1953.

30. International Social Security Association, *Sickness Insurance: National Monographs*, Geneva: 1956.

31. King, Maurice, editor, *Medical Care in Developing Countries*, Nairobi (Kenya): Oxford University Press, 1966.

32. Lynch, Matthew J. and Stanley S. Raphael, *Medicine and the State*, Springfield, Illinois: Charles C. Thomas, 1963.

33. Kenneth W. Newell, editor, *Health By the People*, Geneva: World Health Organization, 1975.

34. Newsholme, A., *International Studies on the Relation between the Private and Official Practice of Medicine, with Special Reference to the Prevention of Disease*, London: George Allen and Unwin, Ltd., 1931.

35. Abdel R. Omran, editor, *Community Medicine in Developing Countries*, New York: Springer, 1974.

36. Paul, Benjamin D., editor, *Health Culture, and Community*, New York: Russell Sage Foundation, 1955.

37. Peters, R.J. and J. Kinnaird, editors, *Health Services Administration*, Edinburgh: E. & S. Livingstone, Ltd., 1965.

38. Purcell, Elizabeth, editor, *World Trends in Medical Education, Faculty, Students, and Curriculum*, Baltimore: Johns Hopkins Press, 1971.

39. Read, M., *Culture, Health, and Disease*, London: Tavistock Publications, 1966.

40. Roemer, Milton I., *Medical Care in Relation to Public Health: A Study of the Relationships between Preventive and Curative Medicine Throughout the World*, Geneva: World Health Organization, 1956.

41. Roemer, Milton I., *Medical Care in Latin America*, Washington: Pan American Union, 1963.

42. Roemer, Milton I., *The Organization of Medical Care under Social Security*, (A Study Based on the Experience of Eight Countries), Geneva: International Labour Office, 1969.

43. Roemer, Milton I., *Evaluation of Community Health Centres*, Geneva: World Health Organization, Public Health Paper No. 48, 1972.

44. Sand, Rene, *The Advance to Social Medicine*, London: Staples Press, 1952.

45. Schoeck, H., editor, *Financing Medical Care*, Caldwell, Idaho: Canton Printers, Ltd., 1962.

46. Sigerist, Henry E., *Civilization and Disease*, Ithaca, New York: Cornell University Press, 1943.

47. Sigerist, Henry E., *On the Sociology of Medicine* (Milton I. Roemer, editor), New York: MD Publications, 1960.

48. Simpson, J., R.G. Thomas, H.N. Willard, and H.J. Bakst, *Custom and Practice in Medical Care, Comparative Study of Two Hospitals in Arboath, Scotland, U.K., and Waterville, Maine, U.S.A.*, London: Oxford University Press, 1968.

49. "Special International Issue," *The Journal of Medical Education*, Vol. 36, No. 9, September 1961.

50. Stampar, A., *Selected Papers of Andrija Stampar* (M.D. Gmek, editor), Andrija Stampar School of Public Health, Zagreb (Yugoslavia): University of Zagreb, 1966.

51. Tabakov, G.A., *Medicine in the United States and the Soviet Union*, Boston: Christopher Publishing House, 1962.

52. Titmuss, R.M., *The Gift Relationship*, New York: Pantheon Books, 1971.

53. U.S. Social Security Administration, *Social Security Throughout the World 1971*, Washington: 1972 (a continuing series).

54. Viel, Benjamin, *La Medicina Socializada y su Aplicacion en Gran Bretaña, Union Sovietica y Chile*, Santiago: Universidad de Chile, 1964.

55. Weinerman, E.R., *Social Medicine in Western Europe*, Berkeley: University of California School of Public Health, June 1951.

56. Weinerman, E.R., *Social Medicine in Eastern Europe, Organization of Health Services and the Education of Medical Personnel in Czechoslovakia, Hungary and Poland*, Cambridge: Harvard University Press, 1969.

57. White, Kerr L. and J.H. Murnaghan, *Interna-*

tional Comparison of Medical Care Utilization: A Feasibility Study, Washington: National Center for Health Statistics, Series 2, No. 33, June 1969.

58. Wilson, Charles M., *One Half the People: Doctors and the Crisis of World Health,* New York: William Sloane Associates, 1949.

59. Wilson, I. Douglas and Gordon McLachlan, editors, *Health Service Prospects: An International Survey,* London: The Lancet and The Nuffield Provincial Hospital Trust, 1973.

60. Winslow, C.-E.A., *The Cost of Sickness and the Price of Health,* Geneva: World Health Organization, 1951.

61. World Congress of Doctors for the Study of Present-day Living Conditions, *Reports and Proceedings,* Vienna: Secretariat du Congres, 1953.

62. World Health Organization, Regional Office for Europe, *Health Services in Europe,* Copenhagen: 1965.

63. World Health Organization, Regional Office for Europe, *Public Health Administration in Europe,* Copenhagen: World Health Organization, 1965.

64. World Health Organization, *Fourth Report of the World Health Situation 1965-68,* Geneva: 1971 (a continuing series).

NATIONAL STUDIES OF HEALTH SERVICES

Australia
65. Dewdney, J.C.H., *Australian Health Services,* Sydney: John Wiley & Sons Australasia, 1972.

66. Sax, Sidney, *Medical Care in the Melting Pot: An Australian Review,* Sydney: Angus and Robertson, 1972.

Belgium
67. International Hospital Federation, *Report of Study Tours of Hospitals in Belgium,* London: 1964.

Canada
68. Badgley, R.F., and S. Wolfe, *Doctors' Strike: Medical Care and Conflict in Saskatchewan,* New York: Atherton Press, 1967.

69. Blishen, B.R., *Doctors and Doctrines,* Toronto: University of Toronto Press, 1969.

70. Royal Commission on Health Services, *The Report of the Royal Commission,* Volumes I and II, Ottawa: Queen's Printer, 1964 and 1965.

71. Task Force on the Cost of Health Services in Canada, *Task Force Reports on the Cost of Health Services in Canada,* Volumes I-III, Ottawa: Department of National Health and Welfare, 1969.

Chad
72. Buck, A.A., R.I. Anderson, T.T. Sasaki, and K. Kawata, *Health and Disease in Chad,* Baltimore: John Hopkins Press, 1970.

China
73. Crozier, R.C., *Traditional Medicine in Modern China,* Cambridge: Harvard University Press, 1968.

74. Horn, Joshua S., *Away with All Pests – An English Surgeon in People's China: 1954-1969,* New York: Monthly Review Press, 1969.

75. Quinn, Joseph R., editor, *Medicine and Public Health in the People's Republic of China,* Washington: Department of Health, Education, and Welfare, Fogarty International Center, June 1972.

76. Sidel, Victor W. and Ruth Sidel, *Serve the People – Observations on Medicine in the People's Republic of China,* New York: Josiah Macy, Jr. Foundation, 1973.

77. Wegman, M.E., T.Y. Ki, and E.F. Purcell, *Public Health in the People's Republic of China,* New York: Josiah Macy, Jr. Foundation, 1973.

Colombia
78. Ministry of Public Health and Association of Medical Schools of Colombia, *Study on Health Manpower and Medical Education in Colombia,* Vol. II: Preliminary Findings, Washington: Pan American Health Organization, 1967.

Cuba
79. Instituto del Libro, *Diez Anos de Revolucion en Salud Publica,* Havana (Cuba): Editorial de Ciencia Sociales, 1969.

Finland
80. Kuusi, P., *Social Policy for the Sixties, Plan for Finland,* Helsinki: Finnish Social Policy Association, 1964.

France
81. Schorr, A.L., *Social Security and Social Services in France,* Research Report No. 7, Washington: U.S. Department of Health, Education, and Welfare, Social Security Administration, Division of Research and Statistics, 1965.

Germany
82. International Hospital Federation, *Report of Study Tour of Hospitals in the German Federal Republic,* London: 1958.

83. Postgraduate Medical School of the German Democratic Republic, *Public Health in the German Democratic Republic,* Dresden: 1972.

Great Britain

84. Abel-Smith, B. and R.M. Titmuss, *The Cost of the National Health Service in England and Wales,* Cambridge: Cambridge University Press, 1956.

85. Eckstein, H., *The English Health Service: Its Origins, Structure, and Achievements,* Cambridge, Massachusetts: Harvard University Press, 1958.

86. Lindsey, Almont, *Socialized Medicine in England and Wales: The National Health Service 1948-1961,* Chapel Hill: University of North Carolina Press, 1962.

87. Medical Services Review Committee, *A Review of the Medical Services in Great Britain,* London: Social Assay, 1962.

88. McLachlan, G., editor, *Problems and Progress in Medical Care,* London: Oxford University Press, 1970

89. Mencher, S., *British Private Medical Practice and the National Health Service,* Pittsburgh: University of Pittsburgh Press, 1968.

90. Powell, J.E., *A New Look at Medicine and Politics,* London: Pitman Medical Publishing Company, Ltd., 1966.

91. Stevens, Rosemary, *Medical Practice in Modern England – The Impact of Specialization and State Medicine,* New Haven, Connecticut: Yale University Press, 1966.

Greece

92. Blum, Richard and Eva Blum, *Health and Healing in Rural Greece,* Stanford, California: Stanford University Press, 1965.

Holland

93. Querido, A., *The Efficiency of Medical Care,* Leiden: H.E. Stenfert, 1963.

India

94. Government of India, Ministry of Health, *Report of the Health Survey and Planning Committee,* Vols. I-IV, New Delhi, 1962.

95. Takulia, H.S., et al., *The Health Center Doctor in India,* Baltimore: Johns Hopkins Press. 1967.

Israel

96. Grushka, T., editor, *Health Services in Israel,* Jerusalem: Ministry of Health, 1968.

Japan

97. Japanese Government, Ministry of Health and Welfare, *A Brief Report on Public Health Administration in Japan,* Tokyo: 1970.

98. Ohtani, F., *One Hundred Years of Health Progress in Japan,* Tokyo: International Medical Foundation of Japan, 1971.

99. Social Insurance Agency, Japanese Government, *Outline of Social Insurance in Japan,* Tokyo: 1971.

Malaysia

100. Jayesuria, L.W., *A Review of Rural Health Services in West Malaysia,* Kuala Lumpur: Ministry of Health, 1967.

New Zealand

101. New Zealand Social Security Department, *The Growth and Development of Social Security in New Zealand,* Wellington: R. E. Owen, 1950.

Norway

102. Evang, Karl, *Health Services in Norway* (3rd edition), Oslo: Hammerstad Boktrykkeri, 1969.

Peru

103. Hall, Thomas L., *Health Manpower in Peru: A Case Study in Planning,* Baltimore: Johns Hopkins Press, 1969.

Sweden

104. Engel, A., *Perspectives in Health Planning,* London: Athlone Press, 1968.

105. Hojer, Karl J., *Social Welfare in Sweden,* Stockholm: The Swedish Institute, 1949.

106. Uhr, C.G., *Sweden's Social Security System,* Research Report No. 14, U.S. Department of Health, Education, and Welfare, Social Security Administration, Office of Research and Statistics, Washington: U.S. Government Printing Office, 1966.

Taiwan

107. Baker, Timothy D. and M. Perlman, *Health Manpower in a Developing Economy: Taiwan, A Case Study in Planning,* Baltimore: John Hopkins Press, 1967.

Tanganyika

108. Titmuss, R.M., et al., *The Health Services of Tanganyika,* London: Pitman Medical Publishing Company, Ltd., 1964.

Turkey

109. Taylor, Carl E., R. Dirican, and K.W. Deuschle, *Health Manpower Planning in Turkey,* Baltimore: Johns Hopkins Press, 1968.

U.S.S.R.

110. Field, M.G., *Soviet Socialized Medicine – An*

Introduction, New York: The Free Press, 1967.

111. Fogarty International Center, *Fundamental Principles of Health Legislation of the U.S.S.R.,* Washington: 1971.

112. Ministry of Health of the U.S.S.R., *The System of Public Health Service in the U.S.S.R.,* Moscow: The Ministry, 1961.

113. Sigerist, Henry E., *Socialized Medicine in the Soviet Union,* New York: Norton, 1938.

114. Sigerist, Henry E., *Medicine and Health in the Soviet Union,* New York: Citadel Press, 1947.

115. World Health Organization, *Health Services in the U.S.S.R.,* Geneva: Public Health Paper No. 3, 1960.

Venezuela

116. Gabaldon, Arnoldo, *Una Politica Sanitaria* (two volumes) Caracas: Ministerio de Sanidad y Asistencia Social, 1965.